AF615635

CHRONIC LEUKEMIA:

APPROACH TO DIAGNOSIS

CHRONIC LEUKEMIA

APPROACH TO DIAGNOSIS

Harold R. Schumacher, M.D.
Director, Clinical Hematology Laboratory,
Hematopathology Fellowship Program
and
Professor of Pathology
University of Cincinnati Medical Center
Cincinnati, Ohio

James D. Cotelingam, M.D.
Head, Hematopathology and Program Director
Triservice Hematopathology Fellowship Program
National Naval Medical Center
Bethesda, Maryland

Published and distributed by

IGAKU-SHOIN Medical Publishers, Inc.
One Madison Avenue, New York, N.Y. 10010

IGAKU-SHOIN Ltd.,
5-24-3 Hongo, Bunkyo-ku, Tokyo

Library of Congress Cataloging-in-Publication Data

Schumacher, Harold R. (Harold Robert)
Chronic leukemia : approach to diagnosis / Harold R. Schumacher, James D. Cotelingam.
p. cm.
Includes bibliographical references and index.
ISBN 0-89640-220-7 (New York). — ISBN 4-260-14220-8 (Tokyo)
1. Leukemia—Diagnosis. I. Cotelingam, James D. II. Title.
[DNLM: 1. Chronic Disease. 2. Leukemia—diagnosis. WH 250 S3922c]
RC643.S377 1993
616.99'419075—dc20
DNLM/DLC
for Library of Congress 92-48717
CIP

ISBN: 0-89640-220-7 (New York)
ISBN: 4-260-14220-8 (Tokyo)

Printed and bound in the U.S.A.

10 9 8 7 6 5 4 3 2 1

Dedicated to
Marilyn, James, and Mercy

PREFACE

The primary objective of this book, like that of its sister volume *Acute Leukemia: Approach to Diagnosis*, is to provide fundamental, up-to-date information on the chronic leukemias that will allow those interested in these diseases to hone their diagnostic skills in this rapidly expanding area of hematology. Like the previous work, this book contains case studies that provide practical information that the diagnostician can utilize to more skillfully diagnose these diseases. We have made a special effort to make the book succinct and totally readable and have retained the requisite knowledge and approach to establish even the most difficult diagnosis. Once more, the multifaceted unified approach has been employed, and like the solving of a jigsaw puzzle, each piece of diagnostic information has been placed in proper perspective to arrive at the correct diagnosis.

The chapter on the morphology of the mundane chronic leukemias may not appear to have a great impact, since frequently the diagnosis is established by the first individual who examines the peripheral blood smear. However, as with acute leukemias, subtly increasing complexities of the chronic leukemias have become evident, and some cases that look like a duck, quack like a duck, and waddle like a duck may not be a duck. The section on cytochemical evaluation does not follow the methodical approach that is used in the acute leukemias, but relies on a few specific techniques that are more supportive than diagnostic. However, terminal deoxynucleotidyl transferase determination in blast crisis of chronic myelogenous leukemia assumes more significance. As in the acute leukemias, the chapter on electron microscopy may assume importance in those difficult cases in which the diagnosis has not been clearly established. The segment on immunophenotypic studies emphasizes the impact made by these techniques in the chronic lymphoid neoplasms and discusses the techniques that have enabled the diagnostician to more clearly understand, diagnose, prognosticate, and treat this multifarious group of disorders. In fact, what previously may have been considered to be banal B-cell chronic lymphotic leukemia by morphology in reality may be something else. This influence of surface marker analysis, as in the acute leukemias, does not carry over into the chronic myeloid leukemias. Nevertheless, cytogenetics becomes absolutely indispensable in establishing the diagnosis of chronic myelogenous leukemia and its numerous evolving subtleties as discussed in this segment. The Philadelphia chromosome has become a landmark in the field of cytogenetics, and its exploration has opened the area of molecular pathology, which has greatly increased our understanding of the biology of this disease. Unfortunately, similar studies have not contributed as greatly to the chronic lymphoid leukemias. Therefore, the cornerstone of diagnosis in the chronic leukemias differs from that of the acute leukemias. However, as before, technically excellent morphology retains major importance, but cytochemistry falls far short of the prominence observed in the acute leukemias. Consequently, morphology and cytogenetics, and morphology and immunophenotypic analysis, seem to deserve preeminence in our diagnostic armamentarium of the chronic myeloid and chronic lymphoid leukemias, respectively.

The application of gene rearrangement analysis, which at its inception was perceived to be the final court of analysis for clonality, has been repeatedly muddied by ambivalent heterogeneous data that in many cases defy logical conclusions. Much is needed to be learned between the interrelationship of immunophenotypic expression and gene rearrangement—an area that currently seems to have eluded even the most astute molecular hematologist and biologist. The polymerase chain reaction, a relative newcomer to the field of molecular hematology, awaits more vigorous testing in the crucible of time before we can determine its exact role in diagnosis and prognosis. The chapter on oncogenes and growth factors is concerned with biological mechanisms that modulate cell growth. These fields of investigation are in their infancy and currently do not possess great practical application in diagnosis; nevertheless, they represent future realms of cell biology that promise to enlighten our understanding of the leukemic process.

The latter portion of the book provides practical information in the case presentation format with accompanying color microphotographs. The case format provides case presentation, screening laboratory results, hospital course, questions, confirmatory laboratory results, diagnosis, discussion, summary, answers to questions, and a current bibliography. The cases encompass the mundane, moderately difficult, and most difficult. The design has been created to present a logical organized analytic approach to the diagnosis of the chronic leukemias.

The authors sincerely hope this minitext, case-oriented format will enable the reader to learn the basic and evolving complexities of diagnosis of the chronic leukemias. This monograph should provide information of interest for those who must deal with the diagnosis and treatment of the chronic leukemias.

Harold R. Schumacher, M.D.
James D. Cotelingam, M.D.

ACKNOWLEDGMENTS

The authors are indebted to a large number of people who have made this book possible.

Secretarial support from Cynthia Jamison and Mickie Husted and assistance from Marlene Armond and Linda Anfield were invaluable.

Pathology residents Drs. Paul Ferbend, Norman Grossl, Paula Kovarik, Surbi Purohit-Buch, Karla Sendelbach, and Pete Candel were most helpful in supplying numerous abstracts, articles, and reviews on chronic leukemia from the Loyola University Medical Center library. Also, we thank Dr. Daniel Pankowsky, hematopathology fellow, for procuring case material, articles, abstracts, reviews, and meeting handout material.

Excellent photographic support was provided by the Loyola University Medical Center photographic unit and Robert E. Vick, Alvin Hayashi, Sharon Haggerty, Dorothy Hennet, Cheryl Fort, and Cathy Hernandez.

Further gratitude is extended to technologists Teresita Mercado, Cindy Blakemore, Michele Niccolai, Marian Hull, Marge Gryzbac, and Kim Plucienik for their expert technical assistance and advice, and for processing all the peripheral blood and bone marrow specimens that are illustrated. Special thanks is given to reference librarian Jean Jacobsen and medical student Marianne Guschwan, and to Holly Simon, Dawn Palka, and Adam Willard for their assistance with reference materials.

We are most grateful to Dr. Kanti Rai for reviewing the chapter on staging and offering many helpful suggestions on improving the text.

We thank Dr. Raoul Fresco for his critical review of the chapter on electron microscopy.

We are greatly indebted to Dr. Kenneth Foon, who edited the chapter on immunophenotyping and provided illustrations. Additionally, Dr. Ruta Radvany furnished basic information relevant to this chapter.

Also, a very special debt of gratitude is extended to Dr. Michelle Le Beau, who edited the chapter on cytogenetics and additionally provided the figures in this section.

A note of appreciation is extended to Dr.George Dizikes, who reviewed the chaper on gene rearrangement and polymerase chain reaction.

We are most thankful also to Dr. Cheryl Willman, who critiqued the chapter on oncogenes and growth factors.

Penultimately, we appreciate greatly the case materials contributed by Dr. Elaine Jaffe, Dr. William Travis, Dr. Chin-Yang Li and Dr. Jacqueline Whang-Peng. Restriction fragment data were provided through the courtesy of Dr. Lynne Abruzzo, Dr. James Lynch, Dr. Francine Foss, Dr. Jeffrey Medeiros, and Dr. Mark Raffeld, and electron micrographs were contributed by Mr. Gavin Riordan and Dr. Mary Shen. Without the generous support of these colleagues, our reference cases could not have been completed.

Finally a great amount of appreciation must be extended to Dr. Areta Kowal-Vern, Dr. Mark Brissette, and Dr. Scott Graham, who read the entire manuscript and offered many helpful and enlightening editorial suggestions. Also, our thanks to Dr. Patricia Miller-Canfield for proofreading the final manuscript.

We sincerely appreciate the above contributions. These have added immensely to improving the quality of this book.

FOREWORD

Diagnostic approaches to the chronic leukemias were once complex and detailed, but of relatively minor importance in the diagnosis, prognosis, and treatment of these diseases. The situation has changed dramatically in recent years with the discovery of therapy that substantially modifies the natural history of these diseases. One striking example is the effectiveness of interferon in controlling the clinical effects of hairy cell leukemia. The interferon effect is relatively specific for hairy cell leukemia, and virtually all correctly diagnosed patients respond. In contrast, patients with B-cell chronic lymphocytic leukemia will have a response rate that is qualitatively different. This striking example illustrates the growing importance of diagnosis to both prognosis and treatment.

The impact of interferon treatment on the natural history of chronic lymphocytic leukemia remains to be fully evaluated. However, the evidence to date indicates that unlike conventional approaches to chronic myelogenous leukemia (CML), interferon induces, in addition to a clinical and cytologic complete remission, a cytogenetic remission as well. In almost 30% of patients in the early benign phase of CML, major cytogenetic remission has been observed, and these patients have a substantially better prognosis than those who fail to respond to interferon. This example of a treatment effect emphasizes the shifting of therapeutic objectives from initial control of the symptoms, which is purely palliative, to control of the cytologic and hematologic manifestations of those diseases, which results in substantial clinical improvements. Such progress has necessitated a diagnostic shift toward cytogenetic evaluation for estimating treatment effectiveness.

In the case of CML, the availability of molecular probes for diagnosing the presence of the *BCR-ABL* gene in diploid patients has also proved to be of prognostic importance, since these patients have a response to interferon that is comparable to that for aneuploid patients. Again, this illustrates a shift from cytogenetic to molecular genetic criteria for response. Thus, adequate diagnosis of CML requires not only cytology and cytogenetics but the ability to effectively detect the *BCR-ABL* gene. For patients in complete remission by cytogenetic and molecular genetic techniques, application of the polymerase chain reaction to the amplification of *c*DNA that is reverse-transcribed from the *BCR-ABL* transcript discovered in the peripheral blood of these patients provides the potential for detection of minimal residual disease and novel approaches to potentially curative therapy.

The knowledge that in addition to cytotoxic chemotherapy and interferon therapy the patients with CML have the potential for curative therapy as a consequence of allogeneic bone marrow transplant in support of intensive cytoreduction has again underscored the importance of accurate diagnosis in staging of CML to assist the physician in recommendations regarding the choice of therapeutic options. For instance, the *BCR-ABL*-negative, Philadelphia chromosome–negative CML patients would have a better prognosis with transplant than with the interferon therapy. But again, the diagnostic approach to such patients is crucial in the appropriate selection of treatments. Thus, for CML, for which less than 20 years ago there was a limited choice of therapies, today there are a substantial number of effective treatments that require accurate diagnosis and staging.

For the chronic lymphoid leukemias the situation is also changing rapidly. The discovery of the halogenated adenosine analogues has provided physicians with a highly effective form of treatment for the common type B-cell chronic lymphocytic leukemia. The adenosine deaminase inhibitor deoxycoformycin and related drugs have also had impressive activity in hairy cell leukemia and other lymphoid malignancies. Finally, the recent description of chlorodeoxyadenosine which has substantially lower toxicity and a high degree of effectiveness in the well-differentiated lymphoid malignancies, has expanded the therapeutic pallet for the physician. These therapeutic options have underscored the need for effective staging of the lymphoid malignancies, precise evaluation of the extent of immunosuppression, and effective utilization of sequential studies for monitoring treatment effects.

It is particularly useful to have available in a single volume in a well-organized format a comprehensive presentation of the available technology for the accurate diagnosis and staging of the chronic leukemias. I think Doctors Schumacher and Cotelingam have assembled well-organized and up-to-date documentation of the available knowledge. In addition, they have provided excellent case studies that illustrate the application of the techniques that are catalogued in the volume. In my opinioin, this is a relatively unique volume; it will make a substantial addition to my library and I am sure to the libraries of many others.

Emil J Freireich, M.D.
Director, Adult Leukemia Research Program
The University of Texas
M. D. Anderson Cancer Center
Houston, Texas

CONTENTS

CHAPTERS

CASE STUDIES

ABBREVIATIONS

A-EST	Alpha naphthyl acetate esterase
AA-EST	Acid alpha naphthyl acetate esterase
ADF	ATLL-derived factor
AEC	Absolute eosinophil count
AEL	Acute erythroleukemia
AIDS	Acquired immune deficiency syndrome
AILD	Angioimmunoblastic lymphadenopathy with dysproteinemia
ALL	Acute lymphocytic leukemia
AM	Aggressive mastocytosis
Am-EST	Aminocaproate esterase
AML	Acute myeloid leukemia
AML-M1	Acute myelomonocytic leukemia without maturation
AML-M4	Acute myelomonocytic leukemia
AML-M5a	Acute monocytic leukemia without diffentiation
AMML	Acute myeloid leukemia
AMoL	Acute monocytic leukemia
ANLL	Acute non-lymphocytic leukemia
AP	Acid phosphatase
ATLL	Adult T-cell leukemia-lymphoma
bcr	Breakpoint cluster region
BCR	Breakpoint cluster region gene
B-EST	Alpha naphthyl butyrate esterase
BFU-E	Erythrocyte burst-forming unit
BL	Basophilic leukemia
C′3	Third component of complement
c-*ABL*	Cellular Abelson protooncogene
CAE	Chloracetate esterase
CALLA	Common acute lymphoblastic leukemic–associated antigen
CBC	Complete blood count
CD	Cluster designation
CDR III	Complementary determining region III
C-EST	Combined esterase
CLC	Circulating lymphoma cells
cIg	Cytoplasmic immunoglobulin
CFU-B	B-cell colony-forming unit
CFU-C	Colony-forming units in culture
CFU-E	Erythroid colony-forming unit

CFU-G	Granulocyte colony-forming unit
CFU-GEMM	Granulocyte-erythrocyte-macrophage-megakaryocyte colony-forming unit
CFU-GM	Granulocyte-macrophage colony-forming unit
CFU-M	Macrophage colony-forming unit
CFU-Me	Megakaryocytic colony-forming unit
CFU-T	T-cell colony-forming unit
cIg	Cytoplasmic immunoglobulin
CLL	Chronic lymphocytic leukemia
CMaL	Chronic mast cell leukemia
CML	Chronic myelogenous leukemia
CMML	Chronic myelomonocytic leukemia
CMML-T	Chronic myelomonocytic leukemia in transformation
CMoL	Chronic monocytic leukemia
CNL	Chronic neutrophilic leukemia
Cμ	Cytoplasmic mμ heavy chain
c-onc	Cellular oncogene
del	Deletion
DCF	2-deoxycoformycin
der	Derivative
DIC	Disseminated intravascular coagulation
DNA	Deoxyribonucleic acid
EL	Eosinophilic leukemia
EM	Electron microscopy
EMA	Epithelial membrane antigen
Ep	Erythropoietin
ET	Essential thrombocythemia
FAB	French-American-British
Fe stain	Iron stain
FF	Form factor
G-6-PD	Glucose-6-phosphate dehydrogenase
GAP	GTPase-activating protein
G-CSF	Granulocyte colony-stimulating factor
GM-CSF	Granulocyte-macrophage colony-stimulating factor
HC	Hairy cell
HCL	Hairy cell leukemia
HCL-v	Hairy cell leukemia, variant
HCT	Hematocrit
HES	Hypereosinophilic syndrome
HGB	Hemoglobin
HIV	Human immune deficiency virus
HLA	Human leukocyte antigens
HTLV	Human T-cell leukemia virus
IDL	Intermediate differentiated lymphoma

Ig	Immunoglobulin
IgH	Immunoglobulin heavy chain
IgL	Immunoglobulin light chain
IL	Interleukin
IM	Indolent mastocytosis
IWCLL	International Workshop on Chronic Lymphocytic Leukemia
JCML	Juvenile chronic myeloid leukemia
JCMML	Juvenile chronic myelomonocytic leukemia
LAP	Leukocyte alkaline phosphatase
LCA	Leukocyte common antigen
LDH	Lactate dehydrogenase
LDT	Lymphocyte doubling time
LGL	Large granular lymphocyte
LSCL	Lymphosarcoma cell leukemia
MALT	Mucosa associated lymphoid tissue
mar	Marker
MBP	Major basic protein
M-BCR	Major breakpoint cluster region
mbcr	Minor breakpoint cluster region
MCH	Mean corpuscular hemoglobulin
MCHC	Mean corpuscular hemoglobin concentration
MCL	Mast cell leukemia
MCV	Mean corpuscular volume
M-CSF	Macrophage-monocyte colony-stimulating factor
MDS	Myelodysplastic syndrome
MF	Mycosis fungoides
MHC	Major histocompatibility
MM	Malignant mastocytosis/multiple myeloma
MOPP	Mustard, oncovin, procarbazine, predisone
MPD	Myeloproliferative disorder
MPV	Mean platelet volume
MPEX	Myeloperoxidase
MRD	Minimal residual disease
mRNA	Messenger ribonucleic acid
NAP-1	Neutrophil attractant-activation protein
NCSWG	National Cancer Sponsored Working Group
NHL	Non-Hodgkin's lymphoma
NI	Nuclear invagination
NK	Natural killer
NRBC	Nucleated red blood cell
ORO	Oil red O
PAS	Periodic acid–Schiff
PCA	Plasma cell antigen

PCL	Plasma cell leukemia
PCR	Polymerase chain reaction
PDW	Platelet distribution width
Ph[1]	Philadelphia chromosome
PHA	Phytohemagglutin
PL	Prolymphocyte
PLL	Prolymphocytic leukemia
PLT	Prolymphocytic transformation
PDGF	Platelet-derived growth factor
ProMACE	Prednisone, methotrexate, adriamycin, cytoxan, etoposide
PUVA	Psoralin, ultraviolet light
PV	Polycythemia vera
RA	Refractory anemia
RAEB	Refractory anemia with excess blasts
RAEB-IT	Refractory anemia with excess blasts in transformation
RARS	Refractory anemia with ringed sideroblasts
RBC	Red blood cell
RDW	Red cell distribution width
RFLP	Restriction fragment length polymorphisms
RLC	Ribosome-lamella complex
RSV	Rous sarcoma virus
SBB	Sudan black B
SCFCCL	Small cleaved follicular center cell lymphoma
sIg	Surface immunoglobulin
sIgA	Surface IgA
sIgD	Surface IgD
sIgM	Surface IgM
sIgG	Surface IgG
sIgM	Surface IgM
SLVL	Splenic lymphoma with villous lymphocytes
SM	Systemic mastocytosis
smIg	Surface membrane immunoglobulin
SS	Sézary syndrome
TBO	Toluidine blue O
TCR	T-cell antigen receptor
Tdt	Terminal deoxynucleotidyl transferase
TGLD	T-gamma lymphoproliferative disease
TRAP	Tartrate-resistant acid phosphatase urticaria
UP	Urticaria pigmentosa
v-onc	Viral oncogene
WBC	White blood cell count
WM	Waldenström's macroglobulinemia

Overview

The classification of the chronic leukemias may seem uncomplicated and elementary when compared with the numerous categories, subcategories, concatenations, and variants of the acute leukemias. However, like most subjects that appear simplistic at first glance, the chronic leukemias have also acquired an increasing degree of complexity with the application of new technologies. Although the gold standard still remains quality high-technological morphology; cytochemical and terminal deoxynucleotidyl transferase analyses do not have the same impact in the diagnosis of the chronic leukemias as in the acute leukemias. However, the same disciplined multifaceted approach must be employed to diagnose the chronic leukemias, including all those parameters that ultimately lead to the best diagnosis.

Unique to the chronic leukemias is the concept of staging, which is addressed in a separate chapter. This concept has been best developed and uniformly accepted in chronic lymphocytic leukemia (CLL), in which both clinical and hematologic data are employed for prognosis. Although similar attempts have been used to stage chronic myelogenous leukemia (CML), such staging systems have not received the wide acceptance received by the Rai and Binet staging criteria utilized in CLL. As in the acute leukemias, electron microscopy has not been a tool implemented with major consequences in the diagnosis of the chronic leukemias. Nevertheless, in special incidences such as blast crisis of CML, mast cell leukemia, hairy cell leukemia, and some of the convoluted nuclear lymphoid disorders, electron microscopy may be a valuable adjunct to diagnosis.

Even though electron microscopy usually does not have a major impact in the diagnosis of the chronic leukemias, immunophenotyping is a quintessential part of the diagnosis of lymphoid disorders. Batteries of surface marker studies are employed routinely to accurately classify the lymphoid malignancies; providing important diagnostic as well as prognostic information. Similar use of surface marker analysis in the CMLs does not assume the important role that it does in the lymphoid neoplasms.

Contrariwise, cytogenetics takes on immense prominence in diagnosing the CMLs, since the Philadelphia chromosome is the sine qua non in establishing the diagnosis of CML. However, recently some additional emphasis is being placed on cytogenetic studies in the CLLs.

The initial surge of interest in immunoglobulin and T-cell receptor gene rearrangement analysis by molecular techniques has been somewhat squelched by the finding of marked heterogeneity among the various leukemias, borderline lesions, and even some so-called benign disorders. This had led investigators to be most cautious in interpreting gene rearrangement data. Despite this, early evidence has suggested that some molecular techniques such as evaluation of *BCR/ABL* by Southern blot analysis seem to have found a place in our diagnostic armamentarium. How the polymerase chain reaction with its molecular multiplicative wizardry will fit into our future diagnostic and prognostic skills is not yet entirely clear.

Other rapidly developing areas include evaluation of oncogenes and growth factors. Again, how these growth modulators will enter into the diagnostic arena remains uncertain. Finally, interphase cytogenetic analysis seems to hold great promise because of simplicity, smallness of sample size, and ability to detect small numbers of malignant cells.

In conclusion, as in the sister volume *Acute Leukemia: Approach to Diagnosis,* the diagnostic approach is a multifaceted unified approach that uses accumulated human knowledge over the past 165 years to diagnose this disease. Our complete understanding remains clouded, but we are beginning to comprehend the complex interactions regulating cell growth that we hope will give us the needed insight to control this disease we call leukemia.

CHAPTER 1

Diagnostic Approach

BACKGROUND

Leukemia, as a distinct disease, was first described by Velpeau in 1827 in a florist and seller of lemonade "who had abandoned himself to the abuse of spiritous liquor and of women, without, however, becoming syphilitic" and who fell ill in 1825 with a pronounced swelling of the abdomen, fever and weakness, and symptoms caused by urinary stones. He died soon after admission to the hospital, and autopsy findings revealed an enormous liver and spleen, and blood thick "like gruel—resembling in consistency and color the yeast of red wine." This description over 160 years ago accurately describes a patient with chronic myelogenous leukemia (CML) in accelerated phase or blast crisis. Examination of such blood from another patient in 1839 by Donne revealed "mucous globules" similar to pus corpuscles. Even though these observations and other similar descriptions were recorded in the literature, leukemia was not recognized as a distinctive entity until Bennett in Scotland and Virchow in Germany published cases within 1 month of each other.

Virchow, the great German pathologist, went on to coin the term *white blood* (*weisses Blut*) to characterize the pathologic findings. Later, Bennett published a monograph on a series of cases in which he used the term *leucocythemia*. However, Virchow had already introduced the term *leukemia* in 1847, and he published a series of articles summarized in 1856 that contained rudimentary elements pertaining to the pathology of leukemia, many of which are still accepted today. He introduced the concept of splenic leukemia (CML) and lymphatic leukemia (chronic lymphocytic leukemia, CLL) based on gross involvement of the spleen and lymph nodes.

Only consolidation of existing knowledge occurred over the next 30 years, except for Neumann's discovery that bone marrow is an important site for the formation of blood corpuscles in health and disease. In the late nineteenth and early twentieth centuries, hematologists used numerous terms to describe leukemia, such as *chloroma, leukosarcoma, myeloma, myelosis,* and *pseudoleukemia.* Many of these terms are used even today. Then as now, problems existed concerning the relationship of lymphoma to leukemia, and terms like *lymphosarcoma, lymphosarcoma cell leukemia,* and *lymphoproliferative diseases* were created and suggest some of the difficulties in our understanding of the interrelationship between these two disorders.

The credit for a much clearer concept of acute and chronic leukemia must be given to Hirschfeld, who identified the source of the granulocytes in the bone marrow. A few years later, Naegeli applied the term *myeloblast* to these progenitor cells, a term destined to be used as a key morphologic element in the separation of acute leukemia from chronic leukemia in modern hematology. Indeed, the French-American-British (FAB) classification employs the presence of 30% or more blast cells in the bone marrow to distinguish the acute leukemias from chronic leukemias and myelodysplastic syndromes.

The great discovery of the modern era of hematology was the Philadelphia chromosome (Ph^1), found in CML cells in 1960 by Nowell and Hungerford. This was the first demonstration that a chromosomal abnormality had a constant association with a distinct malignant entity. Modern cytogenetics and molecular biology have focused on the Ph^1 and have revealed numerous complexities that will be discussed in later chapters.

CLASSIFICATION

The classification of the chronic leukemias at first glance may seem uncomplicated and elementary when compared with the numerous categories, subcategories, and concatenations of the acute leukemias. The FAB classification of the acute leukemias has created a common language that is employed throughout the world and permits hematologists and hematopathologists to communicate on mutual ground in regard to the acute leukemias. Not so with the chronic leukemias, which are further complicated by interrelationships with other entities having pathogenetic similarities.

MYELOPROLIFERATIVE DISORDERS

To emphasize the pathogenetic similarities of CML and other myeloid disorders, Dameshek applied the term *myeloproliferative disorders* (MPDs). This term has been expanded by some hematologists to include chronic, subacute, and acute MPDs. The chronic MPDs are an acquired clonal malignancy characterized by the expansion of the pluripotential stem cell compartment, deranged production of blood cells by one or more myeloid cell lines, and a variably programmed predisposition of affected stem cells to transform into leukemic blast-forming cells. The chronic MPDs include CML, agnogenic myeloid metaplasia with myelofibrosis, polycythemia vera (PV), and essential thrombocythemia (ET). In addition, some authors have included the disorders chronic monocytic, chronic myelomonocytic, and chronic neutrophilic leukemia under this classification. The subacute MPDs include smoldering leukemias, subacute myelomonocytic leukemia, and atypical myeloproliferative syndromes. The acute MPDs include FAB diagnosis M1–M7, and eosinophilic, basophilic, and mixed acute leukemias. The hallmark of these disorders is excessive production and overaccumulation of malignant cells, and/or their progenitors in the peripheral blood and bone marrow. Therefore, the term *myeloproliferative* should be used in this context. However, since frequently the subacute and acute MPDs do not clearly manifest such excessive proliferation, the authors suggest great caution in using these terms. The classification of the MPDs incorporating the above diagnosis are shown in Table 1.1.

MYELODYSPLASTIC SYNDROMES

The myelodysplastic syndromes (MDSs) are depicted in Table 1.2 as classified by the FAB cooperative group. In contrast to the concept of the MPDs, the quintessential features of this classification are ineffective bone marrow maturation and insufficient release of leukocytes, erythrocytes, and platelets or permutations of these elements into the peripheral blood. The indispensable morphologic features are manifested as dyserythropoiesis, dysgranulopoiesis, and dys-

Table 1-1 Myeloproliferative Disorders

Chronic
Chronic myelogenous leukemia (CML)
Agnogenic myeloid metaplasia with myelofibrosis
Polycythemia vera (PV)
Essential thrombocythemia (ET)
Chronic neutrophilic leukemia (CNL)
Chronic monocytic leukemia (CMoL)
Chronic myelomonocytic leukemia (CMML)
Subacute
Smoldering leukemias
Subacute myelomonocytic leukemia
Atypical myeloproliferative diseases
Acute
FAB diagnosis (M1–M7)
Eosinophilic leukemia (EL)
Basophilic leukemia (BL)
Mixed leukemia

megakaryocytopoiesis; the result is maturation arrest within the marrow and cytopenias within the peripheral blood. Within this framework, it is possible for one disease entity, for example, chronic myelomonocytic leukemia (CMML) to manifest itself as an MPD appearing like CML, or as an MDS appearing like a refractory anemia with excessive blasts (RAEB) or a refractory anemia with excessive blasts in transformation (RAEB-IT; referred to as CMML-IT by some groups). Also, CMML, apparently a hybrid disease, may share features of both proliferation and dysplasia within the same case. This contradiction or variability prompted some hematologists to suggest that CMML be separated from the MDSs. In addition, mild to moderate dysplastic changes may occur in typical CML and may progress to severe dysplasia in the later stages, creating diagnostic chaos. Although documentation of the Ph^1 certifies the diagnosis of Ph-positive CML, the appearance of monocytosis in Ph^1-negative CML may erroneously shift the diagnosis to CMML. Furthermore, accentu-

Table 1-2 Myelodysplastic Syndromes

Refractory anemia (RA)
Refractory anemia with ringed sideroblasts (RARS)
Refractory anemia with excess blasts (RAEB)
Chronic myelomonocytic leukemia (CMML)
Refractory anemia with excess blasts in transformation (RAEB-IT)

Table 1-3 Chronic Leukemias

Chronic myeloid leukemias and related disorders
- Chronic myelogenous leukemia (CML)
  - Philadelphia chromosome (Ph^1) positive
  - Philadelphia chromosome (Ph^1) negative
- Chronic neutrophilic leukemia (CNL)
- Chronic monocytic leukemia (CMoL)
- Chronic myelomonocytic leukemia (CMML)
- Eosinophilic leukemia (EL)
- Basophilic leukemia (BL)
- Chronic mast cell leukemia (CMaL)

Chronic lymphocytic leukemia and related disorders
- B-cell disorders
  - B-cell chronic lymphocytic leukemia (CLL)
  - B-cell prolymphocytic leukemia (PLL)
  - B-cell hairy cell leukemia (HCL)
  - Leukemic phase of B-cell lymphomas

T-cell disorders
- T-cell CLL (CD4+) (may not exist)
- T-gamma lymphoproliferative disease (TGLD) (large granular lymphocytosis)
- T-cell prolymphocytic leukemia (PLL)
- Adult T-cell leukemia-lymphoma (ATLL)
- Sézary syndrome (SS)
- T-hairy cell leukemia (HCL)

ation of the maturation arrest, and of dysplastic changes, in advanced presentations of Ph^1-negative CML leads to their reclassification as a subtype of MDS. Currently, the distinction between CMML and Ph^1-negative CML is very controversial, and it is hoped that future investigation into the molecular biology of these disorders will more clearly delineate such classification.

CHRONIC LEUKEMIAS

A scheme presented in Table 1.3 demonstrates the complex interrelationships of the chronic leukemias with other closely related taxonomics such as the MPDs and MDSs. The terminology and classification complexities continue to plague morphologic hematologists and hematopathologists even today in regard to MPDs, MDSs, and the chronic myeloid leukemic disorders. This confusion was not as true for the chronic lymphoid neoplasms until the dawn of surface markers and immunophenotyping. Prior to this era, which had its roots

Table 1-4 Diagnostic Problems with Current Classifications

1. Uniform classification	Lacking throughout literature
2. Diagnostic criteria	Variable
3. MPDs	Confusion exists with subacute and acute leukemias
4. MDSs	Problems with CMML
5. Dysplasia	No WBC defining upper limit
6. Proliferation	No WBC defining lower limit
7. Monocytosis	Absolute rather than relative (see text)

in the 1970s, the small lymphocyte in CLL was considered dull, uninteresting, and morphologically monotonous. Now classification of lymphoid neoplasms has literally exploded into multifarious categories due to the burgeoning impact of immunophenotyping, gene rearrangement, and oncogene analysis.

With the above classifications gleaned and conjured up from the available literature, it became obvious that certain problems exist with the current taxonomy of the chronic leukemias (Table 1.4). Although chronic leukemias have posed fewer classification problems than the acute leukemias in the past, because of their unique morphologic, immunologic, and cytogenetic features, a uniform categorization is needed, especially since sophisticated technology has complicated diagnosis. This categorization has been partly inhibited by degeneracy in codifying the leukemias because of their inherent instability and proclivity to evolve or transform. None of the current classifications for the chronic leukemias are in total agreement!

While the diagnostic criteria do not need to be rigid to establish a diagnosis in most cases of CLL or CML, uniform guidelines for diagnosis should exist. Frequently, many cases of CLL or CML are diagnosed by serendipity when the patient has an elective procedure or is being evaluated for other reasons. Nevertheless, with the increased sophistication of our diagnostic acumen, standardization of the criteria is definitely needed to enable hematologists and hematopathologists throughout the world to communicate in an intelligible, dependable manner. This has transpired to some extent with CLL since the International Workshop met in Barcelona in February 1988, but similar standardized criteria should be extended to the other chronic lymphoid and chronic myeloid malignancies, and related disorders.

Although some uniformity exists in classification of the chronic MPDs, great difficulties arise when authors attempt to classify MPDs into subacute and acute categories. This results in a potpourri of terminology such as oligoblastic (smoldering) leukemia, which is also equated to CMML by some authors. Also, RAEB and myelomonocytic leukemia are placed under the subacute MPDs by some authors, and this further adds to the confusion. Finally, all the acute myeloid leukemias including eosinophilic, basophilic, and even biphenotypic are included under the acute MPDs. Since many of the subacute and acute disorders demonstrate dysplastic features that may coexist or predominate over a myeloproliferative component, such a classification creates confusion. The authors consider the terms *subacute* and *acute MPDs* unsatisfactory because of the mixed dysplastic, myeloproliferative nature of these diseases.

This obfuscation is carried even further because of lack of a functional interpretation of dysplasia or proliferation by a threshold leukocyte count and by the current definition of monocytosis by an absolute rather than a relative value. This is best illustrated by a patient who presents with a white blood count (WBC) 50×10^9/L, 3% blasts and 4% monocytes in the peripheral blood; a hypercellular moderately dysplastic marrow with 7% blasts and 6% monocytes; and a normal karyotype. This depiction could satisfy the criteria of MDS (RAEB), CMML, or Ph^1-negative CML when evaluated by different observers. This problem could be resolved by breakpoint cluster region (bcr) rearrangement analysis, and if positive would indicate a Ph^1-negative bcr+ CML. CMML could be characterized by modifying the criteria for monocytosis to include a relative value of 8% or more monocytes in the peripheral blood or bone marrow in those instances of severe leukocytosis. In CMML patients featuring more myelodysplasia than proliferation, that is, WBC less than 20×10^9/L, an absolute monocyte count of 10^9/L or more would be required. In addition, cytochemistry, immunophenotyping by flow cytometry, and immunoalkaline phosphatase determination would help to differentiate CMML from RAEB. Clearer definitions and classification will evolve when the molecular abnormalities are better understood in relation to the pathophysiologic events.

A disorder in children representing about 2% of childhood leukemias has been designated juvenile CML by some authors. It occurs most often in infants and children under 4 years of age and is similar to adult subacute myelomonocytic leukemia or CMML. As in adult CMML, the Ph^1 is not present.

THE APPROACH

As mentioned earlier, the diagnosis of the chronic leukemias at first assessment appears to be less complicated than that of the acute leukemias. However, with the burgeoning technological advances, new complexities of the chronic leukemias are being uncovered. Even

Table 1-5 Diagnostic Approach

Pertinent clinical data
Peripheral smear
Complete hemogram*
Morphology of bone marrow, aspirate, touch preparations, biopsy, and clot
Cytochemistry and terminal deoxynucleotidyl transferase
Immunophenotype by flow cytometry
Immunoalkaline phosphatase
Cytogenetics†
Electron microscopy‡
Gene rearrangement analysis‡
Oncogenes‡
Tissue culture‡
Polymerase chain reaction‡
Miscellaneous: Uric acid, serum B_{12}, immunoelectrophoresis, serum muramidase, etc.

*Includes differential count, WBC, RBC, HCT, HGB, MCV, MCH, MCHC, RDW, MPV, PDW, reticulocyte, and platelet counts.
†Especially Ph^1 and bcr evaluation.
‡Special cases.

though the diagnosis may be known prior to bone marrow examination, a routine protocol should be established that includes all the diagnostic tests to firmly and clearly establish the correct diagnosis. The diagnostic approach listing the parameters implemented in establishing a diagnosis is depicted in Table 1.5. The diagnostic approach in the chronic leukemias is slightly different from the one implemented in the acute leukemias. Clinical presentation; large spleen; lymphadenopathy; leukocyte alkaline phosphatase levels; acid phosphatase levels with and without tartrate; reticulin and trichrome stains; immunophenotyping; Ph^1 and bcr rearrangement; gene rearrangement; and oncogene analysis assume different implications and significance in the chronic leukemias. Again, as in the acute leukemias, adequate sample material must be obtained and technical procedures must be of the highest quality. Often an easy diagnosis is not established because of inadequate sampling and poor technical quality of the material—the cardinal sin of misdiagnosis!

SUMMARY

Excellent peripheral blood and bone marrow specimens demonstrating good morphology and cytogenetics with bcr rearrangement studies are currently the cornerstone in the diagnosis of the chronic myeloid leukemias. Contrariwise, studies of peripheral blood, bone marrow, and immunophenotyping remain the gold standard for the chronic lymphoid leukemias. As our scientific knowledge progresses, more emphasis will be placed at the molecular level, which has already begun to impact on our diagnostic capabilities. The diagnostic approach is a multifaceted unified compilation of data that should be implemented in all cases.

BIBLIOGRAPHY

Articles

Bennett JH: Case of hypertrophy of the spleen and liver, in which death took place from suppuration of the blood. *Edin Med Surg J* 64:413–423, 1845.

Bennett JM, Catovsky D, Daniel MT, et al: Myelodysplastic syndromes: Is another classification necessary? *Br J Haematol* 56:515–517, 1984.

Bennett JH: Leucocythemia or white cell blood. *Mod J Med Sci* 12:312–326, 1851.

Dameshek W: Some speculation on the myeloproliferative syndromes (editorial). *Blood* 6:372–375, 1951.

Donne A: *Cours de Microscopie.* Paris, Bailliere, 1844, p. 132.

Hirschfeld H: Zur Kenntnis des Histogenese des granuleiten Knochenmarkenzellen. *Arch Pathol Anat* 153:335, 1893.

International Workshop on Chronic Lymphocytic Leukemia: Chronic lymphocytic leukemia: Recommendations for diagnosis, staging and response criteria. *Ann Intern Med* 110:236–238, 1989.

Kantarjian HM, Smith TL, MCredie KB, et al: Chronic myelogenous leukemia: A multivariate analysis of the association of patient characteristics and therapy with survival. *Blood* 66:1326–1335, 1985.

Naegeli O: Ueber rotes Knochenmark und Myeloblasten. *Dtsch Med Wochenschr* 26:287–290, 1900.

Neumann E: Ein Fall von Leukämie mit Erkrankung des Knochenmarkes. *Arch Heilkunde* 11:1–15, 1870.

Nowell PC, Hungerford DA: A minute chromosome in human chronic granulocytic leukemia. *Science* 132:1497, 1960.

Pugh WC, Pearson M, Vardiman J, et al: Philadelphia chromosome-negative chronic myelogenous leukaemia: A morphological reassessment. *Br J Haematol* 60:457–467, 1985.

Travis LB, Pierre RV, DeWald GW: Ph^1-negative chronic granulocytic leukemia: A nonentity. *Am J Clin Pathol* 85:186–193, 1986.

Velpeau A: *Rev Med* 2:218, 1827. Quoted by Virchow R: *Med Z* 16:9 and 15, 1847. Recherches sur l'oeuif humain. *Ann Sci Nat* 12:172–196, 1827.

Virchow R: Weisses Blut. *Neue Notizen aus dem Gebiete der Natur- und Heilkunde,* 136:151–157, 1845.

Virchow R: Weisses Blut und Milztumoren I. *Med Z* 15:157, 1846.

Virchow R: Weisses Blut und Milztumoren II. *Med Z* 16:9, 1847.

Virchow R: Zur pathologischen Physiologie des Blutes II. Weisses Blut. (Leukämie). *Virchows Arch [Pathol Anat Physiol]* 1:547–583, 1847.

Virchow R: Die Leukämie. In Virchow R: *Gesammelte Abhandlungen zur wissenshaftlichen Medizin.* Frankfurt, Meidinger, 1856, p 190.

Review Articles

Bennett JM, Catovsky D, Daniel MT, et al (FAB cooperative group): Proposals for the classification of the myelodysplastic syndromes. *Br J Haematol* 51:189–199, 1982.

Berliner N: T gamma lymphocytosis and T cell chronic leukemias. *Hematol Oncol Clin North Am* 4:473–487, 1990.

Canellos GP: Clinical characteristics of the blast phase of chronic granulocytic leukemia. *Hematol Oncol Clin North Am* 4:359–367, 1990.

Freedman AS: Immunobiology of chronic lymphocytic leukemia. *Hematol Oncol Clin North Am* 4:405–429, 1990

Gale RP: Chronic myelogenous leukemia: A model for human cancers. *Baillieres Clin Haematol* 1:869–886, 1987.

Kantarjian HM, Kurzrock R, Talpaz M: Philadelphia chromosome–negative chronic myelogenous leukemia and chronic myelomonocytic leukemia. *Hematol Oncol Clin North Am* 4:389–404, 1990.

Kurzrock R, Gutterman JU, Talpaz M: The molecular genetics of Philadelphia chromosome positive leukemias. *N Engl J Med* 319:990–998, 1988.

Silver RT: Chronic myeloid leukemia. A perspective of the clinical and biologic issues of the chronic phase. *Hematol Oncol Clin North Am* 4:319–335, 1990.

Silver RT, Gale RP: Chronic myeloid leukemia. *Am J Med* 80:1137–1148, 1986.

Stone RM: Prolymphocytic leukemia. *Hematol Oncol Clin North Am* 4:457–471, 1990.

Strife A, Clarkson B: Biology of chronic myelogenous leukemia: Is discordant maturation the primary defect? *Semin Hematol* 25:1–19, 1988.

CHAPTER 2

Morphology and Classification

GENERAL COMMENTS

The initial diagnostic studies of the chronic leukemias should include high-quality Wright-Giemsa or Romanowsky stains of the peripheral blood, bone marrow aspirate, and touch preparations of the bone marrow biopsy. Clot and biopsy are placed in B5 fixative solution; the biopsy is decalcified in nitric acid; and the specimens are embedded in paraffin, cut at 4μm, and stained with hematoxylin and eosin. As mentioned earlier, the preliminary diagnosis of the chronic leukemias is usually determined from examination of the peripheral blood; however, all pertinent material discussed in Chapter 1 should be collected at the time of the initial examination. The approach should be multifaceted, systematic, and thorough to firmly establish the correct diagnosis. Once treatment is instituted, it will interfere with diagnostic procedures at a later date.

CHRONIC MYELOGENOUS LEUKEMIA (Fig. 2.1)

The diagnosis of chronic myelogenous leukemia (CML) can usually be made without difficulty in most patients by examination of a well stained peripheral blood smear. Bone marrow demonstrates similar,

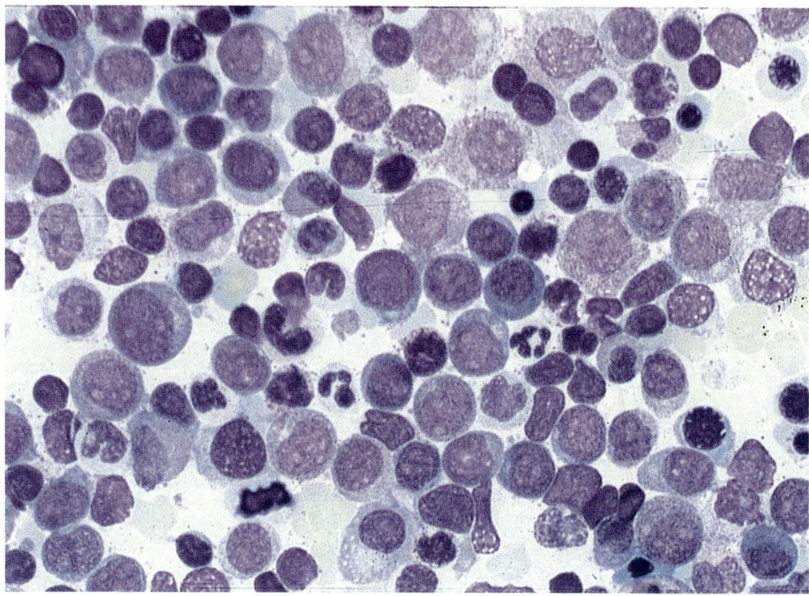

Figure 2-1 Hypercellular bone marrow showing colorful panoply of neutrophils and granulocytic precursors. CML ($\times$400).

usually more concentrated cellularity (Fig. 2.1). Rarely does any other disease produce such an outpouring of colorful myelocytes, metamyelocytes, and mature neutrophils, with variable numbers of eosinophils, basophils, and occasional erythrocyte precursors. The criteria for diagnosis of CML are listed in Table 2.1. The total leukocyte count usually exceeds 100 $\times$ 10^9/L in about 75% of patients at onset. However, some cases may have leukocyte counts as high as 1000 $\times$ 10^9/L, and others surreptitious levels slightly above 10 $\times$ 10^9/L, that may go unrecognized for months or years. In the chronic phase, promyelocytes and myeloblasts do not exceed 15–20% of the total leukocyte population in either the peripheral blood or bone marrow. Immature granulocytic elements increase in peripheral blood and bone marrow as the disease progresses. At diagnosis, most patients with CML have a mild normocytic normochromic anemia, which usually progresses as the leukocyte count increases. Nucleated red blood cells (NRBCs) are commonly observed in small numbers in the peripheral blood. Thrombocytosis is present in roughly 50% of patients at the time of diagnosis. Platelet counts may increase during the chronic phase, and counts over 1000 $\times$ 10^9/L are not unusual. Giant bizarre platelets,

Table 2-1 Diagnostic Criteria for CML

1. Leukocytosis (>25 × 10^9/L)
2. Immature myeloid precursors in peripheral blood with basophilia and eosinophilia
3. Usually normocytic normochromic anemia
4. Elevated levels of serum B_{12}, B_{12}-binding proteins
5. Hyperuricemia
6. Low or absent leukocyte alkaline phosphatase (LAP)
7. Ph^1-positive (95% of cases)
8. Ph^1-negative (5% of cases) (30–50% bcr rearrangement)
9. Hypercellular marrow (fat/cell ratio markedly diminished)
10. Splenomegaly (95%)

abnormal granulation of platelets, micromegakaryocytes, and functional platelet abnormalities may be seen.

Practically all patients demonstrate an acquired pseudo-Pelger-Huët anomaly of granulocytes (Fig. 2.2) that usually occurs late in the disease after myelosuppressive therapy. However, pseudo-Pelger-Huët cells may forecast the clinical onset of CML by months or even years. Besides CML, Pelger-Huët cells may be seen in acute myelogenous leukemia (AML), idiopathic myelofibrosis with certain drugs, infections, and, rarely, CLL and non-Hodgkin's lymphoma.

Other conditions occasionally mimic CML. These conditions are usually associated with leukocyte counts of greater than 50 × 10^9/L. Such conditions are referred to as a leukemoid reaction and are associated with (1) infection, (2) metastatic carcinoma, (3) burns, (4) diabetic ketoacidosis, (5) poisonings, and (6) rhematoid arthritis. The important differences between CML and a leukemoid reaction are depicted in Table 2.2.

Bone marrow in CML is easily aspirated in most cases. The marrow shows predominance of granulocytic elements, and the myeloid/erythroid ratio, which is normally 3:1, may be increased markedly to 20:1 or greater. The granulocytic cell line exhibits the same spectrum of cells observed in the peripheral blood, with a greater preponderance of immature elements in the marrow. Eosinophils and basophils may be increased, usually in proportion to their elevation in the peripheral blood. The erythrocytic cell line usually reveals normoblastic maturation, but megaloblastic maturation and dyserythropoiesis may be seen occasionally in the chronic phase. Megakaryocytes are characteristically increased and show abutment, a common feature of the myeloproliferative disorders (Fig. 2.3). Auer rods are rarely seen and

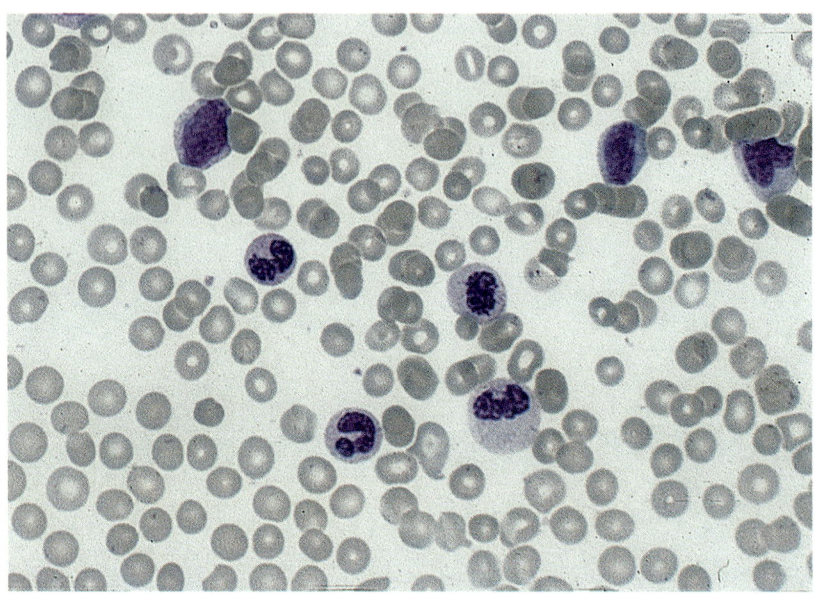

Figure 2-2 Peripheral blood demonstrating pseudo-Pelger-Huët cells in the peripheral blood of patients with CML. Although the spectacle form "pince-nez" nuclear deformations are characteristic of this anomaly, peanut-shaped, dumbbell-shaped, bilobate, and rounded nuclear configurations are observed. The rounded or oblong nuclei are more common in pseudo-Pelger-Huët cells than in the heterozygous hereditary anomaly (×400).

Table 2-2 CML versus Leukemoid Reaction

Parameter	*CML*	*Leukemoid Reaction*
Peripheral blood leukocytes	Blasts and promyelocytes No toxic granulation (Dysgranulopoiesis) Basophilia and eosinophilia	Fewer immature cells Toxic granulation, Döhle bodies Decreased eosinophils and basophils
Erythrocytes	Occasional nucleated red blood cells and Howell-Jolly bodies	May be similar
Platelets	Thrombocytosis or thrombocytopenia; giant platelets	May be similar
LAP	Low or absent	Usually high
Ph^1	Present (95%)	Absent
Physical findings		
Sternal tenderness	May be present	Rarely present
Splenomegaly	Usually prominent (95%)	Rarely prominent

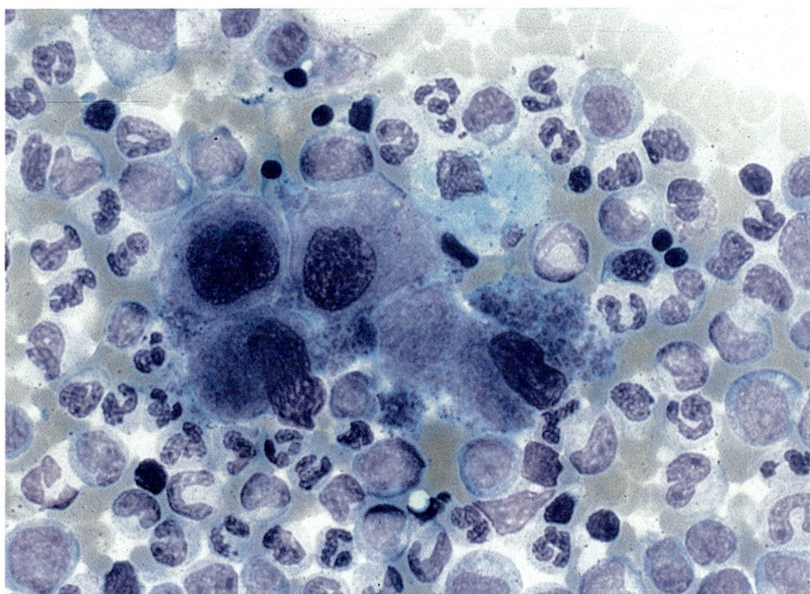

Figure 2-3 Bone marrow of a patient with CML displaying megakaryocytic abutment, a common feature of MPDs. Note sea-blue histiocyte. (×400).

are not nearly as common as observed in the AMLs. Their presence may herald blast crisis. Since morphologic evaluation is of less importance than with the acute leukemias, bone marrow is examined for four other important reasons: (1) cytogenetic studies and bcr rearrangement, (2) in vitro cell growth, (3) oncogenes, that is, *RAS*, and (4) marrow fibrosis.

Reticulin (collagen type 3) is the earliest type of nonbanded collagen fiber associated with early marrow fibrosis. It takes the silver impregnation stain, is commonly increased at the time of diagnosis, and is strikingly increased in nearly half the patients (Fig. 2.4). Marrow fibrosis is associated with a larger spleen size, more severe anemia, higher proportion of marrow and peripheral blood blast cells, additional karyotypic abnormalities, and a poor prognosis. True banded collagen fibrosis usually appears in late stages of CML, indicates a poor prognosis, and is best demonstrated by a Masson trichrome stain (Fig. 2.5).

Approximately one-third of CML patients demonstrate pseudo-Gaucher cells in the spleen and bone marrow (Fig. 2.6). Pseudo-Gaucher cells have been observed in marrow from patients with

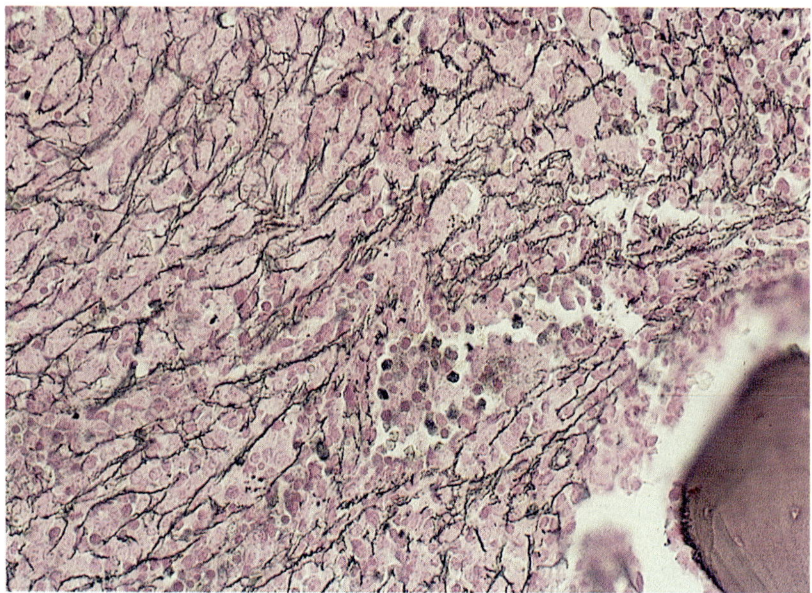

Figure 2-4 Reticulin stain of the bone marrow from a patient with CML showing large numbers of dark-staining precollagen fibers. Such a finding indicates a poor prognosis. (×400).

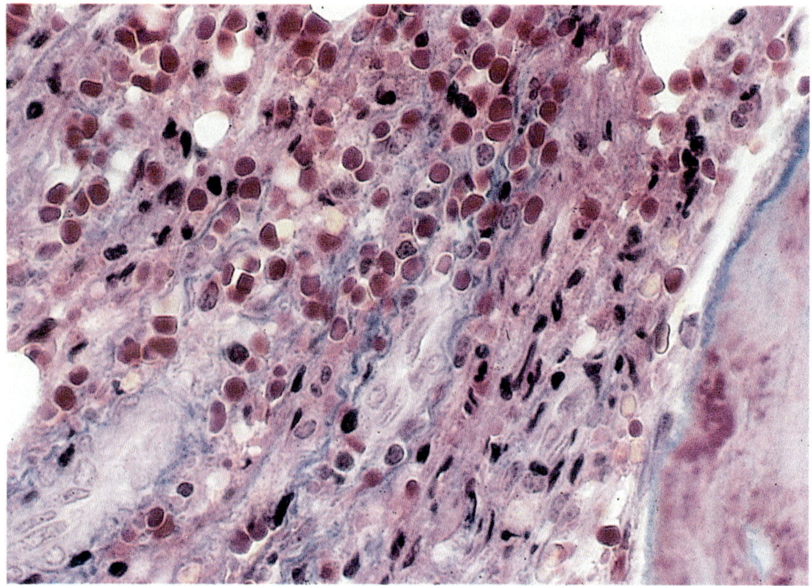

Figure 2-5 Masson trichrome stain of bone marrow from a CML patient exhibiting true banded collagen fibrosis. Note collagen fibers staining blue. This represents permanent collagen, appears in late stages of CML, and indicates a poor prognosis. (×400).

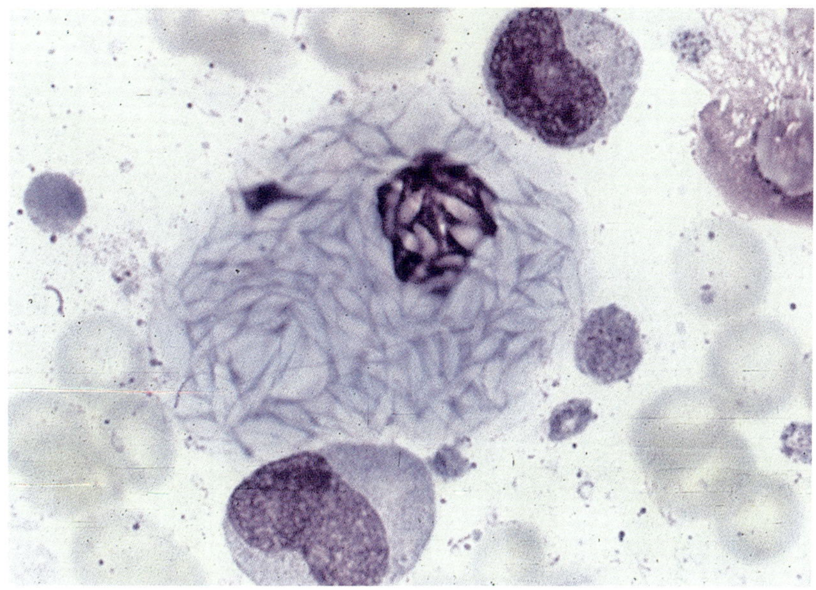

Figure 2-6 (a) Pseudo-Gaucher cell in the bone marrow of a patient with CML. Note "crumpled tissue paper" or "ball of yarn" appearance. Courtesy of Rudolph Ulirsch. (×1000).

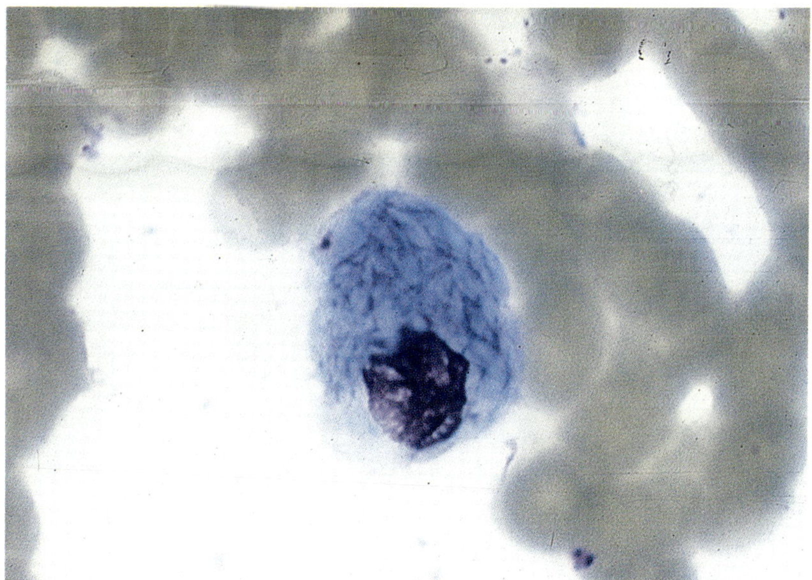

Figure 2-6 (b) Pseudo-Gaucher cell in bone marrow of a patient with CML showing blue fibrillar cytoplasm simulating "ball of yarn" appearance. This cell appears to be a transitional cell between a pseudo-Gaucher cell and sea-blue histiocyte. Courtesy of Rudolph Ulirsch. (×1000).

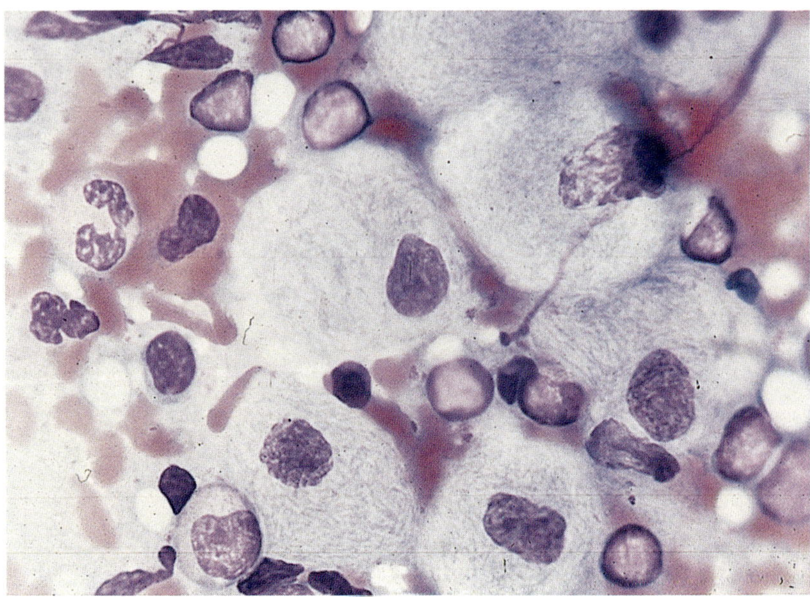

Figure 2-6 (c) Spleen of patient with Gaucher's disease. Contrast these typical Gaucher cells with those hybrids seen in CML. Note colorless cytoplasm. (×400).

thalassemia major, congenital dyserythropoietic anemia, multiple myeloma, immunoblastic lymphoma, and Hodgkin's disease. These cells appear because of the inability of normal cellular glucocerebrosidase activity to degrade the increased glucocerebroside load associated with the markedly increased leukocyte turnover. Pseudo-Gaucher cells appear similar to true Gaucher cells with a fibrillar cytoplasm simulating "crumpled tissue paper" appearance. The cytoplasm stains positive for periodic acid–Schiff (PAS), oil red O (ORO), Sudan black B (SBB), acid phosphatase (AP), and iron.

Sea-blue histiocytes may be observed in CML (Fig. 2.7), AML, acute lymphoblastic leukemia (ALL), idiopathic thrombocytopenic purpura, lymphoma, thalassemia, and sickle cell anemia. They are also observed in a rare primary familial syndrome associated with hepatosplenomegaly and thrombocytopenia, and type B Niemann-Pick disease. These lipid-laden marrow macrophages contain granular and floccular ceroid that is deposited in the cytoplasm and stains blue-green with Wright-Giemsa staining. The cells stain with PAS, ORO, SBB, acid-fast stains, and Baker's acid hematin and show nodular positive autofluorescence.

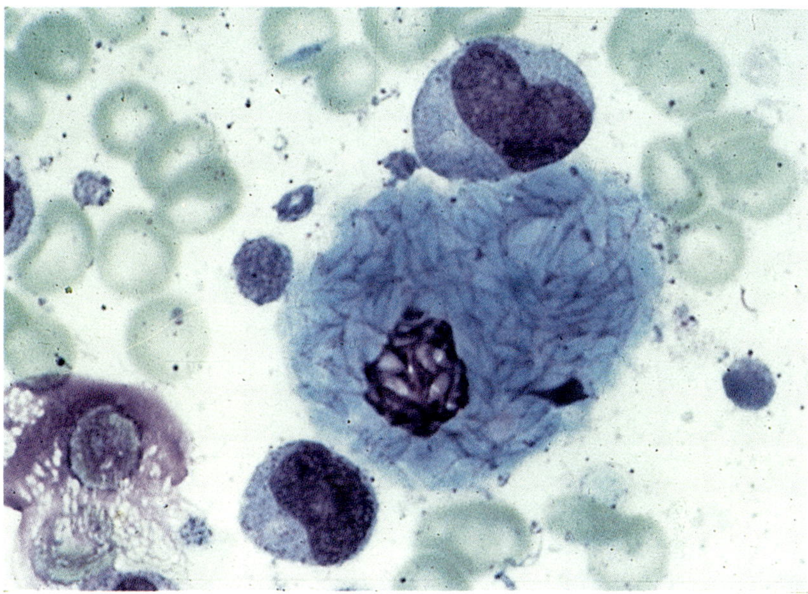

Figure 2-7 Sea-blue histiocyte in the bone marrow of a patient with CML. Note blue-green cytoplasm that still maintains subtle "ball of yarn" appearance. Courtesy of Rudolph Ulirsch. (×1000).

CHRONIC NEUTROPHILIC LEUKEMIA (Fig. 2.8)

Most patients with chronic neutrophilic leukemia (CNL) are over the age of 60, males predominate, splenomegaly occurs in all cases, hepatomegaly is frequent, gouty arthritis common, and lymphadenopathy very infrequent.

The diagnosis is dependent on the clinical findings and examination of peripheral blood and bone marrow. The total leukocyte count is between 25 and 50 $\times$ 10^9/L in the majority of cases and rarely exceeds 100 $\times$ 10^9/L. Neutrophils usually predominate and constitute 90–95% of the leukocytes, although occasional cases may demonstrate 20–50% band forms. Blast cells are usually not present, and rare myelocytes, metamyelocytes, and NRBCs may be present in occasional patients. Toxic granulation and Döhle bodies are not observed. In contrast to CML, the leukocyte alkaline phosphatase (LAP) level is usually increased in all cases, anemia is frequent, but the platelet count is usually normal.

Bone marrow examination reveals marked granulocytic hyperpla-

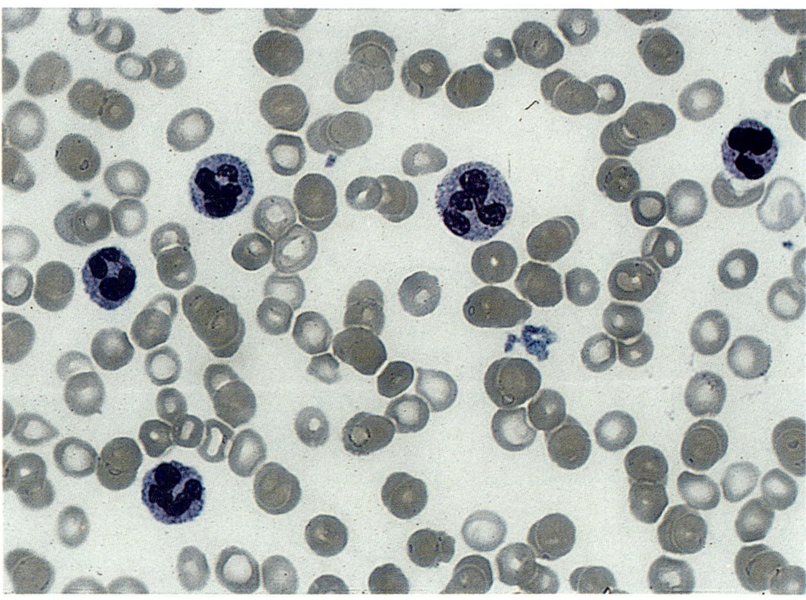

Figure 2-8 Peripheral blood from a patient with CNL. Note predominance of neutrophils and lack of immature elements observed in CML. Also, toxic granulation and Döhle bodies are not seen in the neutrophils. (×400).

sia similar to that found in CML. However, myeloblasts are not overtly increased. Erythropoiesis is usually mildly decreased, and megakaryocyte levels are either normal or increased. Unlike the marrow in CML, reticulin fibrosis is unusual, and the Ph^1 is absent. Most patients have normal karyotypes, but random chromosome abnormalities have been observed. As with CML, levels of serum vitamin B_{12}–binding protein, serum B_{12}, and serum uric acid are increased.

Some patients have developed AML as a terminal event, and a remarkable associated frequency of essential monoclonal gammopathy or muliple myeloma has been seen. The prognosis is much worse than in CML.

CHRONIC MONOCYTIC LEUKEMIA (Fig. 2.9)

Chronic monocytic leukemia (CMoL) is a very rare, poorly documented disorder of the histiomonocytic system. Many cases reported in the literature represent CMML, smoldering leukemia, acute leukemia, and unclassifiable histiomonocytic proliferation.

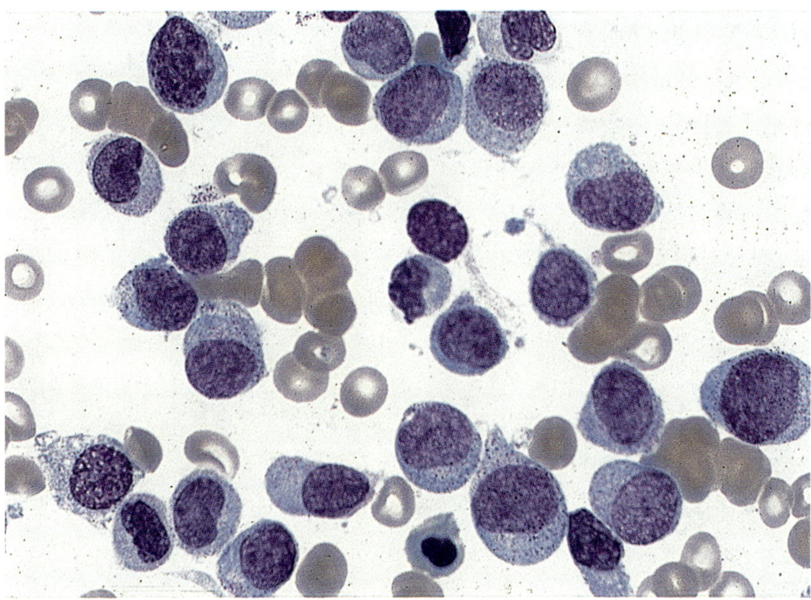

Figure 2-9 Bone marrow from a patient with CMoL. This leukemia is very rare and according to some authors is diagnosed after splenectomy. Monocytes and promonocytes with granules predominate. (×400).

Some authors believe that the disease is diagnosed only after splenectomy. In the authors' opinion, this vague disorder requires additional cases with appropriate documentation utilizing modern technology to create suitable criteria for establishing it as a hematologic entity.

CHRONIC MYELOMONOCYTIC LEUKEMIA (Fig. 2.10)

CMML is a chameleon disorder that may present in infants and children under 4 years of age, or older adults. It manifests itself as an MDS and/or MPD and then frequently explodes terminally into an acute leukemia.

Splenomegaly, sometimes massive, is present in virtually all childhood cases and approximately half of the adult patients.

The FAB group classifies CMML as an MDS that is characterized as follows: (1) absolute monocytosis in the peripheral blood is $>10^9$/L, (2) percentage of blasts in the peripheral blood is $<5\%$ and (3) bone marrow may contain 5–20% blasts, but some patients show a signifi-

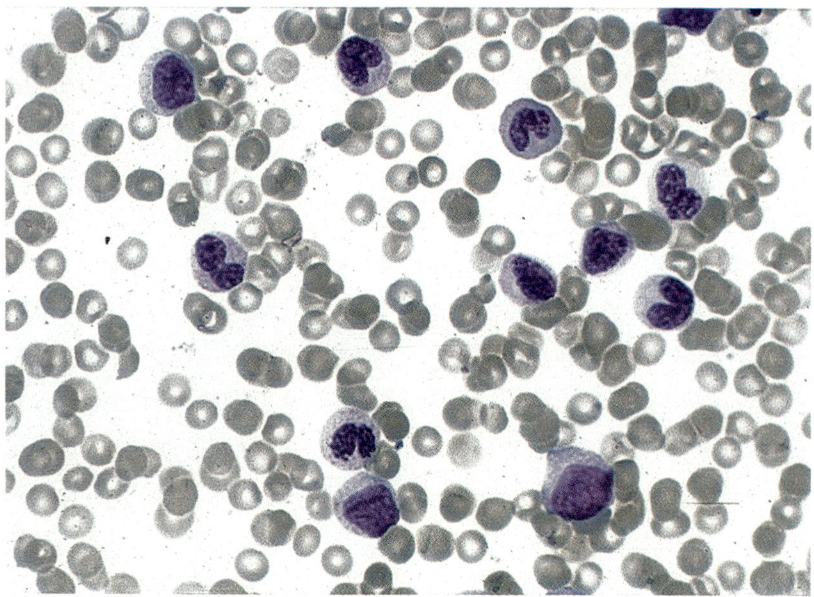

Figure 2-10 Peripheral blood from a patient with CMML. Note cells of both monocytic and myelocytic lineages. (×400).

cant increase in promonocytes and demonstrate <5% blasts in the bone marrow.

At times CMML may be an MPD. Kantarjian et al. (1990) have recommended that myeloproliferative CMML fulfill the following criteria: (1) WBC greater than 20 × 10^9/L and (2) 8% or more monocytes in the peripheral blood or bone marrow. For those cases of CMML featuring more myelodysplasia than proliferation (WBC 20 × 10^9/L or less), an absolute peripheral blood monocyte count of >10^9/L would additionally be required. These criteria help to distinguish CMML from Ph^1-negative CML and RAEB. The authors use this criteria and consider it helpful in difficult cases.

The findings in the marrow depend on the predominance of proliferation, dysplasia, or monocytosis among individual patients. Monocytosis predominates in the marrow and peripheral blood, and dysplastic changes may involve all three cell lines. Qualitative changes include macroblastosis, megaloblastosis, increased sideroblasts, basophilic stippling, and hypo- or hypersegmentation of the myeloid series.

CMML is Ph^1-negative, usually demonstrates elevated blood and urine lysozyme levels, and sometimes demonstrates unexpected polyclonal hypergammaglobulinemia. *RAS* gene mutations occur in

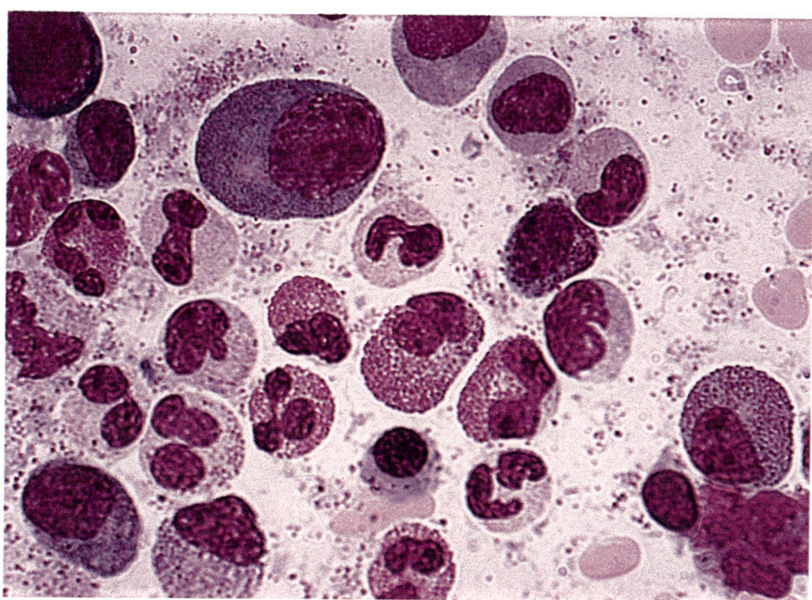

Figure 2-11 Bone marrow from a patient with EL. Note marked eosinophilia, large eosinophilic promyelocyte, and numerous eosinophilic granules in background. (×1000).

30–50% of patients with CMML but are unusual in Ph^1-positive and Ph^1-negative CML. Although Ph^1-positive adult-type CML occurs below the age of 15 years and accounts for 3% of childhood leukemias, a disease different from this disorder designated juvenile CML exists. Juvenile CML accounts for about 2% of childhood leukemias, occurs most often in infants and children under 4 years of age, and is comparable to adult CMML.

EOSINOPHILIC LEUKEMIA (Fig. 2.11)

Early in the course of eosinophilic leukemia (EL) and hypereosinophilic syndrome (HES), it is usually impossible to establish a diagnosis. Both diseases reveal leukocyte counts well over 20×10^9/L and absolute eosinophil counts of greater than 1.5×10^9/L sustained for at least 6 months. Bone marrow examination reveals eosinophilic differentiation from promyelocyte to mature eosinophils with a maturational left shift similar to that of CML. Although almost every organ of the body may be involved, the heart and the lungs frequently demonstrate the most pathologic lesions. Laboratory examination re-

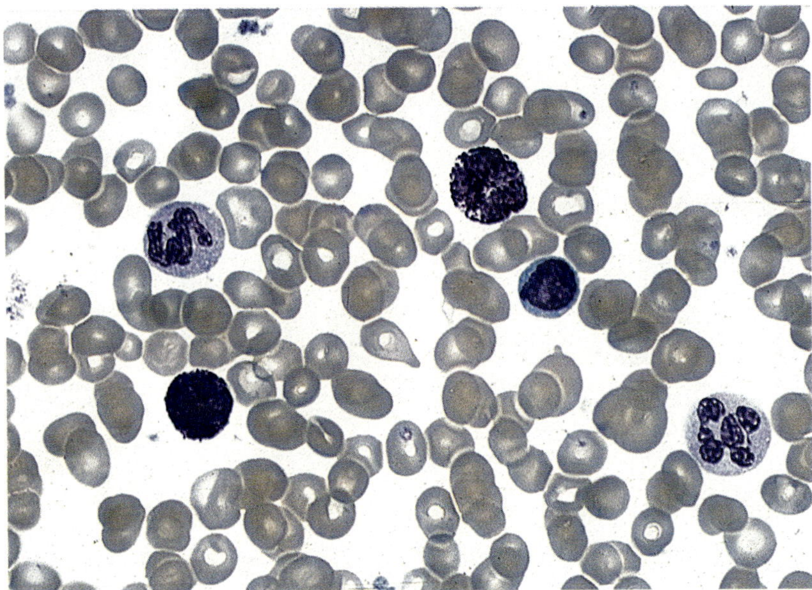

Figure 2-12 Peripheral blood from a patient with CML showing increased basophils. This connotes a poor prognosis, and basophilic leukemia may arise in CML or as de novo acute or chronic leukemia. ($\times 1000$).

veals hyperuricemia, elevated B_{12}-binding capacity, occasionally depressed LAP levels, and increased lysozyme levels consistent with CML. A minority of EL patients are Ph^1+ and should be classified as having a variant of CML. EL must be distinguished from the HES, and from eosinophilia observed occasionally seen in ALL, lymphoblastic lymphoma, and the hypereosinophilic variant of AML (M4Eo) with its associated chromosome-16 abnormalities. Cytogenetic abnormalities support a diagnosis of EL rather than HES. Trisomy 8, 17+, and chromosomal aneuploidy have been reported in some cases of EL.

BASOPHILIC LEUKEMIA (Fig. 2.12)

Basophilic leukemia (BL) is a rare disorder that may occur in the chronic phase of CML or as a manifestation of the accelerated phase of CML. In addition, it may present as a Ph^1-negative, LAP-positive de novo chronic leukemia. Such cases need to be evaluated for bcr rearrangement. Basophilia has been associated with AMLs with t(6;9), t(3;6), and inv(16) chromosomal abnormalities. Furthermore,

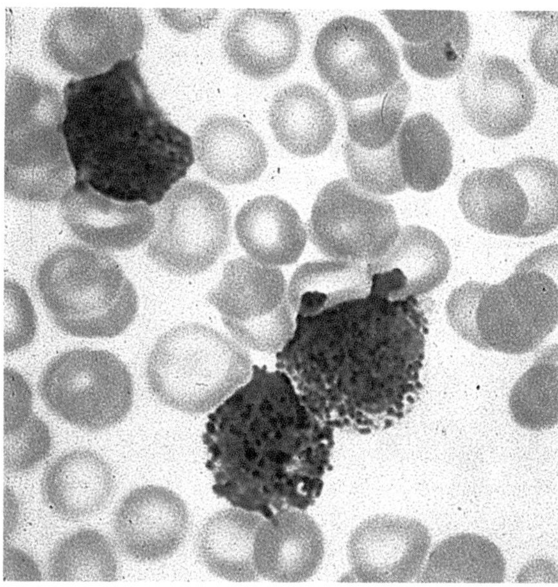

Figure 2-13 Peripheral blood from a patient with mast cell leukemia. Note large mast cells with prominent basophilic granules. These cells differ from basophils in that they are larger and contain hydrolytic enzymes, 5-hydroxytryptamine, and serotonin. (×1000).

cases of acute promyelocytic leukemia with basophilic maturation have been reported. Finally, de novo acute basophilic leukemia exists and may demonstrate symptoms related to histamine release and disseminated intravascular coagulation (DIC). The basophilic circulating cells are peroxidase-negative, but toluidine blue– or Astra blue–positive. With a wide spectrum of presentations, it is most important that all diagnostic parameters be investigated, especially cytochemistries, cytogenetics, bcr rearrangement, and coagulation testing.

CHRONIC MAST CELL LEUKEMIA (Fig. 2.13)

Chronic mast cell leukemia (CMaL) develops in approximately 15% of patients with mast cell neoplasia. Patients may have fever, weight loss, diarrhea, flushing, pruritis, bone pain, and severe abdominal pain. The mast cell, a cell of tissue and bone marrow, differs from the circulating basophil in that it is larger and contains hydrolytic enzymes, 5-hydroxytryptamine, and serotonin; it shows characteristic scroll-like ultrastructural features within granules and discharges its granules exclusively outside the cell (exoplasmosis). Leukocyte

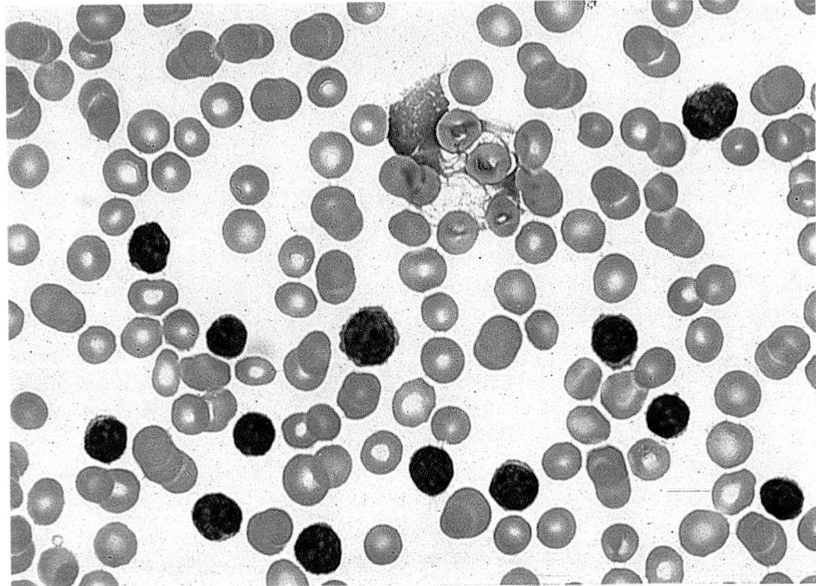

Figure 2-14 Peripheral blood from a patient with CLL. Note characteristic small mature lymphocytes with high nuclear/cytoplasmic ratio. Admixtures of pleomorphic prolymphocytes and prolymphocytes can alter diagnosis and prognosis. ($\times$1000).

counts vary from 10 to 150 $\times$ 10^9/L with 10–90% mast cells. Anemia and thrombocytopenia are invariably present. Bone marrow demonstrates a striking increase in mast cells, some of which may be hypogranular or agranular. Mast cells are negative for myeloperoxidase (MPEX), and alpha naphthyl acetate esterase reactions (A-EST), but usually positive for Giemsa, alcian, Astra, and toluidine blue and aminocaproate esterase (Am-EST). The latter stain is considered by some investigators to be the most specific for mast cells, but special processing of the specimen is required. The malignant form of systemic mastocytosis may develop as a primary disease or may evolve in patients with systemic mastocytosis. This phase may be chronic, but when mast cell leukemia develops, survival is usually less than 6 months.

B-CELL LEUKEMIAS

Chronic Lymphocytic Leukemia (Fig. 2.14)

Most likely all CLLs are of B-cell origin. The various types of lymphocytes observed in the common chronic B-cell leukemias are depicted

Table 2-3 Types of Leukemic B-Lymphoid Cells

*Cell Type (Disease)**	*Size*	*Chromatin*	*Nucleolus*	*Cytoplasm*	*Other Features*
Small lymphocytes (CLL)	<2 RBCs	Clumped in coarse blocks	Absent	Scanty: high nuclear/cytoplasmic ratio	Regular nuclear outline
Large lymphocytes (CLL, mixed cell)	>2 RBCs	Clumped	Inconspicuous or small	Low nuclear/cyto-plasmic ratio, variable	Variable size
Prolymphocytes (PLL)	>2 RBCs	Clumped	One, prominent	Low nuclear/cyto-plasmic ratio	Variable size
Pleomorphic pro-lymphocytes (CLL/PL)	>2 RBCs	Clumped	Central and prominent	Variable nuclear/cy-toplasmic ratio	Variable size
Cleft cells (FL)	1–2 RBCs	Homogeneously coarse	Absent or one or two incon-spicuous	Scanty: not visible or narrow rim	One or two shallow or deep narrow nuclear clefts from angular base

Source: Bennett JM et al: Proposals for the classification of chronic (mature) B and T lymphoid leukemias. *J Clin Pathol* 42:567–584, 1989. Courtesy of John M Bennett and British Medical Association House.

*CLL: Chronic lymphocytic leukemia; PLL: prolymphocytic leukemia; PL: prolymphocyte; FL: follicular lymphoma.

in Table 2.3. Note that the characteristic small lymphocyte of CLL may occur with larger lymphocytes (mixed type). Also, a subtle distinction exists between the pleomorphic prolymphocytes (PLs) of CLL and the more uniform B cells of prolymphocytic leukemia (PLL). However, the PL of CLL may be quite atypical and even mimic infectious mononucleosis cells. Leukemic forms of small lymphocytic lymphoma are similar to the small lymphocytes of CLL. Follicular and diffuse small cleaved lymphomas in their leukemic forms demonstrate distinctive cleaved or clefted cells, the so-called buttock cells.

The diagnosis of CLL established by the International Workshop on CLL (IWCLL) requires (1) lymphocyte counts equal to or greater than 10×10^9/L, (2) bone marrow involvement, and (3) establishment of B-cell phenotype consistent with CLL. If the lymphocyte count is less than 10×10^9/L, both items 2 and 3 are required. In addition to the IWCLL diagnostic criteria, the National Cancer Institute–sponsored working group proposed the following guidelines: (1) mature lymphocytes in the blood should be 5×10^9/L or more, (2) 30% of all nucleated cells should be lymphocytes in the bone marrow aspirate smear, and (3) immunophenotyping of the majority of peripheral blood lymphocytes should be of B-cell type (CD19, CD20, or CD24) that shares one T-cell marker, CD5; the surface immunoglobulin has a low-density expression with only one light chain (either kappa or lambda) preponderance. In typical small cell CLL, small lymphocytes (Fig. 2.14) predominate. Bone marrow aspiration and biopsy both show infiltration with lymphocytes. The extent and pattern of lymphocytic infiltrate on biopsy (i.e., interstitial, nodular, mixed, or diffuse) correlate with the clinical state and prognosis (see Chapter 3).

Besides typical CLL, there are two mixed cell types: (1) CLL/PLL (Table 2.3), which presents a dimorphic picture with small lymphocytes and PLs (>10% and <55%) and (2) CLL with a spectrum of small to large lymphocytes with <10% PLs. Currently the former group may be refractory to treatment and have a poorer prognosis than typical CLL, whereas the second group currently demonstrates no known disadvantage.

B–Prolymphocytic Leukemia (Fig. 2.15)

B-PLL is a distinct disorder characterized by hyperleukocytosis, massive splenomegaly, minimal peripheral adenopathy, and bone marrow infiltration with PLs. PLs are large cells (10–15 μm in diameter) with a thick rimmed nucleolus, moderately dense nuclear chromatin, and pale-blue cytoplasm with a lower nuclear/cytoplasmic ratio than

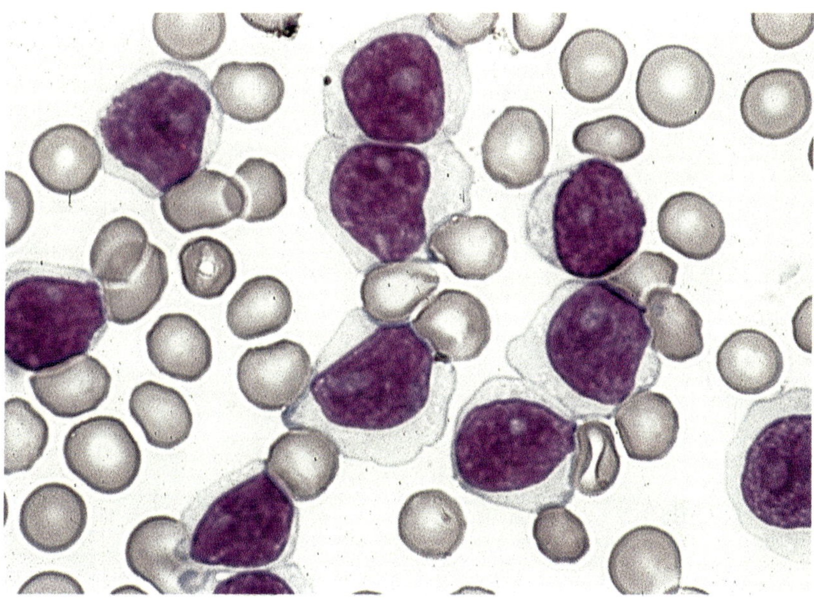

Figure 2-15 Peripheral blood from a patient with B-PLL exhibiting large numbers of PLs. These cells are large and have prominent thick rimmed nucleoli, moderately dense nuclear chromatin, and moderately abundant pale blue cytoplasm. Courtesy of Daniel Catovsky. (×1000).

that of small lymphocytes. Bone marrow involvement may be diffuse or demonstrate a mixed interstitial nodular pattern. Lymph nodes show a diffuse pattern with or without a pseudonodular pattern, and the spleen demonstrates both white and red pulp infiltration by lymphocytes. The white pulp demonstrates a bizonal appearance with follicules showing dense centers and light peripheral zones.

Hairy Cell Leukemia (Fig. 2.16)

Hairy cell leukemia (HCL) is a B-cell malignant lymphoproliferative disorder characterized by pancytopenia, splenomegaly, and the presence of abnormal mononuclear cells with irregular "hairy" cytoplasmic projections in blood, marrow, and other tissues, especially the spleen. On peripheral blood films, the nucleus of the hairy cell is oval, round, or kidney-shaped, frequently exhibiting an inconspicuous small, single nucleolus surrounded by fine diffuse nuclear chromatin. The cytoplasm stains light blue and has a poorly defined outline. In addition, the "hairs" are easily demonstrated in phase-contrast preparations of the peripheral blood. Attempts at bone mar-

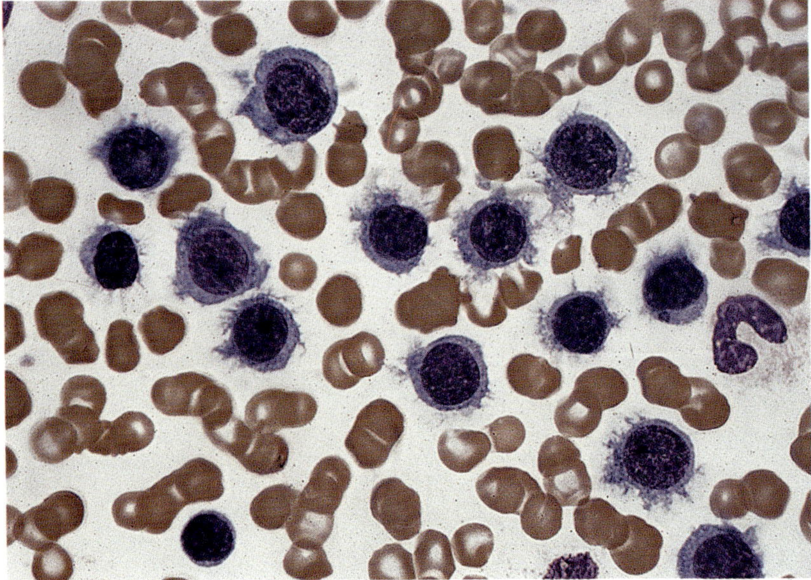

Figure 2-16 Peripheral blood from a patient with HCL who had a previous splenectomy and was in a florid leukemic phase. Note round to oval nucleus, fine diffuse nuclear chromatin, and moderate blue cytoplasm with numerous hairy projections. Such a high count in the peripheral blood is most unusual in HCL. ($\times 1000$).

row procurement usually result in a "dry tap" related to increased reticulin. Bone marrow biopsy is variably infiltrated by hairy cells and reveals a clear zone around the cells, the so-called fried egg appearance. The spleen shows involvement of the red pulp with formation of pseudosinuses, widening of the pulp cords, and numerous fried egg-appearing cells.

Besides classic HCL, a variant exists that has morphologic features combining hairy cells and PLs. The HCL-variant (HCL-v) cell has a moderately condensed nuclear heterochromatin, a single prominent nucleolus, slightly higher nuclear/cytoplasmic ratio, and abundant basophilic cytoplasm, but with the same villous projections as seen in the typical hairy cell (Fig. 2.17). The leukocyte count is greater than 50×10^9/L, an unusual feature of typical HCL. The HCL-v cells infiltrate the red pulp of the spleen causing splenomegaly. The immunophenotype differs from that found in HCL in that the HCL-v cells do not react with CD25 and HC2; however, some cases have been CD11c-positive.

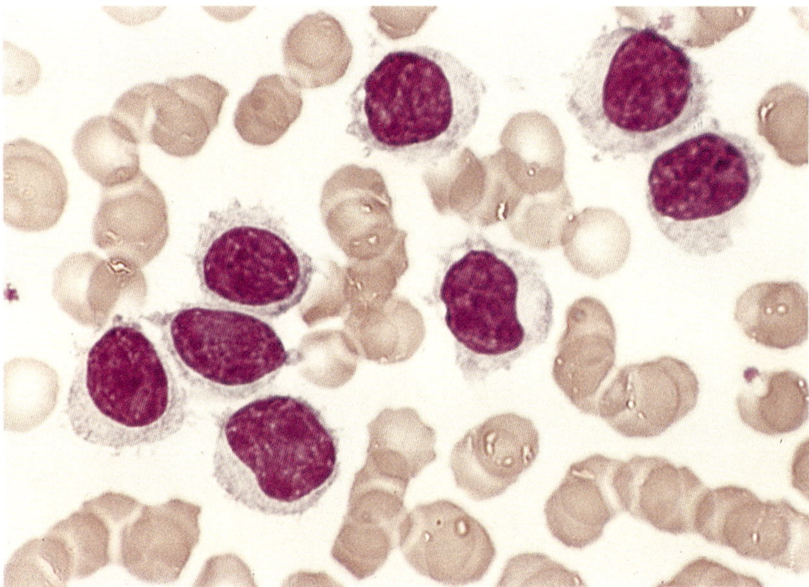

Figure 2-17 Peripheral blood from a patient with HCL-v. The HCL-v cells have moderately condensed nuclear heterochromatin, frequently a single prominent nucleolus, slightly higher nuclear/cytoplasmic ratio, and abundant basophilic cytoplasm with villous projections similar to those of typical hairy cells. Courtesy of Daniel Catovsky. (×1000).

Leukemic Phase of B-Cell Lymphoma

In evaluating a patient with a leukemia, it is always important to keep in mind that leukemias originate in the bone marrow and frequently involve the peripheral blood; however, lymphomas originate in lymph nodes and/or spleen and occasionally involve the peripheral blood and bone marrow. In the past, the term *lymphosarcoma cell leukemia* was applied to the leukemic phase of a lymphoma.

Splenic lymphoma with villous lymphocytes (SLVL) (Fig. 2.18) may be confused with CLL, PLL, HCL, and HCL-v. SLVL cells are characteristically larger than CLL lymphocytes, with short cytoplasmic villi, often localized to one pole. The nuclear/cytoplasmic ratio is greater than that of hairy cells, and a small distinct nucleolus may be present. Rare cells may show lymphoplasmacytic features. Immunophenotype is similar to that of B-cell PLL, and the cells do not react with CD25, CD11c, or HC2. Bone marrow is only involved in approximately half the cases with moderate to extensive nodular and diffuse infiltration. Characteristic of a lymphoma, the white pulp

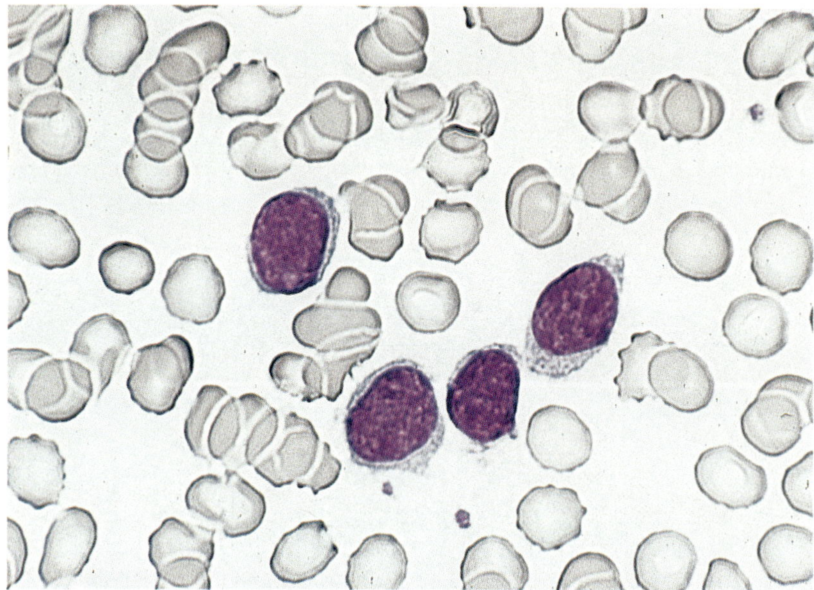

Figure 2-18 Peripheral blood from a patient with splenic lymphoma with villous lymphocytes. These cells are larger than CLL lymphocytes, have short cytoplasmic villi that may be localized to one pole, and demonstrate a greater nuclear/cytoplasmic ratio than hairy cells. Small indistinct nucleoli may be present. Courtesy of Daniel Catovsky. (×1000).

in the spleen is involved, in contradistinction to involvement of the red pulp observed in leukemic disorders (CLL, HCL, HCL-v, PLL).

Follicular lymphomas may demonstrate a leukemic phase with very high WBCs. These small cleaved lymphocytes strikingly demonstrate prominent nuclear clefts or fissures and may divide the nucleus in two (buttock cells) (Fig. 2.19). Contrary to the immunophenotype of B-cell CLL, surface membrane immunoglobulin (SmIg) is strongly positive, FMC7 positive, CD10 often positive, and CD5 usually negative. Bone marrow involvement is common and demonstrates paratrabecular and intertrabecular lymphocytic infiltrate, although occasionally diffuse infiltration is observed.

Intermediate differentiated lymphoma (IDL) (mantle cell) may show leukemic peripheralization in approximately 21% of cases. Apparently the disease may exist as an acute or chronic disorder. Those with absolute lymphocyte counts above 5×10^9/L have a poor prognosis. The lymphocytes are intermediate in size and have condensed chromatin and inconspicuous nucleoli with slight nuclear indenta-

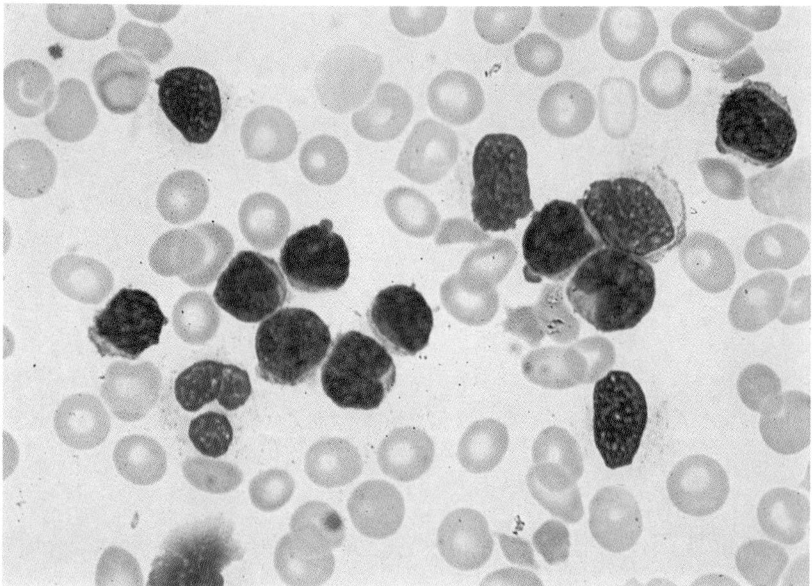

Figure 2-19 Peripheral blood from a patient with follicular lymphoma, small cleaved type in a leukemic phase. Note deep clefts and fissures in some cells forming the so-called buttock cells. (×1000).

tions and clefts (Fig. 2.20). Bone marrow biopsy shows diffuse involvement. Although all the initial cases studied showed a diffuse architectural lymph node pattern, subsequent studies showed the existence of a follicular variant apparently arising in the mantle zone lymphocytes. Hence, the sobriquet *mantle zone lymphoma.* In general, despite the frequent presence of abnormal lymphoid cells in the peripheral blood and often prominent mitoses in tissue sections, intermediate lymphocytic lymphoma may follow a low-grade, relatively indolent clinical course, particularly when a mantle zone rather than a diffuse pattern exists.

Waldenström's macroglobulinemia (WM) may demonstrate a leukemic phase, but leukocyte counts are usually $<10 \times 10^9$/L. WM shows a mélange of lymphocytes in all stages of development that include small and large lymphocytes, atypical lymphocytes, plasma cells, plasmacytoid lymphs, and immunoblasts (Fig. 2.21). The panoply of lymphocytes and plasma cells diffusely infiltrates the marrow. Mast cell numbers are usually increased, and PAS-positive intranuclear bodies (Dutcher bodies) may be observed within the lymphoid elements. Serum IgM elevations are usually >20 g/L.

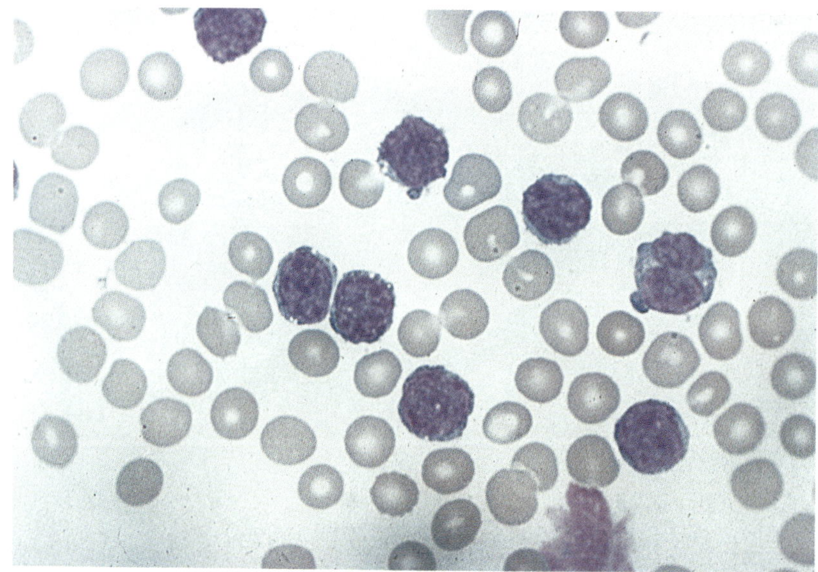

Figure 2-20 Peripheral blood from a patient with IDL (mantle zone lymphoma). Note that the lymphocytes are intermediate in size and have condensed chromatin and inconspicuous nucleoli with slight nuclear indentation and clefts. A rare cell may show buttock-like configuration. (×1000).

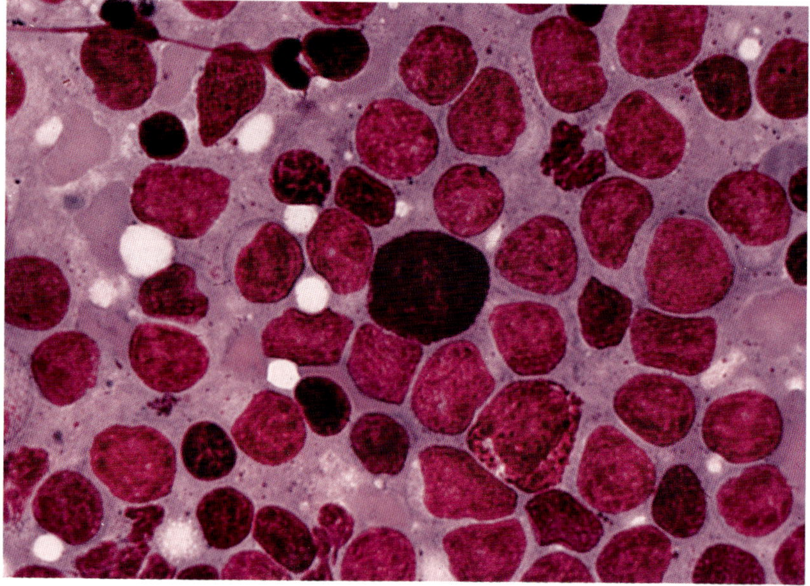

Figure 2-21 Bone marrow from a patient with WM. Note assortment of lymphocytes, plasmacytoid lymphocytes, and immunoblasts in this specimen. Also, notice the mast cell, one of the morphologic hallmarks of this disease. (×1000).

Plasma cell leukemia, a primary leukemia and not the terminal phase of multiple myeloma, is usually an acute leukemia. Two morphologic types seem to exist: one in which the cells are small and the cells range from lymphocytes to plasma cells and the other in which the cells are blastlike. Membrane markers are most helpful in recognizing the latter, and monoclonal cytoplasmic Ig and expression of CD38 are diagnostic. Ultrastructural analysis, Bence Jones proteinuria, and hypercalcemia may contribute in establishing the diagnosis. Primary plasma cell leukemia, unlike the terminal "leukemoid" phase of some myelomas, sometimes responds well to conventional myeloma therapy.

T-CELL LEUKEMIAS

T–Chronic Lymphocytic Leukemia

Most reported series of T-CLL erroneously include a potpourri of the various T-cell chronic lymphoproliferative disorders with at least half representing T-gamma lymphoproliferative disease (TGLD). Some of the lymphocytes of these disorders resemble mature-appearing lymphocytes observed in B-CLL. Some lack granules and usually express the CD4 phenotype, possibly representing cases of adult T-cell leukemia-lymphoma (ATLL). Other cases that are CD8+ probably are cases of TGLD. Their course has varied from fulminating to indolent. In general the natural history of all T-CLLs has been quite variable and probably reflects a spectrum of disease in a relatively rare syndrome as well as the inability of investigators to clearly delineate these T-cell lymphoproliferative disorders. Some authors currently believe that T-CLL does not exist!

T–Gamma Lymphoproliferative Disease (Fig. 2.22)

T-gamma lymphoproliferative disease (TGLD) is a distinct clinical entity that has been obfuscated by a mélange of numerous designations including T-gamma lymphocytosis, T–suppressor cell chronic lymphocytic leukemia, T-cell lymphocytosis with neutropenia, large granular lymphocytic leukemia, and suppressor cell leukemia. The disease is charaterized by large granular lymphocytes in the peripheral blood, a benign clinical course, and a strong association with autoimmune disease. The patients usually demonstrate splenomegaly, occasionally hepatomegaly and lymphadenopathy, and rarely skin involvement. Large granular lymphocytes (LGLs) are a subset of normal circulating cells, constituting 10–15% of peripheral mono-

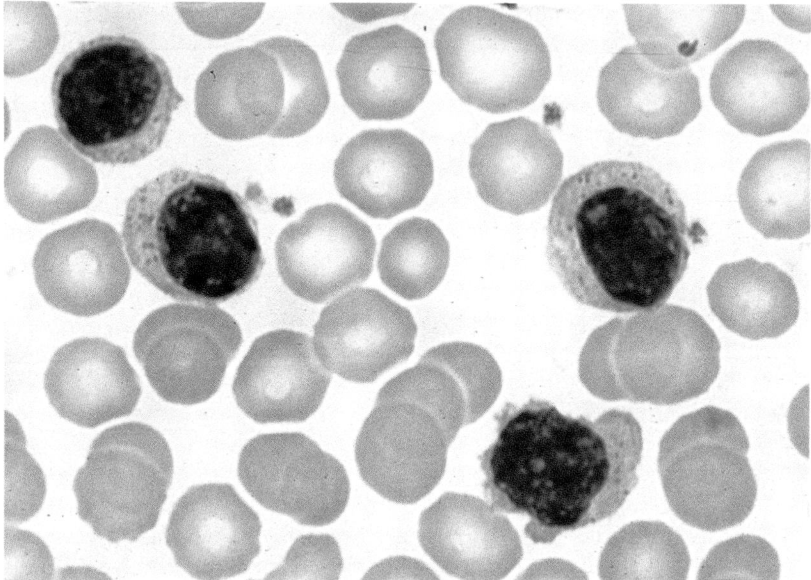

Figure 2-22 Peripheral blood from a patient with T-gamma lymphoproliferative disease. Observe the large lymphocytes with prominent granules. (×1000).

nuclear cells. The total lymphocyte count is elevated but usually less than 20×10^9/L. LGLs have a low nuclear/cytoplasmic ratio and pale-blue cytoplasm that contains azurophilic granules. Nearly all patients have variable degrees of bone marrow infiltration. Most of the cells bear Fc receptors for IgG, and the majority express CD2, CD3, and CD8 and lack CD5. Some authors use lymphoproliferative disorder of granular lymphocytes for these diseases since not all contain the Fc receptor.

T–Prolymphocytic Leukemia (Fig. 2.23)

T-PLL accounts for 20% of the PLLs. T-PLL differs from B-PLL in that the patients usually show lymphadenopthy, skin infiltration, and serous effusions. Both T- and B-PLL patients demonstrate splenomegaly and an aggressive course with WBCs usually in excess of 100×10^9/L. Morphologically, T-PLL is similar to B-PLL in half the cases, but cells in other T-PLL patients have a higher nuclear/cytoplasmic ratio, irregular nuclear outline, and less cytoplasm. Also, some patients may have cells that are small and do not demonstrate a prominent nucleolus by light microscopy. Few case studies show infiltration into the splenic red pulp and obliteration of the white pulp. Bone

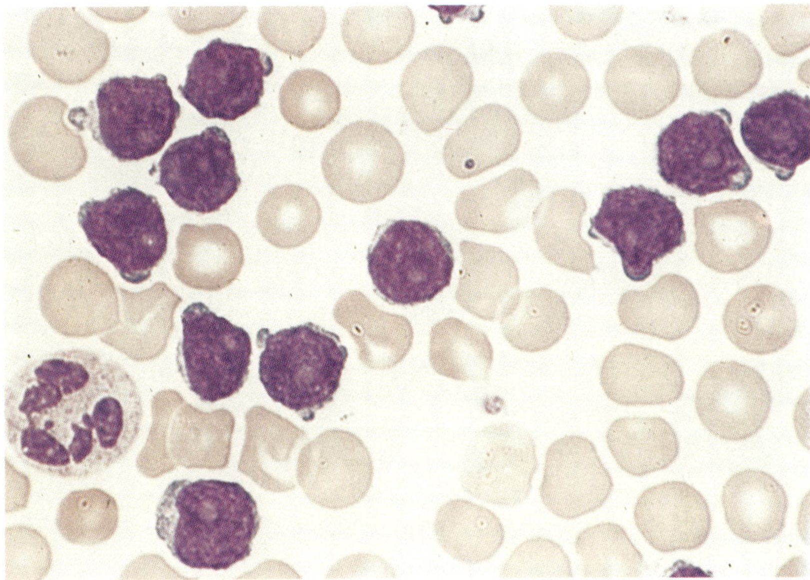

Figure 2-23 Peripheral blood from a patient with T-PLL. These cells may vary from those of B-PLL in that they demonstrate a higher nuclear/cytoplasmic ratio, irregular nuclear outline, and scanty cytoplasm. Note cytoplasmic blebbing. Courtesy of Daniel Catovsky. (×1000).

marrow is usually diffusely infiltrated and shows increased fibrosis. Immunophenotyping shows that the cells have CD2, CD3, CD5, CD4, and/or CD8 on their surface. Patients may respond to splenic radiation or splenectomy, but long-term response to chemotherapy is relatively poor.

Adult T-Cell Leukemia-Lymphoma (Fig. 2.24)

ATLL, first described in Japan over a decade ago, is a spectrum of clinical syndromes that may be acute or chronic. The patients manifest generalized lymphadenopathy associated with circulating polymorphic convoluted abnormal lymphoid cells, bone lesions with bone marrow involvement, hypercalcemia, and skin lesions. The convoluted nucleus may appear like a clover leaf, usually without a nucleolus but if present, small and indistinct. Cytoplasm is moderately abundant, basophilic, and agranular. These cells may be confused with Sézary cells, and those cases of T-PLL without prominent nucleoli. Despite the CD4+ helper phenotype, the cells usually have suppressor activity against mitogen-induced B cells. ATLL has a dis-

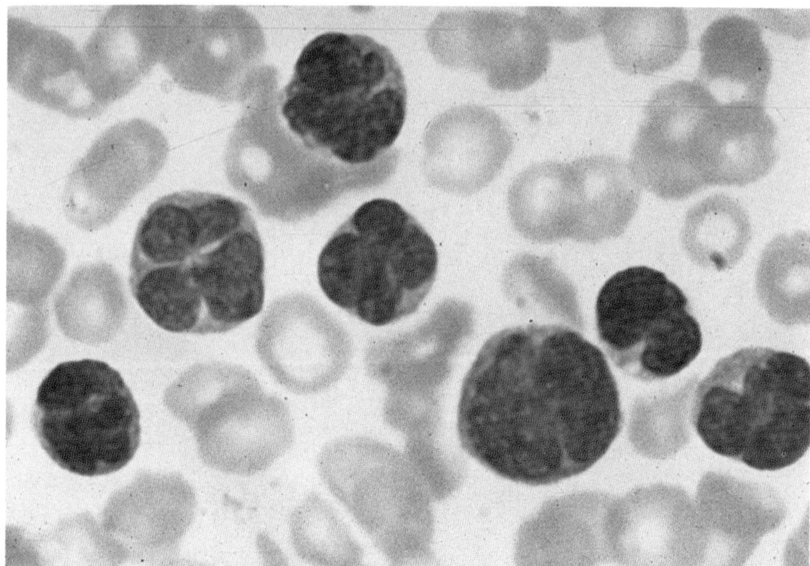

Figure 2-24 Peripheral blood from a patient with ATLL. Note hyperconvoluted lymphoid cells with multiple projecting lobes (propeller cells). (×400).

tinct epidemiology that relates to the first human retrovirus: human T-cell leukemia virus I (HTLV-I), the causative agent. Most cases have been found in southwestern Japan, the Caribbean region, and southeastern United States. The acute form is very aggressive, with a median survival of less than 1 year, whereas patients with the indolent variety may survive for several years.

Sézary Syndrome (Fig. 2.25)

Sézary syndrome (SS) is generally considered to be the leukemic phase of mycosis fungoides and is characterized by generalized exfoliative erythroderma, lymphadenopathy, splenomegaly, and circulating Sézary cells in the peripheral blood. Sézary cells may be (1) atypical small lymphocytes with highly convoluted mulberry-like nuclei, (2) large atypical lymphocytes with hyperchromatic convoluted nuclei surrounded by PAS-positive vacuoles arranged like a string of pearls, and (3) atypical lymphoblasts with cerebriform nuclei and abundant agranular cytoplasm with or without vacuoles. Bone marrow examination is usually normal or may show minimal involvement; however, obvious disease is more apparent as the WBC rises. Skin biopsy

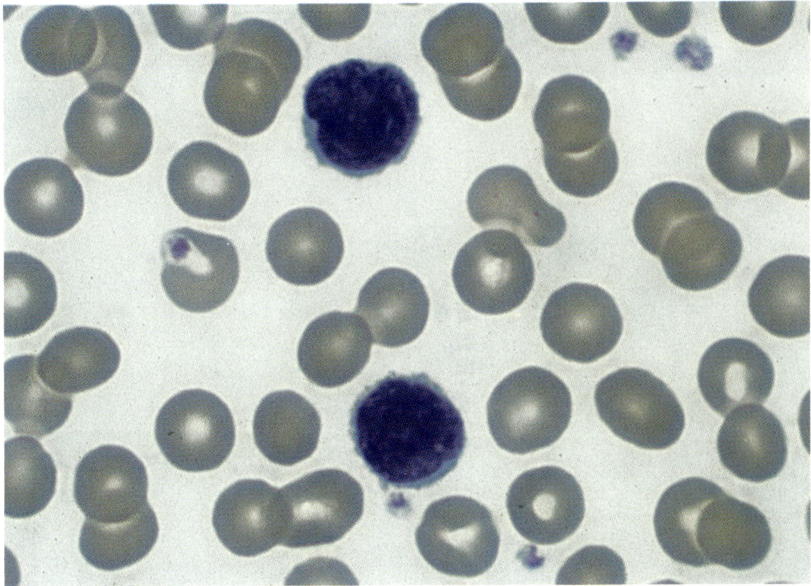

Figure 2-25 Peripheral blood from a patient with SS. Note lymphocytes with highly convoluted cerebriform nuclei and scanty cytoplasm. (×1000).

sections reveal upper dermal infiltration, epidermatropism, and Pautrier's microabscesses. Patients with the SS (median survival 2.5 years) have a poorer prognosis than those mycosis fungoides patients without blood involvement.

T–Hairy Cell Leukemia

T-HCL is rare and accounts for less than 0.01% of all cases of HCL. Most cases have been anecdotal, utilizing older polyclonal antibodies. Also, some hybrid cases demonstrating both B- and T-cell markers have been reported. A multilobular variant of B-HCL with morphologic similarities to T-cell lymphoma has recently been reported. Furthermore, human T-cell leukemia virus II (HTLV-II) has been isolated from rare patients with T-HCL. However, neither this virus nor HTLV-I appears to be associated with classic HCL or its variant, which is more common in Japan. It is doubtful whether this T-cell disease represents a true T-cell variant of HCL or a rare unrelated condition induced by HTLV-II. At this juncture, additional cases are needed to more clearly delineate T-HCL.

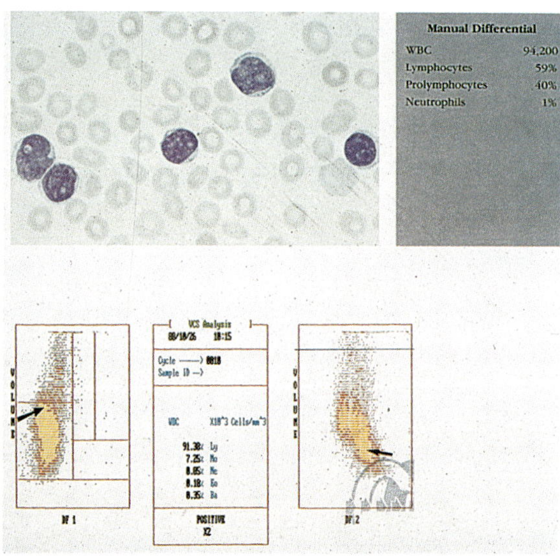

Figure 2-26 Peripheral blood, white cell data, and scatterplot generated by VCS technology from a case of prolymphocytic transformation of CLL. Note volume and DF1 (light scatter) scatterplot showing abnormal population of the larger prolymphocytes (arrow). Also observe volume and DF2 (conductivity) scatterplot, which demonstrates a similar abnormal population of the larger PLs (arrow). Reprinted Courtesy of Coulter Corporation, Hialea, Florida, and with help of Cassandra Boyer, Coulter Corporation.

AUTOMATED HEMATOLOGY ANALYZERS

In addition to light morphology, automated hematology analyzers have begun to impact on diagnosis of leukocytic hematologic disease. These instruments employ a variety of techniques to analyze white blood cells and are now capable of producing an acceptable five-cell population differential. The Coulter STKS analyzer uses a combination of impedance (volume), conductivity, and laser light scatter (VCS technology). The Sysmex NE 8000 combines aperture impedance, radio frequency measurement, and differential cell lysis, whereas the Technicon H1 utilizes tungsten and laser light scatter, peroxidase staining, and differential lysis. The Cell-Dyn, a relative newcomer to the field of automated hematology analyzers, is a fully automated hematology cell counting system utilizing a multi-angle polarized scatter separation to differentiate white blood cells. Cobas Argos 5 Diff, another new arrival, uses electrical impedance, cytochemistry, and optical absorbance for categorizing white cells. Data generated by two of these instruments with microphotographs of the peripheral blood are depicted in Figs. 2.26, 2.27. With this technology, it is

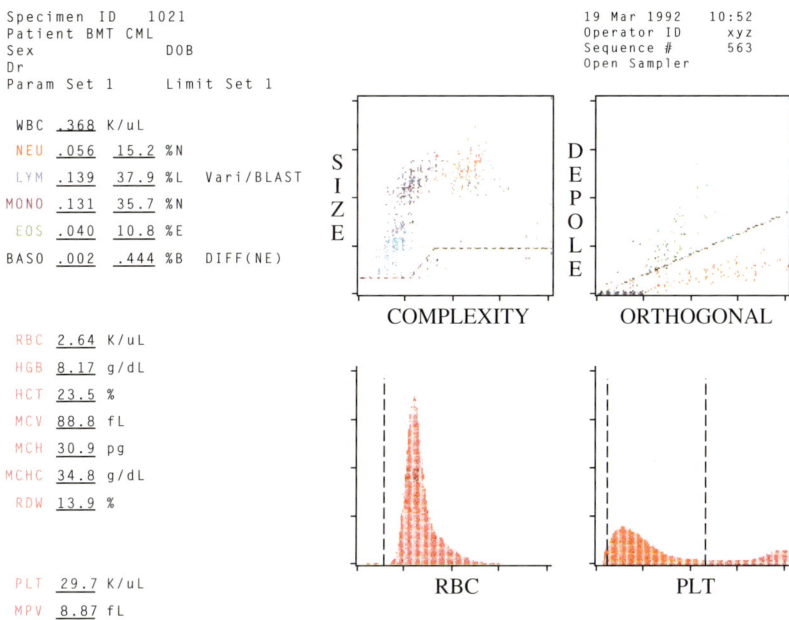

Figure 2-27 Peripheral blood, white cell, red cell, platelet and scatterplot color printout data generated by the Cell-Dyn 3500 from a patient with CML in blast crisis. Note blast flag and distortion of monocyte distribution (lavender) which represent blast cells. Reprinted courtesy of Cell-Dyn, Abbott Diagnostics Division, Mountain View, California and with help of Joseph Orlik, Senior Scientist, Abbott Diagnostics Division.

possible to have presumptive evidence of a leukocytic disorder without first examining the peripheral smear. Needless to say, examination of the peripheral smear with all other data is indicated.

BIBLIOGRAPHY

Articles

Dawson PJ, Dawson G: Adult Niemann-Pick disease with sea-blue histiocytes in the spleen. *Hum Pathol* 13:1115–1120, 1982.

Dekmezian R, Kantarjian HM, Keating MJ, et al: The relevance of reticulin stain-measured fibrosis at diagnosis in chronic myelogenous leukemia. *Cancer* 59:1739–1743, 1987.

Di Donato C, Croci G, Lazzari S, et al: Chronic neutrophilic leukemia: Description of a new case with karyotypic abnormalities. *Am J Clin Pathol* 85:369–371, 1986.

Dorr AD, Moloney WC: Aquired pseudo-Pelger anomaly of granulocytic leukocytes. *N Engl J Med* 261:742–746, 1959.

Hanson CA, Ward PC, Schnitzer B: A multilobular variant of hairy cell leukemia with morphologic similarities to T-cell lymphoma. *Am J Surg Pathol* 13:671–679, 1989.

Hayhoe FGJ, Flemans RJ, Cowling DC, et al: Acquired lipidosis of marrow macrophages: Birefringent blue crystals and Gaucher-like cells, sea blue histiocytes, and grey-green crystals. *J Clin Pathol* 32:420–428, 1979.

Hirsch-Ginsberg C, Le Maistre AC, Kantarjian H, et al: RAS mutations are rare events in Philadelphia chromosome-negative/bcr gene rearrangement-negative chronic myelogenous leukemia, but are prevalent in chronic myelomonocytic leukemia. *Blood* 76:1214–1219, 1990.

Katayarna I, Hirashima K, Maruyama K, et al: Hairy cell leukemia in Japanese patients: A study with monoclonal antibodies. *Leukemia* 1:301–305, 1987.

Kornberg A, Goldfarb A, Shaler O, et al: Pseudo Pelger-Huët anomaly in chronic lymphocytic leukemia. *Acta Haematol* 66:127–128, 1981.

Lee RE, Ellis LD: The storage cells of chronic myelogenous leukemia. *Lab Invest* 24:261–264, 1971.

Le Maistre A, Lee MS, Talpaz M, et al: *RAS* oncogene mutations are rare late stage events in chronic myelogenous leukemia. *Blood* 73:889–891, 1989.

Liesveld-Liesveld J, Smith BD: Acquired Pelger-Huët anomaly in a case of non-Hodgkin's lymphoma. *Acta Haematol* 79:46–49, 1988.

McDaniel HL, MacPherson BR, Tindle BH, et al: Lymphoproliferative disorder of granular lymphocytes. *Arch Pathol Lab Med* 116:242–248, 1992.

O'Donnell JR, Farrell MA, Fitzgerald MX, et al: Agnogenic myeloid metaplasia preceded by repeated leukemoid reactions and persistent acquired Pelger-Huët anomaly of granulocytes. Case report with review of acquired Pelger-Huët anomaly. *Cancer* 50:1498–1505, 1982.

Rosenblatt JD, Gassan JC, Glaspy J, et al: Relationship between human T cell leukemia virus-II and atypical hairy cell leukemia: A serological study of hairy cell leukemia patients. *Leukemia* 1:397–401, 1987.

Wahlin A, Nordenson I, Roos G: Chronic monocytic leukemia terminating in blastic transformation. *Blut* 53:405–409, 1986.

Warner BA, Reardon DM, Marshall DP: Automated haemotology analysers: A four way comparison. *Med Lab Sci* 47:285–296, 1990.

Weisenburger DD: Non-Hodgkin's lymphomas of primary follicle/mantle zone origin. *Leukemia* 5(1):26–29, 1991.

Wick MR, Li CY, Pierre RV: Acute nonlymphocytic leukemia with basophilic differentiation. *Blood* 60:38–45, 1982.

Youman JD, Taddeini L, Cooper T: Histamine excess symptoms in basophilic chronic granulocytic leukemia. *Arch Intern Med* 131:560–562, 1973.

Review Articles

Bearman RM, Kjeldsberg CR, Pangalis GA, et al: Chronic monocytic leukemia in adults. *Cancer* 48:2239–2255, 1981.

Benevenisti DS, Ultmann JE: Eosinophilic leukemia. Report of five cases and review of the literature. *Ann Intern Med* 71:731–745, 1969.

Bennett JM, Catovsky D, Daniel MT, et al: Proposals for the classification of chronic (mature) B and T lymphoid leukaemias. French-American British (FAB) Cooperative Group. *J Clin Pathol* 42:567–584, 1989.

Berline N: T gamma lymphocytosis and T cell chronic leukemias. *Hematol Oncol Clin North Am* 4:473–487, 1990.

Chang KL, Stroup R, Weiss L: Hairy cell leukemia: Current status. *Am J Clin Path* 97:719–738, 1992.

Cheson BD, Bennett JM, Rai KR, et al: Guidelines for clinical protocols for chronic lymphocytic leukemia: Recommendations of the NCI (National Cancer Institute)-sponsored working group. *Am J Hematol* 29:152–163, 1988.

Denburg JA: Basophil and mast cell lineages in vitro and in vivo. *Blood* 79:846–860, 1992.

Dighiero G, Travade P, Chevret S, et al: B-cell chronic lymphocytic leukemia: Present status and future directions. *Blood* 78:1901–1914, 1991.

Fauci AS, Harley JB, Roberts WC, et al: NIH Conference. The idiopathic hypereosinophilic syndrome. Clinical pathophysiologic and therapeutic considerations. *Ann Intern Med* 97:78–92, 1982.

International Workship on Chronic Lymphocytic Leukemia: Chronic lymphocytic leukemia: Recommendations for diagnosis, staging and response criteria. *Ann Intern Med* 110:236–238, 1989.

Kantarjian HM, Kurzrock R, Talpaz M: Philadelphia chromosome negative chronic myelogenous leukemia and chronic myelomonocytic leukemia. *Hematol Oncol Clin North Am* 4:389–404, 1990.

Kulo A, Kawonami M, Matsuyama E, et al: Chronic neutrophilic leukemia associated with monoclonal gammopathy (IgA, kappa type). *Rinsho Ketsueki* 30:858–862, 1989.

Quattrin N: Follow up of sixty-two cases of acute basophilic leukemia. *Biomedicine* 28:72–79, 1978.

Rai KR, Han T: Prognostic factors and clinical staging in chronic lymphocytic leukemia. *Hematol Oncol Clin North Am* 4:447–456, 1990.

Sausville EA, Eddy JL, Makuch RW, et al: Histopathologic staging at initial diagnosis of mycosis fungoides and the Sézary syndrome. Definition of three distinctive prognostic groups. *Ann Intern Med* 109:372–382, 1988.

Schumacher HR, Garvin DF, Triplett DA: *Introduction to Laboratory Hematology and Hematopathology.* New York, Alan R Liss, 1984, pp 75–86.

Silver RT: Chronic myeloid leukemia. A perspective of the clinical and biologic issues of the chronic phase. *Hematol Oncol Clin North* 4:319–335, 1990.

Silver RT, Gale RP: Chronic myeloid leukemia. *Am J Med* 80:1137–1148, 1986.

Sokal JE, Baccarani M, Russo D, et al: Staging and prognosis in chronic myelogenous leukemia. *Semin Hematol* 25:49–61, 1988.

Spiers AS: Chronic granulocytic leukemia. *Med Clin North Am* 68:713–727, 1984.

Swaim W: Laboratory and clinical evaluation of white blood cell differential counts. Comparison of the Coulter VCS, Technicon H-1, and 800-cell manual method. *Am J Clin Pathol* 95:381–388, 1991.

Tharp MD: The spectrum of mastocytosis. *Am J Med Sci* 289:119–132, 1985.

Travis WD, Li CY, Hoagland-Hoagland HC, et al: Mast cell leukemia: Report of a case and review of the literature. *Mayo Clin Proc* 61:957–966, 1986.

Watanabe S, Mukai K, Shimoyama M: Peripheral T-cell lymphoma. *Cancer Metastasis Rev* 7:243–261, 1988.

Webb TA, Lin CY, Yam LT: Systemic mast cell disease: A clinical and hematopathologic study of 26 cases. *Cancer* 49:927–938, 1982.

CHAPTER 3

Staging

GENERAL COMMENTS

The heterogenous nature of CML and the continuous accumulation of functionally incompetent lymphocytes in CLL involving blood, bone marrow, lymph nodes, and spleen have compelled numerous investigators to create prognostic staging systems to predict outcome in these chronic leukemias. Although numerous CML staging systems have been proposed by various investigators for CML, none have received the wide acceptance enjoyed by the Rai and Binet CLL staging schemes. Both CLL staging systems are simple to utilize in the clinic and are accurate predictors of survival for the majority of CLL patients. Recently, the International Workshop on Chronic Lymphocytic Leukemia (IWCLL) has recommended integrating the Binet and the Rai staging systems.

CHRONIC MYELOGENOUS LEUKEMIA AND RELATED DISORDERS

An accurate understanding of patient prognosis is essential for the evaluation of clinical trials aiming to improve treatment strategies in CML. Earlier efforts in this direction identified a number of disease

Table 3-1 Staging of Metamorphosis in CML

I.	Extramedullary metamorphosis without bone marrow invasion
II.	Accelerated myeloproliferative phase without overt blastic change
III.	Blasts over 30% but confined to bone marrow
IV.	Invasion of the peripheral blood: blast cells over 20% of the differential count (1) with anemia, (2) with thrombocytopenia, (3) with neutropenia
V.	Extensive organ involvement

Source: Spiers ASD: Metamorphosis of chronic granulocytic leukemia: Diagnosis, classification, and management. *Br J Haematol* 41:1–7, 1979. Courtesy of Alexander SD Spiers and Blackwell Scientific Publications, Ltd.

features associated with a poor outlook. There is general agreement regarding the validity of most of these ominous signs, but difficulty arises in identifying prognostic criteria permitting prediction of the course of patients still in the chronic stage of disease. Conventionally, CML is divided into three general stages: (1) chronic, (2) accelerated, and (3) blast crisis. However, the term *metamorphosis,* or change from the chronic stable phase to a more aggressive form, has been introduced and used to an advantage by some investigators. The metamorphosis, or change, that occurs in the disease is far more intricate than is implied by the restricted term *blast crisis.* Indeed, the wary clinician should suspect metamorphosis with any deviation in clinical or hematologic features during the chronic phase of CML. In spite of the high index of suspicion, it is not uncommon for weeks or even months to elapse between the appearance of the first atypical features and the firm conclusion that the disease has undergone metamorphosis and become refractory. The stages of metamorphosis are shown in Table 3.1 In stage I, dissemination of disease to blood and bone marrow occurs early. Stage II is heterogenous; the process departs from CML and may mimic any of the MPDs. Findings vary widely, the most common being failure of erythrocyte, platelet, and/or, less frequently, neutrophil production. This stage has a much greater propensity to convert to the blastic phase (approximately 80%) than any other MPD. Stage III probably represents an earlier phase than stage IV, in which the peripheral blood is involved. Peripheral blood from a patient with a myeloblastic and a lymphoblastic crisis of CML is shown in Figs. 3.1 and 3.2. Stage V is distinguished by a massive body load of leukemic cells, which may or may not represent progression from stage IV.

Besides stages of metamorphosis of CML in individual patients, some investigators have attempted to stage all patients with CML

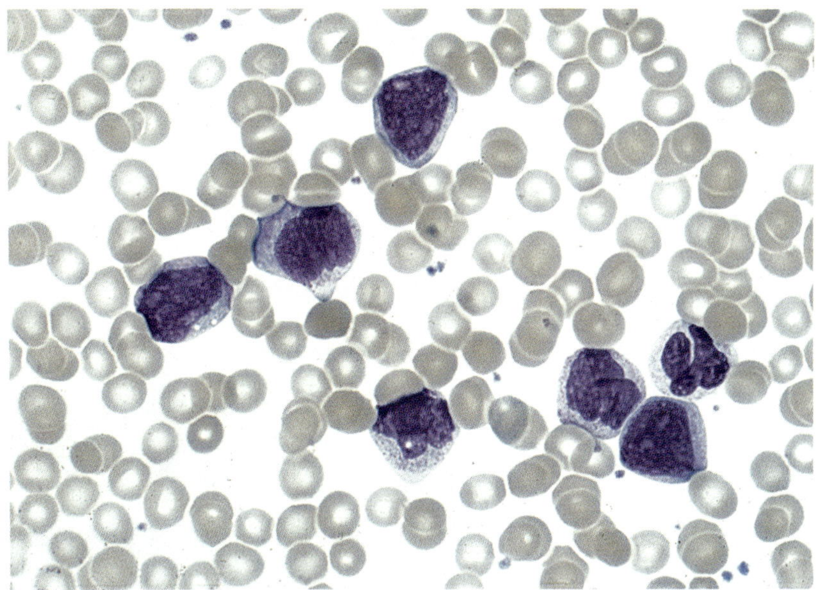

Figure 3-1 Peripheral blood from a patient with CML in myeloblastic crisis. Note increased numbers of blasts and promyelocytes. Some mature residual granulocytic elements remain. (×1000).

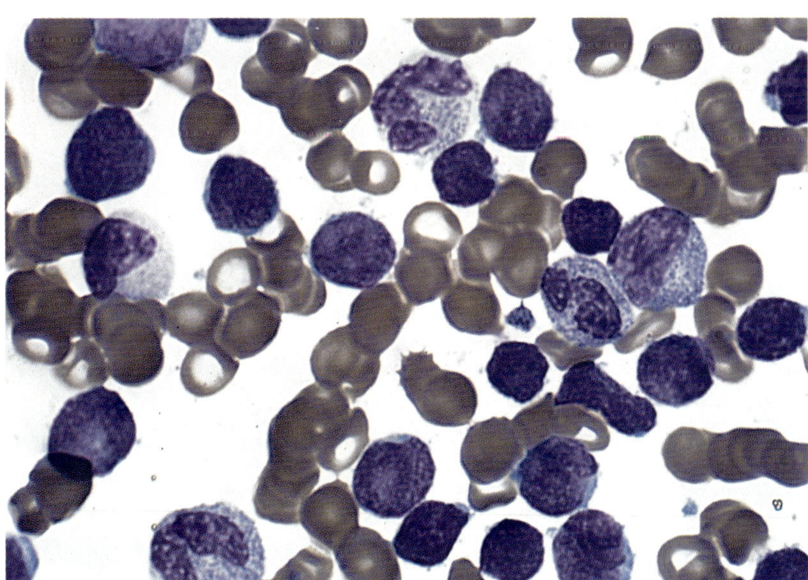

Figure 3-2 Peripheral blood from patient with CML in lymphoblastic crisis. Note large numbers of blasts with high nuclear/cytoplasmic ratio lacking distinct nucleoli. Some residual granulocytic elements are also present. (×1000).

Table 3-2 Summary of the Staging Systems for CML

Reference	*Poor Prognostic Factor**	*Method of Classification*
Tura et al. (1981)	Spleen ≥ 15 cm bcm Liver ≥ 15 cm bcm Plt > 500 or < 150 × $10^3/\mu L$ WBC ≥ 100 × $10^3/\mu L$ Blood blasts ≥ 1% Blood promyelocytes + myelocytes ≥ 20%	Stage 1 = 0 or 1 factor Stage 2 = 2 or 3 factors Stage 3 = ≥ 4 factors
Cervantes, Rozman (1982)	Spleen > 0 cm bcm Liver > 0 cm bcm Marrow blasts > 5% Nucleated red cells ≥ 1%	Stage 1 = 0 or 1 factor Stage 2 = 2 factors Stage 3 = ≥ 3 factors
Sokal et al. (1984)	Older age High platelet counts Englarged spleen High blood blasts percentage	Solve regression equation, assign to stage based on value of hazard ratio
Kantarjian et al. (1985)	Blood basophils ≥ 7% Black race Chromosome abnormality other than Ph^1 Age ≥ 60 years Marrow basophils ≥ 3%	Solve regression equation, assign to stage based on value of hazard ratio

Source: Kantarjian HM, et al: Chronic myelogenous leukemia: A multivariate analysis of the associations of patient characteristics and therapy with survival. *Blood* 66:1326–1335, 1985. Courtesy of Hagop M Kantarjian and Cahners Publishing Company Medical Health.

*bcm = below costal margin; Plt = platelets; WBC = white blood cells.

into different risk groups at onset. These are depicted in Table 3.2. All use a three-stage system that includes chronic, accelerated, and blastic stages. Unfortunately, there is no agreement on the definition of these stages. A patient might be classified as "blastic" at one center and "accelerated" at another. Furthermore, differentiation between "chronic" and "accelerated" disease may be difficult, especially among untreated patients. The Kantarjian et al. (1985) criteria for "new synthesis prognostic staging system" for CML were based on literature results, clinical experience, and an earlier study by these authors that defined the characteristics of the accelerated-phase CML. This new synthesis prognostic staging system designed by Kantarjian

Table 3-3 Proposed Synthesis Staging System for CML

Stage	*Median Definition*	*Parameters*	*Survival (Months)*
1	0 or 1 characteristic parameter at right	Age ≥ 60 years Spleen ≥ 10 cm below costal margin	56
2	2 characteristic parameters at right	Blasts ≥ 3% in blood or ≥ 5% in marrow Basophils ≥ 7% in blood or ≥ 3% in marrow	45
3	≥ 3 characteristics including parameter at right	Platelets ≥ 700 × $10^3/\mu L$	30
4	≥ 1 characteristic parameter(s) at right (regardless of features listed above)	Cytogenetic cloncal evolution Blasts ≥ 15% in blood Blasts + promyelocytes ≥ 30% in peripheral blood Basophils ≥ 20% in blood Platelets < 100 × $10^3/\mu L$	30

Source: Kantarjian HM, et al: Proposals for a simple synthesis prognostic staging system in chronic myelogenous leukemia. *Am J Med* 88:1–8, 1989. Courtesy of Hagop M Kantarjian and Cahners Publishing Company Medical Health.

et al. (1989) is depicted in Table 3.3. Note that stage 3 and 4 both demonstrate 30 months' median survival; however, stage 4 was associated with a higher mortality rate (29%) at 1 year, compared with stage 3 (9%). The new synthesis prognostic staging system has two objectives: (1) to test the proposed CML staging systems and (2) to develop a more accurate and simple staging system based on the existing knowledge of prognostic factors, clinical experience, and the experience with accelerated-phase CML. Kantarjian et al. make the claim that their new synthesis prognostic staging system is superior to the other CML staging systems. However, only time will tell whether this staging system for CML will enjoy the same worldwide acceptance as have the Rai and Binet staging systems for CLL.

CHRONIC LYMPHOCYTIC LEUKEMIA AND RELATED DISORDERS

Based on the observations of Dameshek (1967) and Galton (1966) that CLL is a disease of continuous accumulation of functionally incompe-

Table 3-4 Clinical Staging System for Chronic Lymphocytic Leukemia

Stage	*Findings at Diagnosis**	*Median Survival (Months)*
0	Lymphocytes in blood 15 × 10^9/L (15,000/μL) or higher, and 40% or more lymphocytes in marrow†	150
I	Above plus enlarged lymph nodes	101
II	Above plus splenomegaly, hepatomegaly, or both	71
III	Above plus anemia (HGB less than 11 g/dL)	19
IV	Above plus thrombocytopenia (platelets less than 100 × 10^9/L 100,000/μL)	19

Source: Rai KR, et al: Clinical staging of chronic lymphocytic leukemia. *Blood* 46:219–234, 1975. Courtesy of Kanti R Rai and WB Saunders Company.

*In stages II to IV, lymph node enlargement may be present or absent; in stages III and IV, splenomegaly and hepatomegaly are not essential features.

†Threshold has been lowered by NCSWG to 5000/μL, and by the IWCLL to 10,000/μL.

tent lymphocytes, Rai et al. proposed a staging system in which the tumor burden correlated directly with the stage of the disease, that is, minimum tumor burden correlated with earliest stage, heavy tumor burden correlated with later stages. Initially, they used five stages, which are shown in Table 3.4. However, after several years of use, it became difficult to apply this staging classification in adequately planning prospective therapeutic trials. Therefore, only three groups of survival curves that differed from each other were utilized: (1) stage 0, (2) stages I and II combined, and (3) stages III and IV combined. The Rai et al. (1975) criteria proposed a 15 × 10^9/L lymphocytosis in the peripheral blood. In 1981, Binet et al. presented a method of staging that incorporated anemia, thrombocytopenia, and lymphadenopathy (Table 3.5). Recently, the IWCLL recommended that the Rai and Binet staging systems be combined, with the Binet stage designated first as a letter and the Rai stage to follow given in Roman numerals in parenthesis: A(0) or A(I) or A(II), B(I) or B(II), and C(III) or C(IV). Although Rai and Binet set the threshold for absolute lymphocytosis at ≥ 15 × 10^9/L, the National Cancer Institute Sponsored Working Group (NCSWG) and the IWCLL placed these thresholds at 5 × 10^9/L, and 10 × 10^9/L, respectively. Albeit that the staging systems of Rai and Binet have been both simple and easy to apply to clinical medicine and are accurate predictors of survival, both fail to prospectively identify those patients whose disease will remain

Table 3-5 International Clinical Staging Scheme for Chronic Lymphocytic Leukemia

		Median Survival (Years)
Stage A	Lymphocytosis in blood, 15 × 10^9/L (15,000/μL) or higher,* and 40% or more marrow lymphocytes. No anemia or thrombocytopenia, and less than three areas of nodal involvement.†	>7
Stage B	Lymphocytosis in blood and marrow as above with three or more areas of lymphoid involvement, enlarged lymph nodes, spleen, or liver. No anemia or thrombocytopenia.	<5
Stage C	Lymphocytosis in blood and marrow as above with anemia (HGB less than 10 g/dL in women) or thrombocytopenia (less than 100 × 10^9/L (100,000/μL)) regardless of lymphoid involvement.	<2

Source: Binet JL, Anguier A, Dighero G, et al: A new prognostic classification of chronic lymphocytic leukemia derived from a multivariate survival analysis.*Cancer* 48:198–206, 1981.

*Threshold has been lowered by NCSWG to 5000/μL, and by the IWCLL to 10,000/μL.

†Each cervical, axillary, and inguinal area (whether unilateral or bilateral), spleen, and liver count as one area. The number of areas of lymphoid involvement thus ranges from one to five.

quiescent with an indolent course and those with a rapidly progressive clinical course.

In an attempt to better predict the clinical course, other promising parameters have been evaluated. Blood lymphocyte count seems to correlate with survival; those patients with lymphocyte counts below 50 × 10^9/L have an indolent course, whereas those with higher counts demonstrate a more aggressive course. Blood lymphocyte doubling time (LDT) has been used to predict outcome. If the LDT is longer than 12 months, as in the low and intermediate risk groups, the patients tend to have a benign indolent course, whereas those with shorter LDT usually have a more aggressive clinical course.

Bone marrow biopsy pattern of the lymphocytic infiltrate can offer prognostic information. Four patterns have been recognized: (1) diffuse, (2) nodular, (3) interstitial, and (4) mixed nodular and diffuse (Fig. 3.3). These can be broadly classified into two groups—diffuse and nondiffuse. Patients with a diffuse lymphocytic infiltrate tend to

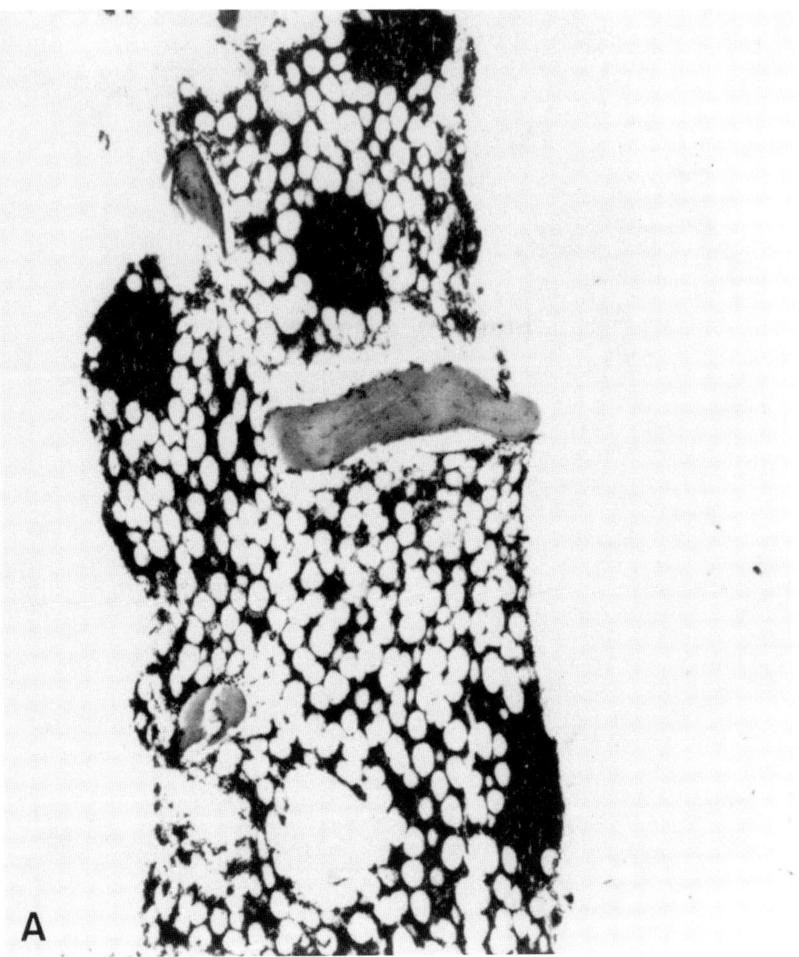

Figure 3-3 (A) Bone marrow biopsy from patient with CLL showing nodular pattern of infiltration.

have an aggressive course, while those with a nondiffuse pattern have an indolent course.

Combined LDT and bone marrow pattern may be used to predict outcome. Those with a long LDT and nondiffuse bone marrow pattern have an indolent course, whereas those with a short LDT and diffuse bone marrow pattern have an aggressive course.

CLL can undergo three transformations that alter staging criteria and predict an unfavorable prognosis. These are (1) prolymphocytic transformation of CLL and hybrid CLL/PLL, (2) Richter transforma-

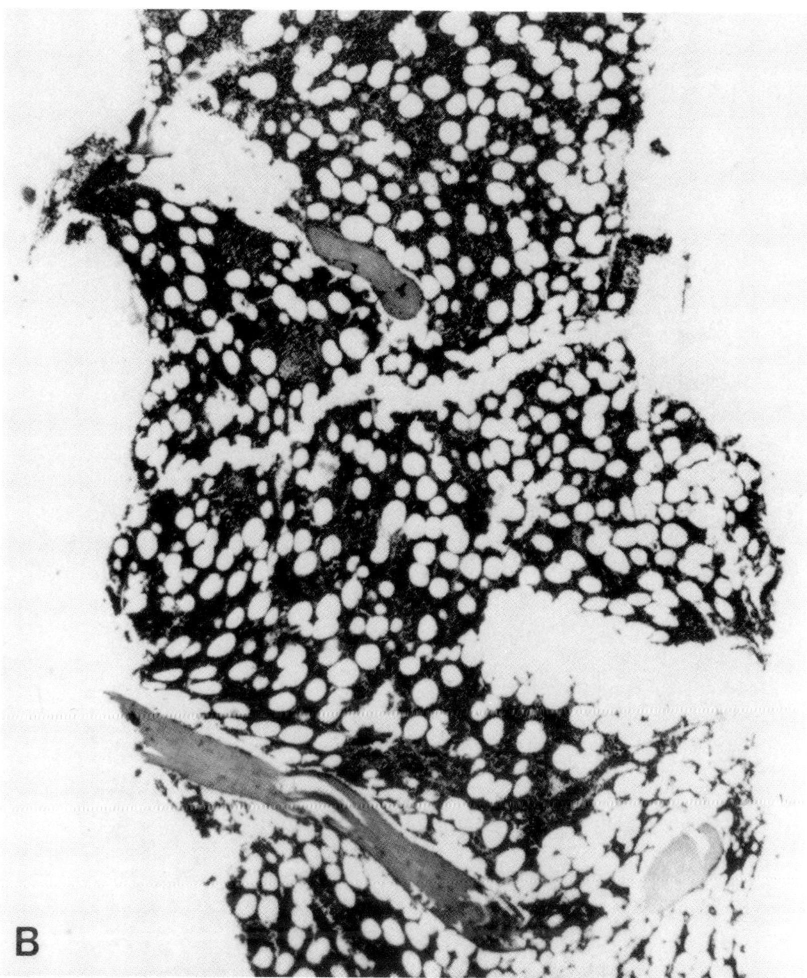

Figure 3-3 (B) Bone marrow biopsy from patient with CLL showing interstitial pattern of infiltration.

tion, and (3) acute lymphoblastic leukemia. Prolymphocytic transformation is an insidious and sometimes progressive change in the disease, in about 10% of cases. Progressive splenomegaly is a feature of PLL and may be an acquired abnormality in prolymphocytic transformation. In about 15% of CLL patients, there is a population of small lymphocytes and prolymphocytes (11–55% of lymphoid cells). These patients are designated hybrid CLL/PLL and have more pronounced splenomegaly. Some have a more aggressive course than the usual CLL patient. Fever, weight loss, rapid lymph node enlargement, ab-

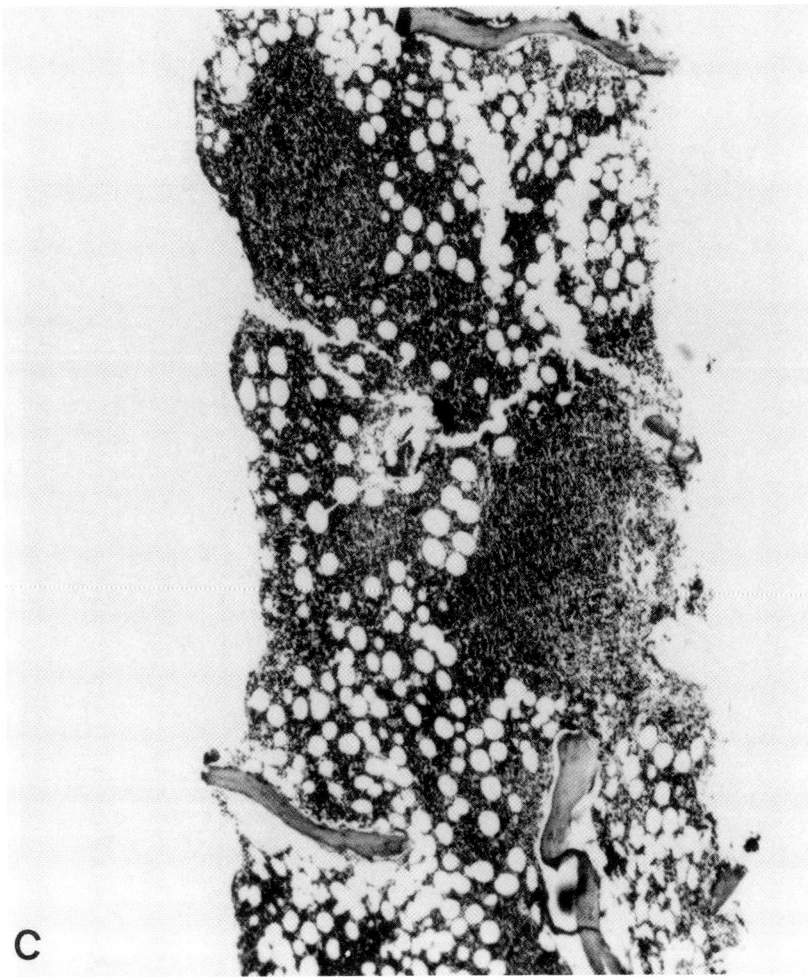

Figure 3-3 (C) Bone marrow biopsy from patient with mixed nodular and interstitial pattern of infiltration.

dominal symptoms, hepatosplenomegaly, central nervous system symptoms, and clinical deterioration are suggestive of Richter syndrome. This transformation represents an aggressive lymphoproliferative disorder resembling large cell lymphoma. Lymph node biopsy is essential and reveals architecture effaced by large immunoblasts with abundant basophilic cytoplasm, irregular nuclei, and prominent nucleoli (Fig. 3.4). Response to chemotherapy is poor, and median survival is usually about 4 months; however, intensive multiagent

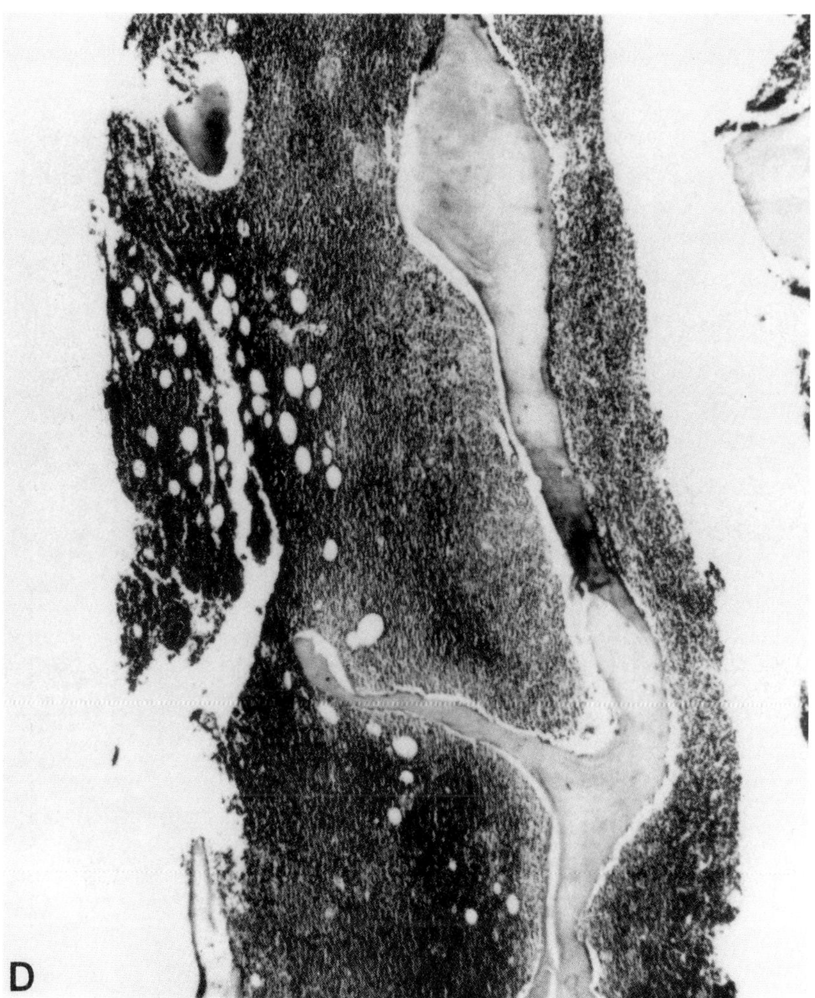

Figure 3-3 (D) Diffuse patterns of infiltration. (×35). Reproduced with permission from Pangalis GA, et al: Patterns of bone marrow involvement in chronic lymphocytic leukemia and small lymphocytic (well differentiated) non-Hodgkin's lymphoma. *Cancer* 54:702–708, 1984. Courtesy of GA Pangalis and JB Lippincott.

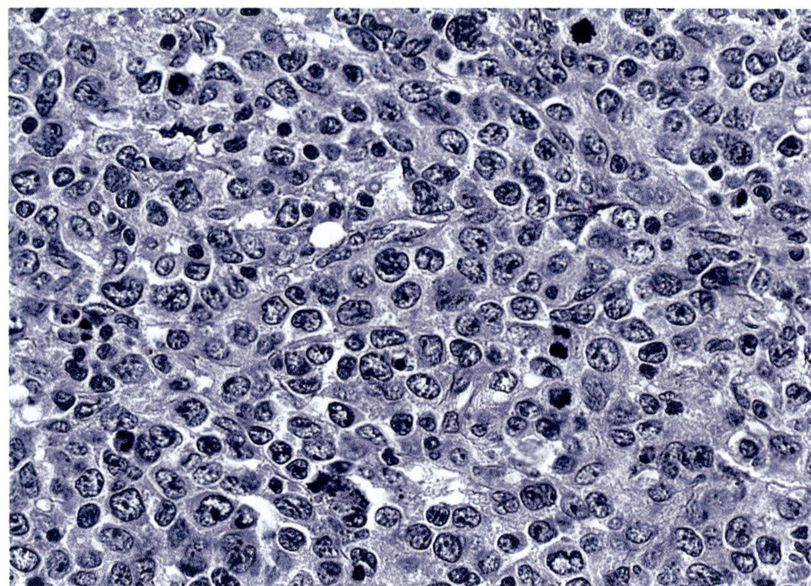

Figure 3-4 Lymph node from a patient with Richter's transformation in a CLL. Note sheets of large immunoblastic cells. ($\times 400$). Courtesy of Elaine Jaffe.

regimens have resulted in occasional long-term remission. ALL transformation in CLL is extremely rare. Cases described have demonstrated FAB L2 morphology, and the blast cells bear intense surface Ig, HLA-DR activity, and strong terminal deoxynucleotidyl transferase (Tdt) positivity. The increased simultaneous expression of the c-*MYC* and μ chain genes in ALL transformation in CLL has been reported.

Occasionally, non-Hodgkin's lymphomas (NHLs) may involve peripheral blood in a leukemic manner. The staging of the NHLs uses the Ann Arbor staging classification. The clinical staging is based solely on physical examination and laboratory results, whereas pathologic staging is based on biopsies. Only those lymphomas that involve the peripheral blood in a leukemic phase, arbitrarily defined as greater than 5×10^9/L abnormal lymphocytes in the peripheral blood, will be considered here. Such cases may or may not demonstrate bone marrow involvement. They represent stage IV disease and can be further subdivided as those without symptoms (A), or those with symptoms (B). B symptoms include (1) unexplained weight loss of more than 10% of the body weight in 6 months before admission, (2) unexplained fever with temperatures above 38°C, and

(3) night sweats. Most NHLs in the leukemic phase have B symptoms and would be staged IVB.

Splenic lymphoma with villous lymphocytes involves the peripheral blood (WBC 3–38 × 10^9/L), white pulp of the spleen, and bone marrow in 50% of the cases in a moderate to pronounced diffuse or nodular infiltration.

Prior to the era of immunologic markers, several conditions (B- and T-derived) were broadly described as *lymphosarcoma cell leukemia.* The most common NHL to produce a stage-IV leukemic phase is follicular lymphoma. The WBC may be as high as 45–220 × 10^9/L. The lymphocytes are small, cleaved, sometimes splitting the nucleus, earning them the name *buttock cells.* Bone marrow involvement is common and characteristically shows paratrabecular localization; however, diffuse infiltration can be observed.

Intermediate NHL (mantle zone lymphoma) involves the peripheral blood in 21% of cases at initial presentation. Those cases with leukemic involvement of the peripheral blood (absolute lymphocyte counts > 5 × 10^9/L have a poorer prognosis than those with no or slight peripheralization. However, the disease may follow a relatively indolent course, particularly when a mantle zone rather than a diffuse architectural pattern predominates. Bone marrow biopsy may show diffuse disease, especially when a diffuse lymph node pattern exists.

Lymphoplasmocytic lymphoma, including WM, may demonstrate a leukemic phase. In WM, the paraprotein concentrations are usually greater than 20 g/L and the WBC less than 10 × 10^9/L. However, in those cases considered here, the abnormal lymphoid population must be greater than 5 × 10^9/L. Both peripheral blood and bone marrow are infiltrated with a heterogenous array of lymphocytes, plasmacytoid lymphocytes, immunoblasts, and plasma cells. Mast cells are frequently observed in the bone marrow.

SS, a T-cell disorder, is characterized by generalized exfoliative erythroderma, an epidermal infiltrate of atypical mononuclear cells, and greater than 20% Sézary cells circulating in the peripheral blood. Staging is complex, and the reader is referred to Sausville et al. (1988) for more details (see Case 14). The median survival is 40 months, versus 10 years or more in patients with a negative smear. Furthermore, a positive peripheral smear is not uniformly associated with visceral disease, as only 16 of 51 patients with a positive smear in the review by Sausville et al. had visceral involvement. The median survival was 25 months for patients with visceral disease and 90 months for those without. Therefore, those with both peripheral blood involvement and visceral disease have a poor prognosis. Surprisingly, of the patients with peripheral blood involvement, only about 10% showed evidence of bone marrow disease. In contrast, circulating neoplastic cells are strongly correlated with advanced histopathologically determined lymph node disease. This supports the concept that Sézary cells probably arise from these involved lymph nodes. The clinical usefulness of the Sausville staging system remains to be utilized to demonstrate its true clinical usefulness!

BIBLIOGRAPHY

Articles

Brouet JC, Fermand JP, Laurent G, et al: The association of chronic lymphocytic leukaemia and multiple myeloma: A study of eleven patients. *Br J Haematol* 59:55–66, 1985.

Bunn PA Jr., Lamberg SI: Report of the Committee on Staging and Classification of Cutaneous T-Cell Lymphomas. *Cancer Treat Rep* 63:725–728, 1979.

Carbone PP, Kaplan HS, Musshoff K, et al: Report of the Committee on Hodgkin's Disease Staging Classification. *Cancer Res* 31:1860–1861, 1971.

Cervantes F, Rozman C: A multivariate analysis of prognostic factors in chronic myeloid leukemia. *Blood* 60:1298–1304, 1982.

Cheson BD, Bennett JM, Rai KR, et al: Guidelines for clinical protocols for chronic lymphocytic leukemia: Recommendations of the National Cancer Institute Sponsored Working Group. *Am J Hematol* 29:152–163, 1988.

Dameshek W: Chronic lymphocytic leukemia—An accumulative disease of immunologically incompetent lymphocytes. *Blood* 29:566–584, 1967.

Fermand JP, James JM, Herait P, et al: Associated chronic lymphocytic leukemia and multiple myeloma: Origin from a single clone. *Blood* 66:291–293, 1985.

Foucar K, Rydell RE: Richter's syndrome in chronic lymphocytic leukemia. *Cancer* 46:118–134, 1980.

Galton DA: The pathogenesis of chronic lymphocytic leukemia. *Can Med Assoc J* 94:1005–1010, 1966.

Kantarjian HM, Smith TL, McCredie KB, et al: Chronic myelogenous leukemia: A multivariate analysis of the associations of patient characteristics and therapy with survival. *Blood* 66:1326–1335, 1985.

Kantarjian HM, Dixon D, Keating MJ, et al: Characteristics of accelerated disease in chronic myelogenous leukemia. *Cancer* 61:1441–1446, 1988.

Pangalis GA, Roussou PA, Kittos C, et al: B-chronic lymphocytic leukemia. Prognostic implication of bone marrow histology in 120 patients: Experience from a single hematology unit. *Cancer* 59:767–771, 1987.

Rozman C, Montserrat E, Rodríguez-Fernández JM, et al: Bone marrow histologic pattern—The best single prognostic parameter in chronic lymphocytic leukemia: A multivariate survival analysis of 329 cases. *Blood* 64:642–648, 1984.

Sausville EA, Eddy JL, Makuch RW, et al: Histopathologic staging at initial diagnosis of mycosis fungoides and the Sézary syndrome. Definition of three distinctive prognostic groups. *Ann Intern Med* 109:372–382, 1988.

Shaw MT: Clinical and haematological manifestations of the terminal phase. In Shaw MT: *Chronic Granulocytic Leukemia.* Eastbourne, Praeger, 1982, pp 169–188.

Sokal JE, Cox EB, Baccarani M, et al: Prognostic discrimination in "good-risk" chronic granulocytic leukemia. *Blood* 63:789–799, 1984.

Spiers ASD: Metamorphosis of chronic granulocytic leukemia: Diagnosis, classification, and management. *Br J Haematol* 41:1–7, 1979.

Torelli UL, Torelli GM, Emilia G, et al: Simultaneously increased expression of the *c-myc* and mu chain genes in the acute blastic transformation of a chronic lymphocytic leukaemia. *Br J Haematol* 65:165–170, 1987.

Tura S, Baccarani M, Corbelli G, et al: Staging of chronic myeloid leukaemia. *Br J Haematol* 47:105–119, 1981.

Review Articles

Binet JL, Auquier A, Dighiero G, et al: A new prognostic classification of chronic lymphocytic leukemia derived from a multivariate survival analysis. *Cancer* 48:198–206, 1981.

Binet JL, Catovsky D, Chandra G, et al: Chronic lymphocytic leukemia: Proposals for a revised prognostic staging system. *Br J Haematol* 48:365–367, 1981.

Dighiero G, Travade P, Chevret S, et al: B-cell chronic lymphocytic leukemia: Present status and future directions. *Blood* 78:1901–1914, 1991.

International Workshop on Chronic Lymphocytic Leukemia. Chronic lymphocytic leukemia: Recommendations for diagnosis, staging and response criteria. *Ann Intern Med* 110:236–238, 1989.

Kantarjian HM, Keating MJ, Smith TL, et al: Proposal for a simple synthesis prognostic staging system in chronic myelogenous leukemia. *Am J Med* 88:1–8, 1990.

Rai KR: A critical analysis of staging in CLL. In Gale RP, Rai KR: *Recent Progress and Future Direction*. UCLA symposia on molecular and cellular biology. New Series, vol. 59. New York, Alan R Liss, 1987, pp 253–264.

Rai KR, Sawitsky A, Cronkite EP, et al: Clinical staging of chronic lymphocytic leukemia. *Blood* 46:219–234, 1975.

Weisenburger DD, Nathwani BN, Diamond LW, et al: Malignant lymphoma, intermediate lymphocytic type: A clinicopathologic study of 42 cases. *Cancer* 48:1415–1426, 1981.

CHAPTER 4

Cytochemistry, Terminal Deoxynucleotidyl Transferase, Histochemistry and Miscellaneous Abnormalities

GENERAL COMMENTS

In contrast to the acute leukemias, cytochemical stains and terminal deoxynucleotidyl transferase (Tdt) do not, with some exceptions, play as important a role in diagnosing the chronic leukemias. On the other hand, histochemical stains such as chloracetate esterase (CAE), reticulin, and trichrome may be more helpful in certain situations in the chronic leukemias than in the acute leukemias. Also, miscellaneous abnormalities involving uric acid, serum B_{12}-binding proteins, serum B_{12}, serum lactic dehydrogenase, serum potassium, serum calcium, skeletal defects, and serum and urine immunoglobulins may be helpful in diagnostic evaluations.

LAP activity in neutrophils, a key cytochemical stain, has been used to differentiate between CML and leukemoid reaction. It will be discussed in detail later.

AP activity may help provide initial immunophenotypic information since it is localized in the Golgi area and has a characteristic dotlike appearance in T cells. All nonerythrocytic isoenzymes of AP except isoenzyme 5 are sensitive to tartrate. Hairy cells of HCL contain isoenzyme 5 and are resistant to tartrate inhibition. This finding, usually performed on peripheral blood, constitutes an important diagnostic parameter in this disorder.

The PAS reaction is not specific for any of the chronic leukemias. In CML, the PAS reaction in the granulocytes is less than that of the normal granulocytes. This stain is not helpful in the chronic lymphoid leukemias, but a granular and block positivity arranged in a rosary-bead pattern with clear areas of cytoplasm between the granules supports a diagnosis of ALL. Controversy concerning both diagnostic and clinical significance of the PAS reaction exists among hematologists and hematopathologists.

The CAE reaction, or Leder's stain, is most useful as a specific marker for the granulocytic series with some exceptions. Mast cells and histiocytes show strong CAE activity. Since it is not entirely specific and does not begin to accumulate until the promyelocytic stage, it lacks the importance of MPEX in the acute leukemias. However, since it can be used to stain tissue, it is used to great advantage to diagnose granulocytic sarcoma and extramedullary hematopoiesis. In addition, cytochemical preparations on touch material may be utilized.

The nonspecific esterases utilized in our laboratory include alpha naphthyl acetate esterase (A-EST) and alpha naphthyl butyrate esterase (B-EST). Both A-EST and B-EST reactions are positive for monocytes; however, megakaryocytes are strongly positive with A-EST but negative or weakly positive with B-EST. Both may be used with advantage to help diagnose myelomonocytic, monocytic, and megakaryocytic leukemias. If the A-EST is reacted in an acidic environment with prolonged incubation, the enzyme revealed is called acid A-EST (AA-EST). The acid A-EST reacts with helper T cells and has been useful in identifying chronic T-lymphoid leukemias, mycosis fungoides, and SS. Combined esterase (C-EST) as used in our laboratory consists of both CAE and A-EST. It allows one to evaluate both the granulocytic and monocytic series simultaneously on one slide. Therefore, C-EST becomes valuable in evaluating myelomonocytic leukemias.

MPEX activity is found in the primary granules of the granulocytic series and the lysosome granules of the monocytic series. It is not normally found in lymphoid cells. Although the MPEX reaction is a key cytochemical reaction employed in the acute leukemias, it is not used as extensively in diagnosing the chronic leukemias. Nevertheless, it plays a significant role in differentiating myeloblastic and lymphoblastic crisis of CML. Furthermore, the MPEX reaction may be used on touch preparations of tissue to establish the diagnosis of granulocytic sarcoma and extramedullary hematopoiesis, especially when immature granulocytic elements are present, which sometimes are not readily discerned by the CAE reaction.

The SBB reaction is similar to the MPEX reaction in the spectrum of cells stained. It is as sensitive as the MPEX reaction but is more sensitive than CAE in identifying myeloblasts. One caveat is that cases of Burkitt's lymphoma and rare cases of ALL may have cells with lipid-containing cytoplasmic vacuoles that stain positively with SBB. The toluidine blue O (TBO) reaction is a specific marker for both basophils and mast cells. It is most useful in the diagnosis of basophilic and mast cell leukemia.

Gomori's silver impregnation stain employs a histochemical technique for evaluation of marrow fibrosis. This technique is helpful in confirming myelofibrosis in CML and agnogenic myeloid metaplasia, and in demonstrating fine intercellular reticulin networks characteristic of HCL and mast cell disease.

The Tdt determinations performed by indirect immunofluorescence, immunoperoxidase, or flow cytometry are positive in ALL blast crisis of CML. These cases constitute approximately 30% of blast crisis in CML; the remaining 70% are myeloid and usually Tdt-negative. In all other chronic leukemias, the Tdt test is negative.

The stains that may be employed to assist in diagnosing the chronic leukemias include the following:

1. Leukocyte alklaine phosphatase (LAP)
2. Acid phosphatase (AP) with and without tartrate
3. Chloroacetate esterase (CAE)
4. Nonspecific and acid alpha naphthyl acetate esterase (AA-EST) reactions
5. Reticulin stain
6. Myeloperoxidase (MPEX)
7. Toluidine blue (TBO)

Cell specificity and clinical utilization of the various cytochemical reactions used in the chronic leukemias are shown in Table 4.1.

LEUKOCYTE ALKALINE PHOSPHATASE

The most useful stain in the diagnosis of CML is the reaction for activity of LAP. The precise function and subcellular localization of LAP in neutrophils remains unclear. LAP is a zinc-containing phosphomonoesterase with a pH optimum near 10 that catalyzes the hydrolysis of a wide variety of phosphoester substances. The activity of LAP, which is limited to the granulocytic series, first appears in

Table 4-1 Cell Specificity and Clinical Application of Cytochemical and/or Histochemical Reactions in the Chronic Leukemias

Cytochemical and/or Histochemical Reaction	*Cell Specificity*	*Clinical Application*
Leukocyte Alkaline Phosphatase (LAP)	Neutrophils, Osteoblasts, Mantle zone B lymphocytes	CML, CNL, MPD, Mantle zone lymphoma
Acid Phosphatase (AP)	T cells	T-lymphoid leukemias, T-PLL, T-lymphomas, T-ALL
Tartrate-resistant AP (TRAP)	Hairy cells, ATLL cells, Sézary cells	HCL, ATLL, Sézary syndrome
Chloroacetate esterase (CAE)	Neutrophils	Granulocytic sarcoma in CML, MPD
Alpha-naphthyl acetate esterase (A-EST)	Monocytes, Histiocytes, Megakaryocytes, Plasma cells	CMML, CMoL
Alpha-naphthyl butyrate esterase (B-EST)	Monocytes, Histiocytes	CMML, CMoL
Acid alpha-naphthyl acetate esterase (AA-EST)	Helper T cells	T-lymphoid leukemias, T lymphomas, Sézary syndrome
Reticulin	Precollagen	CML, HCL, Mast cell disease
Myeloperoxidase (MPEX)	Granulocytes, Monocytes	Blast crisis CML
Toluidine Blue O (TBO)	Basophils, Mast cells	Mast cell disease

myelocytes and rapidly increases with maturation of the cell to the neutrophil stage.

Most techniques for evaluation of LAP employ an azo dye coupling procedure using a substituted naphthol compound as the substrate and fast violet B or fast blue RR salt as the coupler. Fresh peripheral blood slides are stained and a reaction product (fast violet B) (fast blue RR) within the neutrophils is observed. The slides are counterstained with hematoxylin. LAP stain of a normal control (Fig. 4.1a), a CML (Fig. 4.1b), and a leukemoid reaction (Fig. 4.1c) are depicted in the figures. One hundred consecutive neutrophils are counted, and each cell is graded from 0 to 4 (Table 4.2). The score of 100 neutrophils is calculated by multiplying the number of neutrophils at a particular grade by that grade. The sum of all grades is the total and represents the score (Table 4.3). In our laboratory a score from 22 to 118 is considered normal.

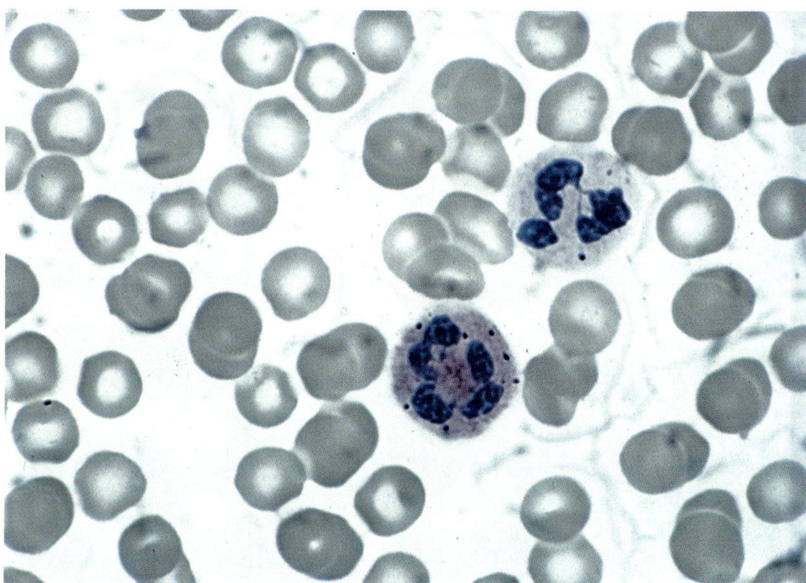

Figure 4-1 (a) Normal control peripheral blood stained for LAP. Coupler fast violet B. Note 1+ and 3+ neutrophils. (×1000).

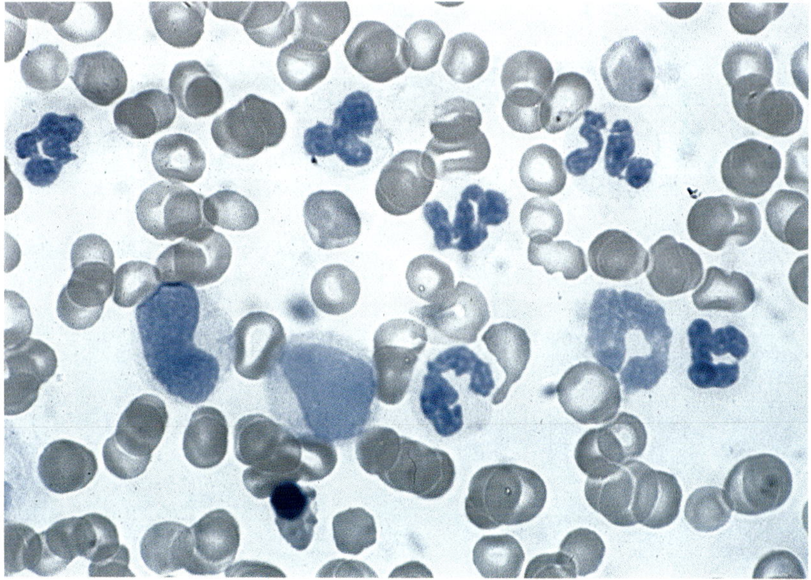

Figure 4-1 (b) Peripheral blood from a patient with CML stained for LAP. Note lack of staining in neutrophils. (×1000).

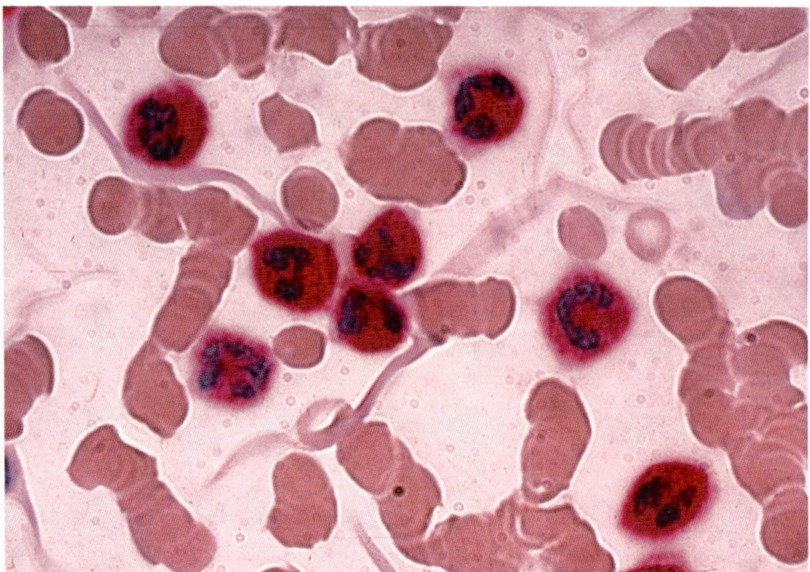

Figure 4-1 (c) Peripheral blood from a patient with a leukemoid reaction stained for LAP. Coupler fast violet B. Notice strong red 3+ reaction in all the neutrophils. (×1000).

Decreased LAP scores occur in about 90% of patients with CML. Low LAP activity is not unique to CML but may be found in paroxysmal nocturnal hemoglobinuria, hypophosphatemia, sickle cell anemia, infectious mononucleosis, and on rare occasions in normal people.

High LAP activity is frequently present in polycythemia vera, bacterial infections, pregnancy, and in patients receiving steroids. LAP

Table 4-2 LEUKOCYTE ALKALINE PHOSPHATASE Scoring Criteria

Cell Rating	*Amount* (%)*	*Size of Granules*	*Staining Intensity*	*Background of Cytoplasm*
0	None	None	None	None
1+	50	Small	Faint–moderate	Colorless to very pale pink
2+	50–80	Small	Moderate–strong	Colorless to pale pink
3+	80–100	Medium–large	Strong	Colorless to pink
4+	100	Medium–large	Brilliant	Not visible

*Percentage of volume of cytoplasm occupied by Azo dye precipitate.

Table 4-3 LEUKOCYTE ALKALINE PHOSPHATASE Scoring Calculation

Grade		*Number of Neutrophils Classified*		*Score*
0	×	20	=	0
1	×	20	=	20
2	×	20	=	40
3	×	20	=	60
4	×	20	=	80
		100		200

may be a good indication for inflammatory reactions of tissue; and in Hodgkin's disease, the LAP score closely parallels the progression of the disease. The LAP score is normal or elevated in CML in blastic crisis and usually markedly elevated in CNL. It may be normal or high in some patients with CML who are infected.

A rare subset of human lymphocytes also possess LAP activity. They are found in the mantle zone of lymph node follicles and account for the fact that lymphomatous mantle zone lymphocytes frequently contain LAP activity.

ACID PHOSPHATASE

The acid phosphatases (APs) are a group of enzymes capable of hydrolyzing monophosphate esters in acidic environments. Blood and bone marrow smears are exposed to a substrate containing naphthol AS-BI phosphoric acid and fast garnet GBC. The naphthol released by the enzymatic hydrolysis couples with the fast garnet GBC and forms a red dye complex at sites of activity. In human blood cells, seven different nonerythrocytic isoenzymes exist, and all except isoenzyme 5 are sensitive to tartrate inhibition. Nearly all nucleated cells and platelets show varying degrees of diffuse granular red reaction product when stained with AP. The red reaction product will disappear or contain only minute amounts after reaction with tartrate in all nucleated cells and platelets. The quintessential exception to this is HCL, in which cells contain isoenzyme 5 and are resistant to tartrate. Nonetheless, both Sézary cells and polylobated cells of ATLL can show polar AP positivity and tartrate-resistant AP (TRAP).

In addition to the value of AP in the above disorders, the stain provides important clues in other T-cell disorders such as T-lymphoid

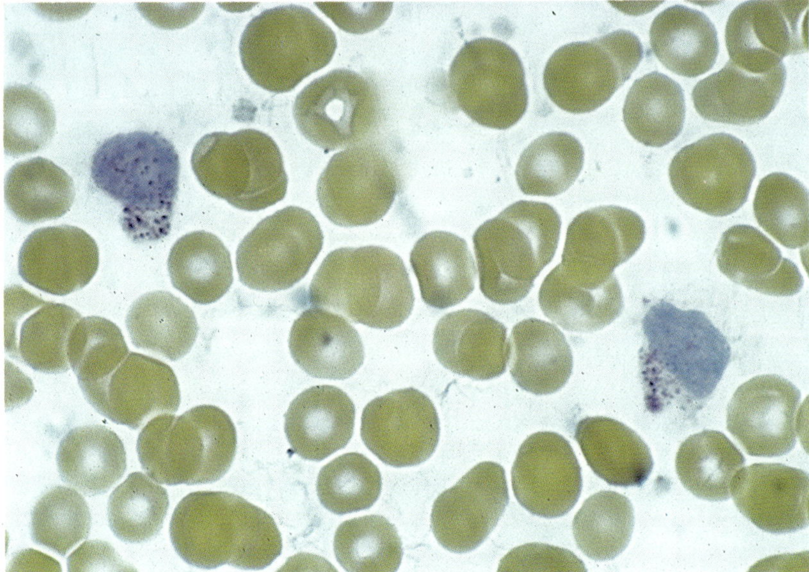

Figure 4-2 TRAP reaction on peripheral blood from a patient with HCL. Notice two hairy cells with red granular reaction product. (×1000).

leukemias, T-PLL, and especially T-ALL, since the AP activity is localized in the Golgi area and assumes a dotlike appearance. Therefore, this stain is of definite value in T-cell disorders, particularly when complete immunologic evaluation is not possible. A HLC showing TRAP is depicted in Fig. 4.2. In blood smears, a positive reaction is denoted by the presence of more than two cells with diffuse and intense activity.

CHLOROACETATE ESTERASE

CAE activity is most useful as a specific marker for cells of the granulocytic series and to a lesser extent for mast cells. However, the stain is less sensitive than peroxidase in demonstrating that leukemic blasts are of myeloid origin. This is most likely because CAE usually begins accumulating in promyelocytes. The esterase reaction begins when blood, bone marrow, or tissue containing granulocytic cells is incubated with naphthol AS-D chloroacetate in the presence of a stable diazonium salt. We use fast Corinth V salt, but fast garnet GBC, hexazotized pararosaniline, and hexazotized new fuchsin have been employed by others. Enzymatic hydrolysis of ester linkages liberates free naphthol compounds. These couple with the diazonium salt to form highly colored deposits at the sites of enzyme activity. Eosinophils, basophils, monocytes, and lymphocytes show weak to negative activity. Megakaryocytes and platelets have weak variable activity. Erythroblasts and plasma cells do not show CAE activity. Mast cells and histocytes show strong CAE activity. Evaluation of CAE activity by histochemical and cytochemical methods may be used to advantage in the diagnosis of granulocytic sarcoma, which may herald blastic transformation in CML and other myeloproliferative disorders. Granulocytic sarcoma most commonly affects skin, soft tissues, lymph nodes, bone, and periosteum. Also, antilysozyme immunoperoxidase should be used in conjunction with CAE stain since some cases of granulocytic sarcoma may be CAE-negative. Since rare CAE positivity may be seen in ALL, AMoL, and acute erythroleukemia (AEL), specificity may be increased by adding fluoride to the reaction, which will show sensitivity in ALL and AMoL, but not in AML. A CAE reaction on a granulocytic sarcoma is shown in Fig. 4.3.

NONSPECIFIC AND ACID ALPHA NAPHTHYL ACETATE ESTERASE REACTIONS

Nonspecific esterases (NSEs) are enzymes that hydrolyze several synthetic substrates, show strong positivity in monocytes and histiocytes, and show weaker or negative activity in other normal or pathologic cells. Alpha naphthyl acetate and alpha naphthyl butyrate are used as substrates in our laboratory; and fast blue RR salt for A-EST, and pararosaniline for B-EST, are employed as dye couplers. The A-EST stain produces punctate black dots, whereas the B-EST reaction creates a reddish-brown stain product. The addition of sodium fluoride will abolish esterase activity in the monohistiocytic series. Since the A-EST reaction is usually positive and the B-EST reaction usually negative in megakaryocytes, they may be used as presumptuous evidence to differentiate monocytic and megakaryocytic leukemias. A combined esterase using both CAE and A-EST or B-EST has been used in some laboratories. This enables the hematopathologist to evaluate both the monocytic and granulocytic series on the same slide. These esterase stains may be implemented with advantage in CMML, monocytic and megakaryocytic crisis of CML, and in the rare cases of CMoL. A B-EST stain on a CMoL is shown in Fig. 4.4.

The AA-EST reaction is best demonstrated in an acidic environment with prolonged incubation. This enzyme (AA-EST) is present

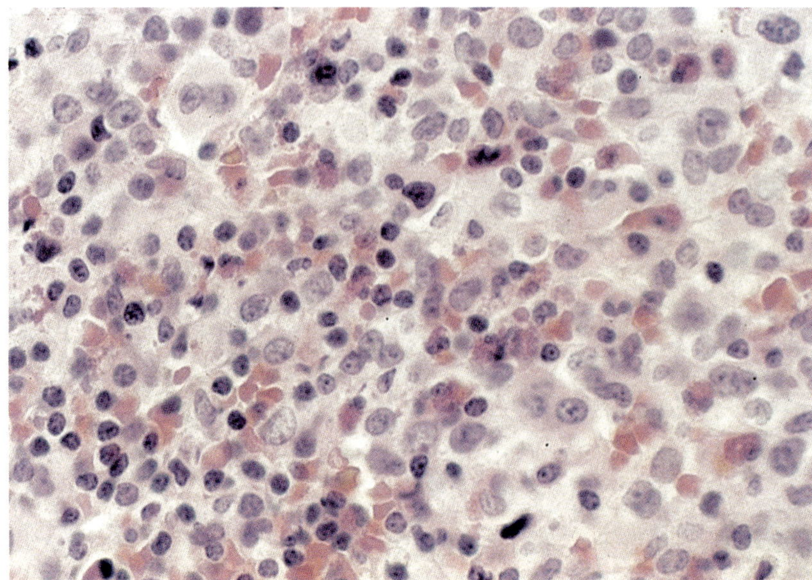

Figure 4-3 (a) CAE reaction on lymph node preparation from a patient with granulocytic sarcoma. Observe numerous pink-staining granulocytes. (×100).

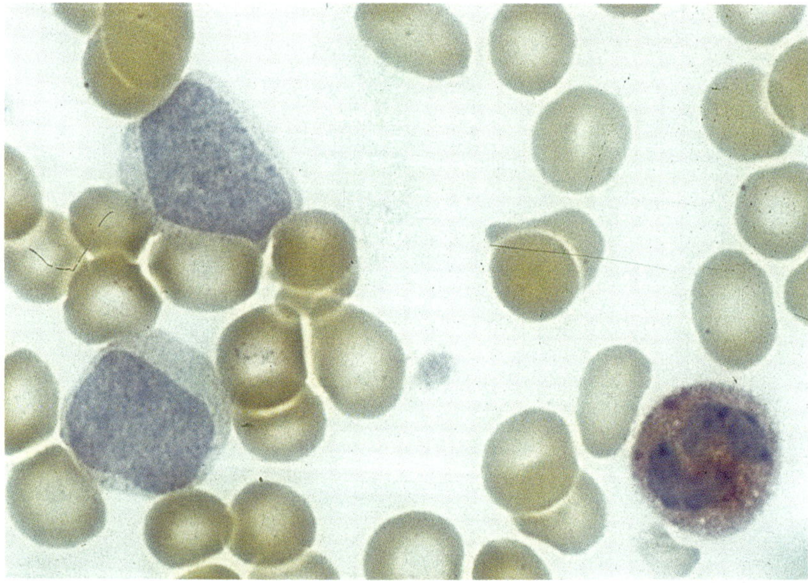

Figure 4-3 (b) CAE reaction on peripheral blood from a patient with granulocytic sarcoma in lymph node who later demonstrated myeloblasts in peripheral blood and bone marrow. Notice positive-staining neutrophil and two negative-staining blasts. The CAE reaction is poor in detecting myeloblasts. However, in this case electron microscopy MPEX was needed to determine the myeloid nature of these cells. (×1000).

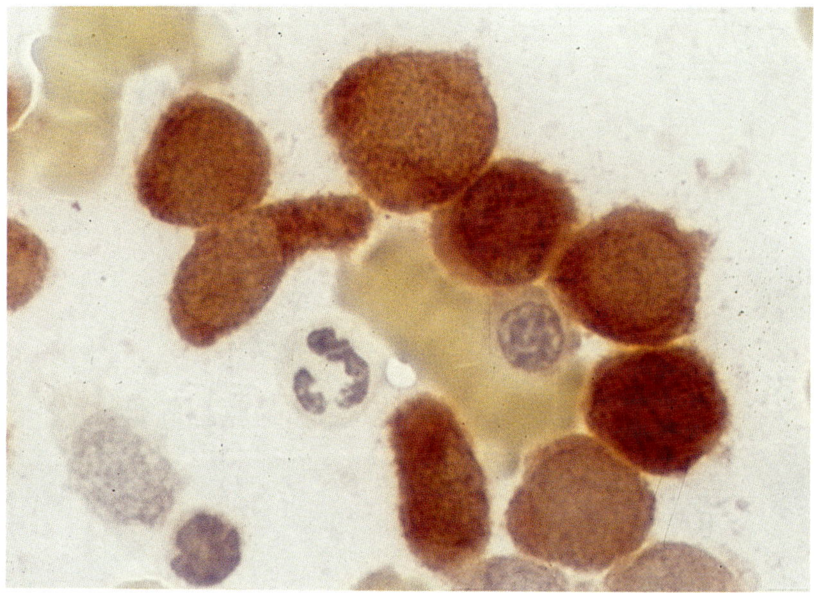

Figure 4-4 (a) B-EST reaction on a bone marrow preparation from a patient with CMoL. This patient had a prolonged chronic course. Many of the monocytic elements were promonocytes and monocytes and stained a strong reddish-brown, a feature observed in more mature monocytic elements. (×1000).

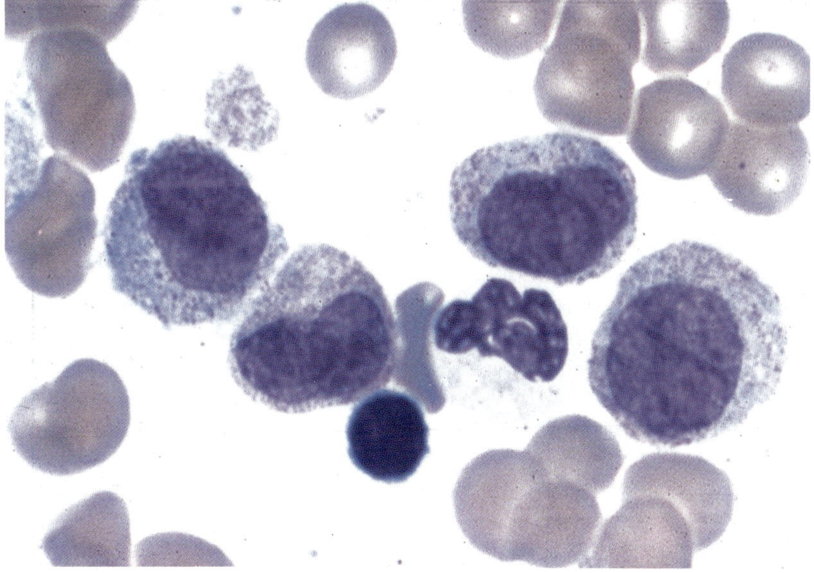

Figure 4-4 (b) Bone marrow from same patient as Figure 4.4a stained with May-Grünwald-Giemsa. Note maturing monocytic elements. (×1000).

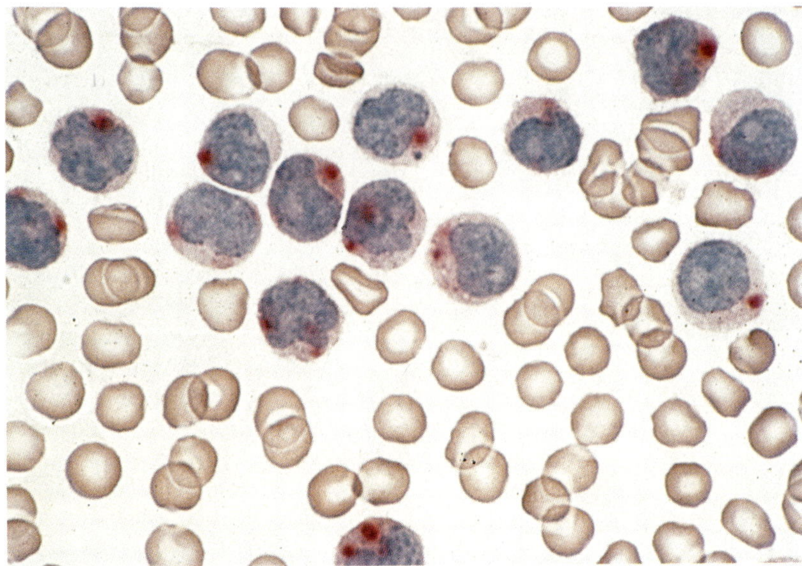

Figure 4-5 AA-EST stain on a peripheral blood smear from a patient with helper T-cell lymphoid leukemia. Note single and multiple dotlike staining (×320). Courtesy of Chin-Yang Li.

almost exclusively in helper T lymphocytes. Therefore, the AA-EST reaction is clinically useful in identifying chronic T-lymphoid leukemias, and T-cell lymphomas including mycosis fungoides and SS. When stained, the enzyme assumes a well-demarcated intense dot-like pattern in the cytoplasm in more mature T-cell disorders. However, it may be variable in T-ALL, and the activity may be weak or negative in lymphoblasts. The enzyme is resistant to sodium fluoride. Surprisingly, hairy cells of HCL show a characteristic pattern of activity consisting of small, medium-sized, or large distinct granules often distributed in a semicircle or crescent in the cytoplasm but sparing the nucleus. A similar positive crescentic pattern is observed with the B-EST reaction, and the positivity is not inhibited by sodium fluoride. A dotlike reaction product in chronic T-lymphoid leukemias using the AA-EST reaction is shown in Fig. 4.5.

RETICULIN STAIN

Gomori's silver impregnation, a histochemical reaction, is used to evaluate precollagen-type fibrosis in the bone marrow biopsy. Significant reticulin fibrosis occurs in nearly 50% of patients with CML at onset and is associated with greater splenomegaly, more severe anemia, greater weight loss, more marrow blasts, and additional karyotypic abnormalities. Prognostically, median survival was significantly shorter for those newly diagnosed CML patients with prominent reticulin fibrosis. The development of myelofibrosis late in the disease is also a poor prognostic feature, since it heralds blastic transformation. Approximately 25% of CML patients develop extensive collagen fibrosis that can be detected by Masson's trichrome stain. Both reticulin fibrosis (precollagen) and collagen fibrosis in CML resolve rapidly during remission in response to chemotherapy or following successful marrow transplantation. In addition to demonstrating marrow reticulum in CML and other MPDs, the Gomori method may be used to demonstrate reticulin fibrosis in HCL and mast cell disease. Reticular fibrosis and collagen fibrosis in CML were shown in Chapter 2 (Figs. 2.4 and 2.5).

MYELOPEROXIDASE

Although the MPEX reaction is the cornerstone of cytochemistry in the acute leukemias, it does not have the diagnostic impact on the chronic leukemias. Originally, the MPEX stain employed benzidine dihydrochloride, which permitted transfer of hydrogen ions from the benzidine to hydrogen peroxidase, leaving a black derivative dye. Since benzidine has well-known carcinogenicity, we use 4-chloro-1-naphthol as a chromogen and counterstain with May-Grünwald-Giemsa. The MPEX reaction may be used to differentiate myeloblastic from lymphoblastic crisis in CML. It is used in conjunction with Tdt determination. A myeloblastic and lymphoblastic crisis of CML showing MPEX activity is depicted in Figs. 4.6a and 4.6b, respectively.

TOLUIDINE BLUE O

TBO is a basic dye that reacts with the acid mucopolysaccharides in human blood cells. This cytochemical reaction is a specific marker for both basophils and mast cells. Therefore, it is very useful in the diagnosis of mast cell leukemia and basophilic leukemia. In neoplastic disorders, the acid mucopolysaccharides in the neoplastic basophils and mast cells may be scarce and not demonstrable. Hence, a negative TBO reaction should not be considered as an absolute criterion

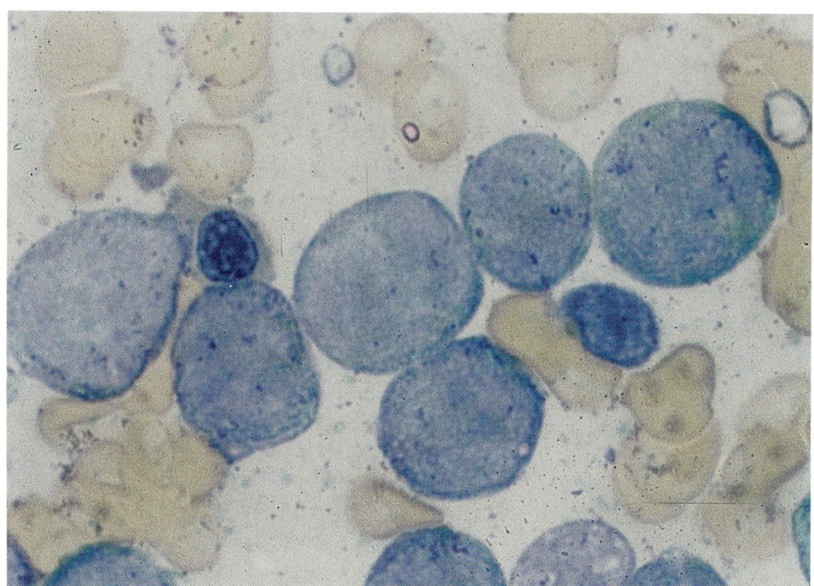

Figure 4-6 (a) MPEX-reaction on bone marrow from a patient with a myeloblastic crisis of CML. Note subtle positive black granules in blasts. This was further confirmed by SBB, which was positive, and Tdt, which was negative. (×1000).

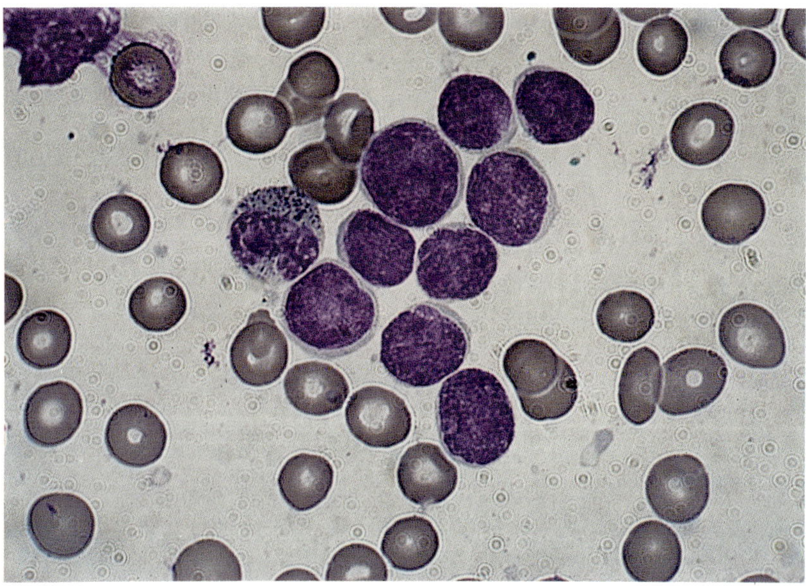

Figure 4-6 (b) MPEX reaction on bone marrow from a patient with a lymphoblastic crisis of CML. Note negative lymphoblasts and MPEX-positive neutrophilic band. (×1000).

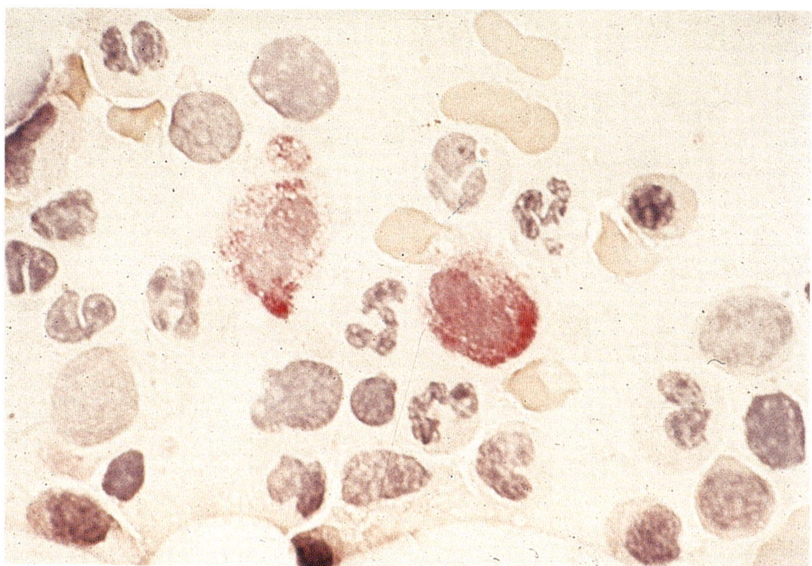

Figure 4-7 Bone marrow smear in a case of systemic mast cell disease stained with Am-EST. Note positive staining in two atypical mast cells. (×320). Courtesy of Chin-Yang Li.

to exclude such neoplasms. The aminocaproate esterase (Am-EST) reaction to identify mast cells has been used by some investigators. It is sensitive to storage and heat, and the incubation is unduly prolonged; therefore, Am-EST has not gained popularity as a mast cell stain (Fig. 4.7). The PAS reaction in basophils at all stages of maturity may be much increased in CML and MPDs, with coarse granularity and block-type positivity. PAS is also positive in mast cells. Also, SBB reaction may show a peculiar reddish metachromatic hue with only occasional black granules in abnormal basophils, even when their granules are inconspicuous. A TBO reaction of a systemic mastocytosis is shown in Fig. 4.8. Basophils and mast cells can be further characterized by monoclonal antibodies and electron microscopy.

TERMINAL DEOXYNUCLEOTIDYL TRANSFERASE

Tdt is an unusual deoxynucleotide-polymerizing enzyme that catalyzes the addition of deoxynucleotide triphosphates to the 3′-hydroxyl ends of the oligo- and polydeoxynucleotides without template instruction. It has been utilized as an indirect immunofluo-

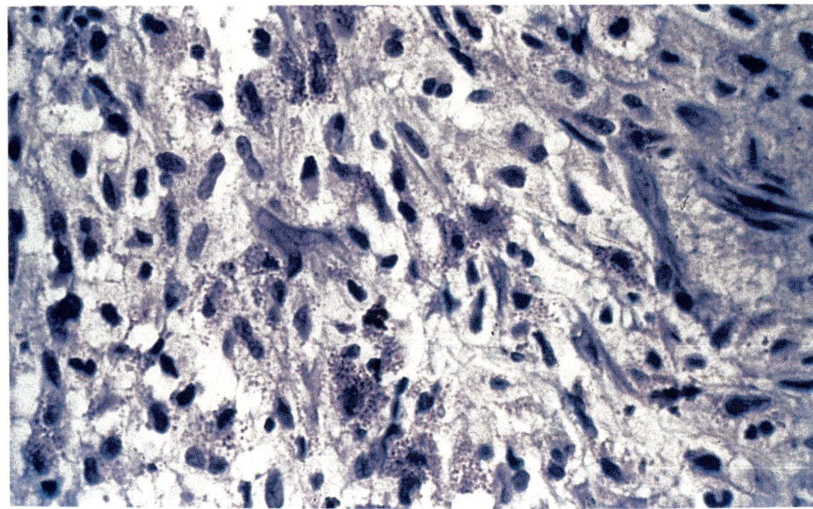

Figure 4-8 TBO stain of biopsy section from a patient with systemic mastocytosis showing metachromatic staining of granules in many cells—typical of mast cells. (×400). From McKenna RW, Hernandez J: Systemic Mastocytosis. *ASCP Hematology Check Sample,* H 87-10 (H-189). Chicago, IL. American Society of Clinical Pathologists, 1987. Reprinted with permission.

rescent and immunoperoxidase slide procedure. Also, it has been evaluated by flow cytometry. Tdt is an invaluable marker in the acute leukemias, and equally important in blast crisis of CML. Approximately 30% of blast crisis of CML are of lymphoid origin and Tdt-positive (Fig. 4.9); the remaining 70% are usually myeloid and generally Tdt-negative.

MISCELLANEOUS ABNORMALITIES

Hyperuricemia and hyperuricuria occur in untreated CML. Uric acid excretion is often two to three times normal in patients with active CML; and rapid cell lysis from therapy may lead to urinary urate stones, acute gouty arthritis, or uric acid nephropathy.

Levels of serum vitamin B_{12}–binding proteins and vitamin B_{12} are increased in patients with MPDs. Since neurotophils contain vitamin B_{12}–binding proteins including transcobalamin I and III, the increase in transcobalamin level and the resultant increase in vitamin B_{12} con-

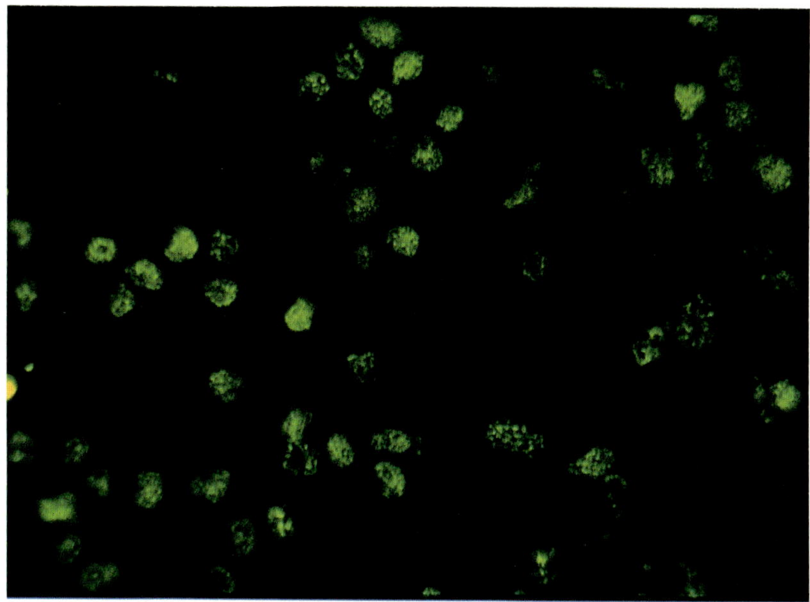

Figure 4-9 Tdt detected by indirect immunofluorescent slide technique on bone marrow from a patient with CML in lymphoblastic crisis. Note apple-green nuclear positivity. (×400).

centration are particularly notable in CML. In fact, the serum B^{12} level in some CML patients is increased to over 10 times normal. Also, any increase in the number of granulocytes such as in other MPDs and leukemoid reactions can be accompanied by an increase in serum B_{12}-binding protein and B_{12} levels.

The serum lactic dehydrogenase level is elevated in CML. Pseudohyperkalemia due to the release of potassium from leukocytes during clotting may occur, and spurious hypoxemia or pseudohypoglycemia from in vitro utilization of oxygen or glucose by granulocytes can occur. Hypercalcemia and lytic bone lesions are uncommon but ominous accompaniments of acute blast crisis, heralding rapid deterioration.

Hypogammaglobulinemia occurs in 50–75% of patients with CLL at some point in their disease. The degree of hypogammaglobulinemia correlates with the clinical stage of the disease, and virtually all patients with advanced disease are so affected. This decline in gamma globulin is a major contributor to the associated increased risk of infection, especially with encapsulated organisms. Although hypogammaglobulinemia is the most common finding by serum protein electrophoresis, 5% of cases demonstrate a monoclonal pattern. If the immunoglobulin is IgM and high levels are present, hyperviscosity may ensue and produce a clinical picture that may be confused with WM. CLL B cells have a lower density of surface membrane IgM, but higher concentrations within the cytoplasm in comparison to normal lymphocytes. The Coombs' test is positive in 20% of CLL patients at some time during the course of their disease. However, only one-third of these develop serious hemolysis. This is probably due to the low avidity of the IgG class warm antibody.

BIBLIOGRAPHY

Articles

Catovsky D, Cherci M, Greaves MF, et al: Acid-phosphatase reaction in acute lymphoblastic leukaemia. *Lancet* 1:749–751, 1978.

Clough V, Geary CG, Hashmi K, et al: Myelofibrosis in chronic granulocytic leukaemia. *Br J Haematol* 42:515–526, 1979.

Dekmezian R, Kantarjian HM, Keating MJ, et al: The relevance of reticulin stain–measured fibrosis at diagnosis in chronic myelogenous leukemia. *Cancer* 59:1739–1743, 1987.

Doe KA, Gryzbac M, Schumacher HR: A new modified rapid noncarcinogenic myeloperoxidase staining technique using 4-chloro-1-naphthol. *Lab Med* 19:374–375, 1988.

Gittin RG, Scharfman WB, Burkart PT: Granulocytic sarcoma: Three unusual patients. *Am J Med* 87:345–347, 1989.

Higgy KE, Burns GF, Hayhoe FG: Identification of the hairy cells of leukaemic reticuloendotheliosis by an esterase method. *Br J Haematol* 38:99–106, 1978.

Huhn D, Thiel E, Rodt H: Classification of normal and malignant lymphatic cells using acid phosphatase and acid esterase. *Klin Wochenschr* 58:65–71, 1980.

Kaplow LS: A histochemical procedure for localizing and evaluating leukocyte alkaline phosphatase activity in smears of blood and marrow. *Blood* 10:1023–1029, 1955.

Li CY, Yam LT: Cytochemical characterization of leukemic cells with numerous cytoplasmic granules. *Mayo Clin Proc* 62:978–985, 1987.

McCarthy DM: Annotation. Fibrosis of the bone marrow: Content and causes. *Br J Haematol* 59:1–7, 1985.

Rutenburg M, Rosales CL, Bennett JM: An improved histochemical method for the demonstration of leukocyte alkaline phosphatase activity: Clinical application. *J Lab Clin Med* 65:698–705, 1965.

Sigma Technical Bulletin, No. 85 (7/77).
Tolksdorf G, Stein H: Acid alpha-naphthyl acetate esterase in hairy cell leukemia cells and other cells of the hematopoietic system. *Blut* 39:165–176, 1979.
Wehinger H, Möbius W: Cytochemical studies on T and B lymphocytes and lymphoblasts with special reference ot acid phosphatase. *Acta Haematol* 56:129–136, 1976.

Review Articles

Chang KL, Stroup R, Weiss L: Hairy cell leukemia: Current status. *Am J Clin Pathol* 97:719–738, 1992.
Dighiero G, Travade P, Chevret S, et al: B-cell chronic lymphocytic leukemia: Present status and future directions. *Blood* 78:1901–1914, 1991.
Hayhoe FG, Quaglins D: *Haematological Cytochemistry,* ed 2. Edinburgh, Churchill Livingstone, 1988.
Kass L: Cytochemistry of esterases. In: *CRC Critical Reviews in Clinical Laboratory Sciences.* West Palm Beach, CRC Press, 1979, pp 205–222.
Kass L: *Leukemia: Cytology and Cytochemistry.* Philadelphia, JB Lippincott, 1982.
Li CY, Yam LT, Lam KW: Acid phosphatase isoenzyme in human leukocytes in normal and pathological conditions. *J Histochem Cytochem* 18:473–481, 1970.
Li CY, Yam LT, Lam KW: Studies of acid phosphatase isoenzymes in human leukocytes: Demonstration of isoenzyme cell specificity. *J Histochem Cytochem* 18:901–910, 1970.
Schumacher HR: *Acute Leukemia: Approach to Diagnosis.* New York, Igaku-Shoin, 1990, pp. 33–50.
Sun T, Li CY, Yam LT: *Atlas of Cytochemistry and Immunochemistry of Hematologic Neoplasms.* Chicago, American Society of Clinical Pathology Press, 1985, pp 22–40.
Webb TA, Li CY, Yam LT: Systemic mast cell disease: A clinical and hematopathologic study of 26 cases. *Cancer* 49:927–938, 1982.

CHAPTER 5
Electron Microscopy

INTRODUCTION

As with the acute leukemias, electron microscopy (EM) has not played a major role in the diagnosis of the chronic leukemias. However, EM may be of value in those difficult cases in which light microscopy, light cytochemical analysis, immunophenotyping, cytogenetics, and gene rearrangement studies do not provide the essential information for diagnosis. Recently, EM has played a more important role in these cases because of technological advances in specimen preparation. What formerly took several days, now takes only a few hours. Since it is imperative for the clinician to obtian the correct diagnosis as quickly as posssible to institute appropriate therapy, EM has become an integral part of the diagnosis in many cases.

EM has been of great vlaue in those cases in which the diagnosis cannot be established with certainty. These cases are always difficult and may require all the supportive diagnostic techniques available. Some EM findings such as Auer rods and splinter-forms, bull's eyes, and basophilic granules clearly define the myeloid nature of leukemia. Ultrastructural MPEX staining is of great vlaue in difficult undifferentiated myeloid blast crises of CML. Also, mast cell disease and chronic mast cell leukemia (CMaL) can be more fully characterized by EM. Other ultrastructural changes such as ribosome-lamellae bodies, hairy cytoplasmic projections, and marked nuclear convolutions assist in establishing lymphoid lineage.

DIAGNOSTIC ELECTRON MICROSCOPY

EM may be used to advantage in the chronic leukemias and related disorders in the following ways:

1. To determine MPEX activity of blasts in CML blast crisis
2. To detect basophils in a basophilic blast crisis of CML
3. To detect mast cells of CMaL and systemic mast cell disease
4. To offer diagnostic support in hairy cell leukemia (HCL)
5. To offer diagnostic support in the convoluted nuclear lymphoid disorders

The MPEX activity can be used at the ultrastructural level to detect myeloblastic cells that are extremely undifferentiated. Since the number of granules is small or absent, they are not identifiable by light microscopy. MPEX, which can be detected by EM, first appears in the perinuclear space and later in the endoplasmic reticulum and finally on the concave surface of the Golgi zone. There, it is packaged into primary granules. Besides identifying blast cells, ultrastructural MPEX cytochemistry helps to define complex cellular subpopulations that occur in blast crisis of CML. In addition to bone marrow diagnosis, EM and ultrastructural MPEX stain may be used to detect the type of blasts in blast crisis in CML evolving in lymph nodes by use of fine needle aspirate. An early myeloblast from a CML blast crisis showing MPEX activity is depicted in Fig. 5.1.

Basophilic leukemia may be observed in CML with exaggerated basophilia; acute basophilic transformation of CML; AML with t(6;9), t(3;6), or inv(16) and marrow basophilia; acute promyelocytic leukemia with basophilic maturation; or acute basophilic leukemia. Basophils participate in initial responses dependent on circulating blood, whereas mast cells participate in localized tissue-bound reactions. Both cells originate in the bone marrow from a morphologically unidentifiable precursor, which may be the same as the one for other granulocytes and monocytes (GM-CFU). Basophils stain with toluidine blue O (TBO), alcian blue, and AP. They may stain very weakly for MPEX, Sudan black B (SBB), and chloroacetate esterase (CAE). Basophils synthesize and store histamine and heparin. Unlike mast cells, they contain the major basic protein and lysophospholipase

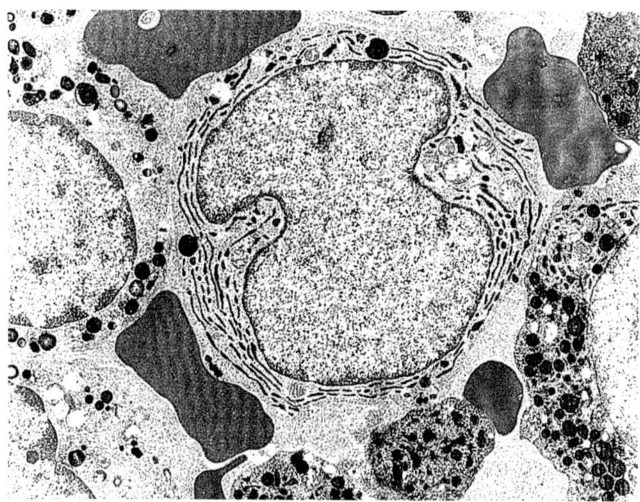

Figure 5-1 Transmission electron micrograph showing MPEX reaction in a myeloblast from a myeloblastic crisis of CML. Note accumulation of MPEX reaction product in perinuclear cistern, endoplasmic reticulum, and two primary granules. BM ($\times$ 12,000). From Schumacher HR: *Acute Leukemia: Approach to Diagnosis*. New York, Igaku-Shoin, 1990.

that are also found in eosinophils. Lysophospholipase is present in Charcot-Leyden crystals. Although EM has not been used frequently to diagnose basophilic leukemia or basophilic crisis of CML, it has been used to identify immature basophilic precursors such as basophilic promyelocytes, myelocytes, and metamyelocytes in blast crisis of CML. Bone marrow EM in such cases shows immature and mature types that contain granules characteristic of basophils. Also, Butler et al (1982) studied 13 cases of CML in blast crisis in which 1 case demonstrated basophilic granules by EM and EM MPEX studies. This was particularly true for those cases classified as M1. Apparently, the basophils in CML exhibit a variety of ultrastructural and biochemical abnormalities, and the distinction between basophils and mast cells may be difficult because of overlapping features. These findings support the concept of lineage promiscuity and infidelity observed so frequently in all varieties of leukemias. A blood cell from CML showing hybrid basophilic and mast cell ultrastructural features is depicted in Fig. 5.2.

Mast cell diseases include a spectrum of disorders that encompasses localized mastocytosis, urticaria pigmentosa, systemic mastocytosis, malignant mastocytosis, and mast cell leukemia. Mast cell

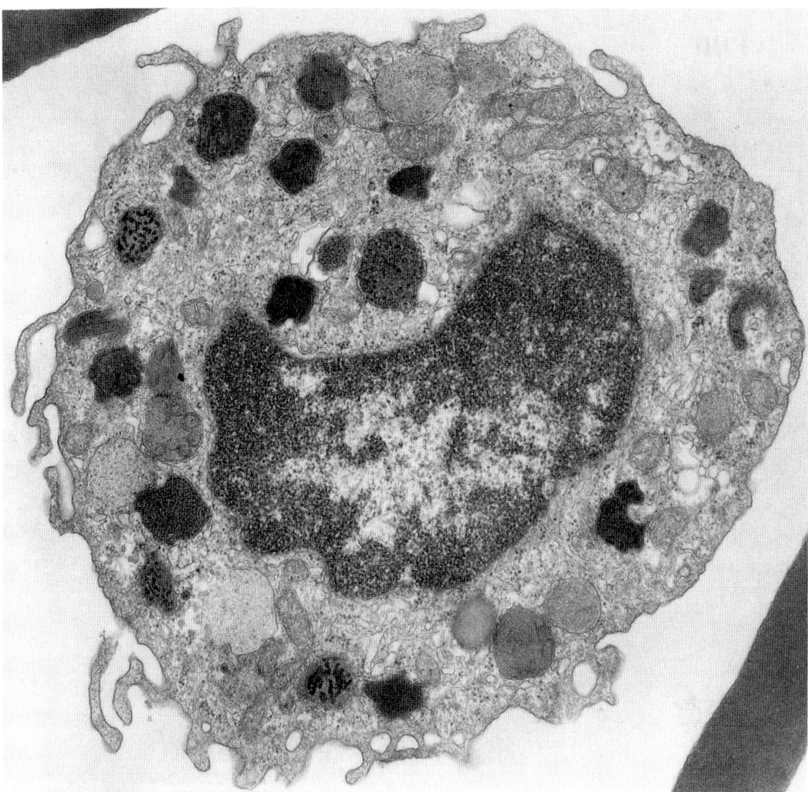

Figure 5-2 Transmission electron micrograph of peripheral blood from a patient with CML demonstrating a "basophil" that is not distinguishable from a mast cell. Some of the granules have "scrolls" and other crystalloid structures. The nucleus is not lobulated like that of a mature basophil and has the chromatin distribution of a less differentiated cell. From Zucker-Franklin D: In Zucker-Franklin D, Greaves MF, Grossi CE, Marmont AM: *Atlas of Blood Cells: Function and Pathology,* ed 2. Milan, Philadelphia, E. Edi-eremes, Lea & Febiger, 1988, pp 287–320. (×30,000).

leukemia develops in about 15% of patients with malignant mast cell disorder. Mast cells are of monocyte-macrophage lineage, respond to the lymphokine interleukin-3 (IL-3), and synthesize and store within metachromatic granules arachindonate derivatives, histamine, and heparin. In response to membrane receptor–bound IgE to a specified antigen, mast cell granules fuse with the cell membrane, dissolve, and release their anaphylatoxic contents into the surrounding area. Leukemic mast cells are stained with Sudan black, TBO and alcian blue, CAE, and AP. They are negative for peroxidase and A-EST. EM

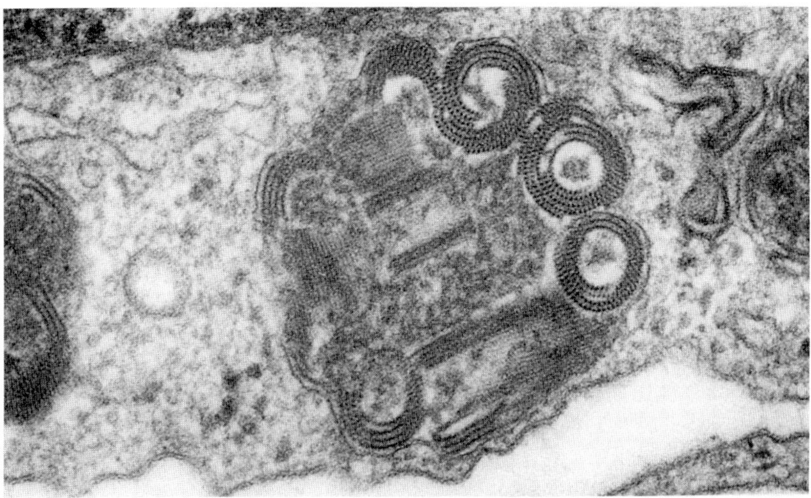

Figure 5-3 Transmission electron micrograph of typical mast cell granule showing "scrolls" consisting of several coils of a crystalline or fibrillar structure, as well as parallel lines, which probably represent scrolls cut along their long axis. From Zucker-Franklin D: Ultrastructural evidence for the common origin of human mast cells and basophils. *Blood* 56:534–540, 1980. (×150,000).

may show the characteristic scroll-like ultrastructural features of mast cell granules, shown in Fig. 5.3.

HCL, or leukemic reticuloendotheliosis, is a chronic LPD originating as a lymphoma of splenic B cells and rarely T cells that eventually causes splenomegaly, pancytopenia, and the appearance of unique "hairy" lymphocytes in blood and bone marrow. Hairy cells display a set of features that collectively are diagnostic and distinguish HCL from other B-cell lymphomas and leukemias. These features are (1) TRAP, (2) ribosome-lamellae bodies by EM, (3) HC1, HC2, CD19, CD20, CD25 (Tac), PCA-1 positivity, but CD21, PC-1 negativity, (4) strong surface receptors for C3b, (5) receptors for Fc portion of IgG, (6) frequent expression of monoclonal surface lgG (SIgG). A hairy cell variant exists that is intermediate between HCL and PLL. The irregular cytoplasmic processes that characterize the cells are particularly well demonstrated by phase-contrast microscopy and scanning and transmission EM. In about 50% of cases, a ribosome-lamella body or complex can be found in the cytoplasm by transmission EM (Fig. 5.4). This cytoplasmic inclusion is a cylindrical structure composed of a central hollow space and an outer sheath of multple parallel lamellae, with ribosome-like granules in the interlamellar space.

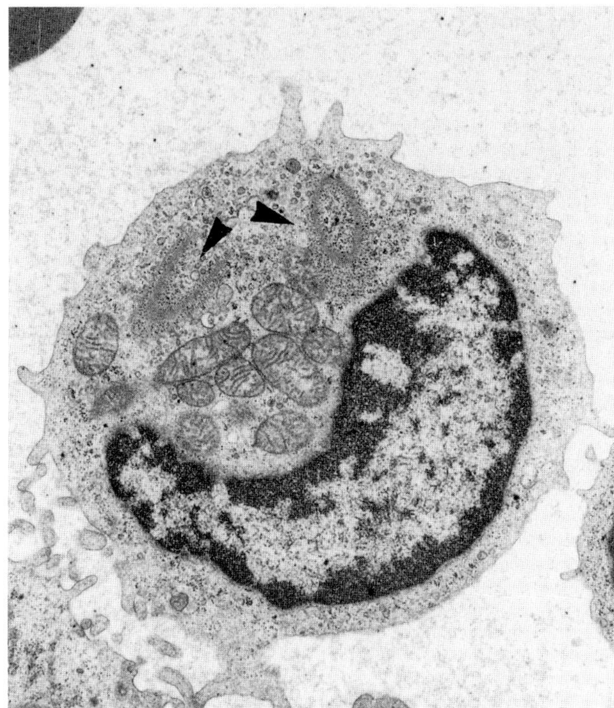

Figure 5-4 This transmisison electron micrograph of a "hairy cell" shows two obliquely cut ribosome-lamella complexes (arrowheads). Only a few microvilli are present in this section. Courtesy of Raoul Fresco. (×11,000).

These structures may be seen by light microscopy as rod-shaped inclusions, which may be helpful in diagnosis. These inclusions are highly suggestive of the diagnosis of HCL but may be observed occasionally in other lymphoid and nonlymphoid neoplastic cells, and even benign plasma cells accompanying malignant infiltrates.

The Sézary syndrome (SS), which represents the leukemic phase of mycosis fungoides (MF), a cutaneous T-cell lymphoma, can present a cytologic challenge. Sézary cells, especially when present in small numbers in the peripheral blood, can be confused with reactive lymphocytes, including viral-induced lymphocytosis. Even when present in large numbers, Sézary cells can be mistaken morphologically for other types of chronic leukemias such as CLL, plasma cell leukemia, and the leukemic phase of nodal-based lymphomas with their characteristic buttock cells. Since the presence of Sézary cells in the peripheral blood of patients with MF carries a poor prognosis, quantitation

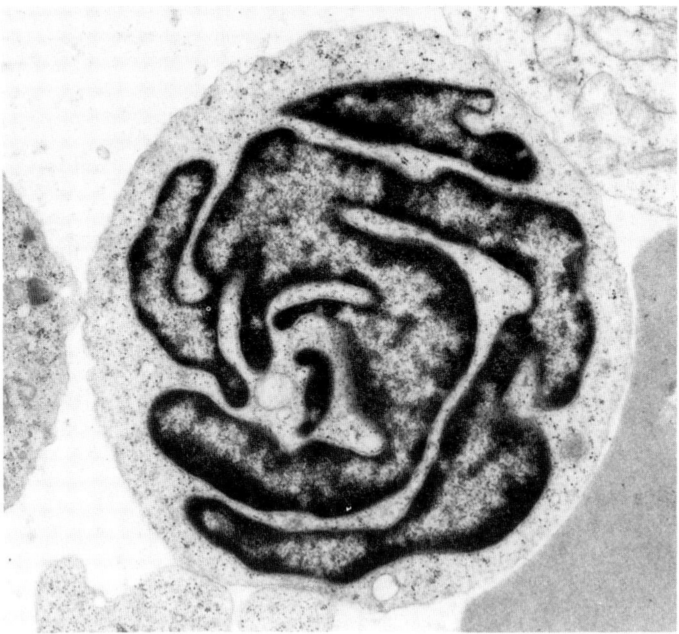

Figure 5-5 The cerebriform nucleus of a Sézary cell, as seen in blood smears, appears serpentine in an ultrathin section examined with the electron microscope. Courtesy of Raoul Fresco. (×11,000).

of these lymphoid cells with cerebriform nuclei is most important. In fact, the diagnosis of SS requires greater than 15–20% circulating Sézary cells. The characteristic convoluted nucleus of a Sézary cell is depicted in Fig. 5.5.

Apparently, the Sézary cell originates in lymph nodes but has a marked homing mechanism for the epidermis and dermis, an epidermotropism that sets SS apart from other T-cell disorders. The malignant cells almost always have a phenotype of mature helper-inducer CD4+ cells: E rosette+, CD2+, and CD3+. Cytochemistry reveals the Sézary cells to be AP and beta-glucuronidase-positive, and MPEX and CAE-negative. The PAS reaction may be positive or negative. Tdt determinations are always negative.

Recent EM studies by Payne and Glasser (1990) utilizing a bivariate graphic analysis to establish morphometric domains have been most useful in the diagnosis of SS. The bivariate technique uses a sensitive shape analytic formula ($4\pi A/P^2$, where A = area and P = perimeter that defines the form factor (FF). The FF ($4\pi A/P^2$) is a measurement that bears an inverse linear relationship to the degree of deviation

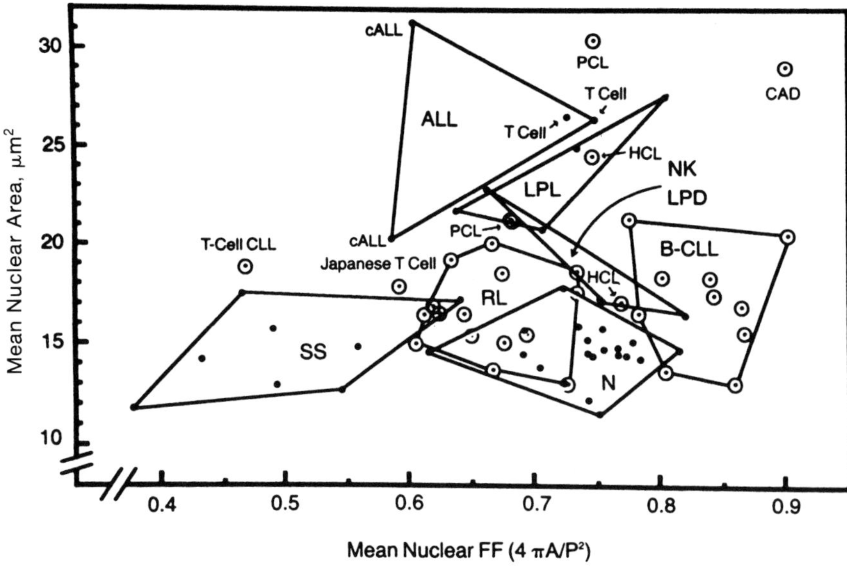

Figure 5-6 Morphometric domains of normal subjects and patients with reactive lymphocytosis, leukemias, and natural killer cell lymphoproliferative disorders (NK LPDs). cALL indicates common acute lymphocytic leukemia; PCL, plasma cell leukemia; CAD, cold agglutinin disease; LPL, leukemic phase of lymphoma; HCL, hairy cell leukemia; CLL, chronic lymphocytic leukemia; Japanese T Cell, Japanese T-cell leukemia; RL, reactive lymphocytosis; B-CLL, B-cell chronic lymphocytic leukemia; SS, Sézary syndrome; N, normal; FF, form factor; *A*, area; and *P*, perimeter. From Payne CM, et al: Sézary syndrome. *Arch Pathol Lab Med* 114:667, 1990. Copyright 1990, American Medical Association.

from a circle. The FF value of a perfect circle is 1.0. The measurement used in the bivariate graphic analysis is the mean nuclear area *A*. The morphometric domains for normal and reactive lymphocytes and various lymphoid malignancies are depicted in Fig. 5.6. Although T-cell CLL and ATLL were distinguished by the morphometric domain generated by bivariate graphic analysis, and not by histogram analysis, the authors suggest the use of the simpler histogram method for everyday practice to diagnose SS. This technique employs evaluation of sharply angled nuclear invaginations (NIs). Those readers who wish to use the histogram method are referred to the additional article of Payne, Nagle, and Lynch (1984).

In summary, transmission EM may be used with and without cytochemical techniques and with morphometric analysis to help diagnose the more difficult cases of the chronic leukemias and related entities.

BIBLIOGRAPHY

Articles

Bartl R, Frisch B, Hill W, et al: Bone marrow histology in hairy cell leukemia. Identification of subtypes and their prognostic significance. *Am J Clin Pathol* 79:531–545, 1983.

Butler AE, Vardiman JW, Golomb HM: Ultrastructural characterization of de novo and secondary leukemias. *Virchows Arch [Cell Pathol]* 39:239–257, 1982.

Dunphy CH, Katz RL, Fanning, CV, et al: Leukemic lymphadenopathy: Diagnosis by fine needle aspiration. *Hematol Pathol* 3:35–44, 1989.

Gabriel LC, Escribano LM, Marie JP, et al: Peroxidase activity in circulating mast cells in blast crisis of chronic granulocytic leukemia. Comparative studies with basophils and cutaneous mast cells. *Am J Clin Pathol* 86:212–219, 1986.

Hewson JW, Bradstock KF, Kerr A, et al: Characterizing "difficult" acute leukemias. A combined electron microscopic and immunological marker study. *Pathology* 18:99–110, 1986.

Katayama I, Nagy GK, Balogh K Jr.: Light microscopic identification of the ribosome-lamella complex in "hairy cells" of leukemic reticuloendotheliosis. *Cancer* 32:843–846, 1973.

Kuto F, Nagaoka T, Watanabe Y, et al: Chronic myelocytic leukemia: Ultrastructural histopathology of bone marrow from patients in the chronic phase. *Ultrastruct Pathol* 6:307–317, 1984.

Ozaki M, Kanemitsu N, Yasukawa M, et al: Basophilic crisis of chronic myelogenous leukemia. *Jpn J Med* 28:67–71, 1989.

Parkin JL, McKenna RW, Brunning RD: Philadelphia chromosome-positive blastic leukaemia: Ultrastructural and ultracytochemical evidence of basophil and mast cell differentiation. *Br J Haematol* 52:663–677, 1982.

Payne CM, Glasser L: Ultrastructural morphometry in the diagnosis of Sézary syndrome. *Arch Pathol Lab Med* 114:661–671, 1990.

Payne CM, Nagle RB, Lynch PJ: Quantitative electron microscopy in the diagnosis of mycosis fungoides. A simple analysis of lymphocytic nuclear convolutions. *Arch Dermatol* 120:63–75, 1984.

Rosner MC, Golomb HM: Ribosome-lamella complex in hairy cell leukemia. Ultrastructure and distribution. *Lab Invest* 42:236–247, 1980.

Soler J, O'Brien M, de Castro JT, et al: Blast crisis of chronic granulocytic leukemia with mast cell and basophilic precursors. *Am J Clin Pathol* 83:254–259, 1985.

Weiselberg L, Teichberg S, Vinciguerra V, et al: Electron microscope cytochemical analysis of chronic myelocytic leukemia: A case report. *Cancer* 47:533–536, 1981.

Zimmerman KG, Payne CM, Nagle RB: Ribosome-lamellae complexes in benign plasma cells accompanying neoplastic infiltrates. *Am J Clin Pathol* 81:364–367, 1984.

Review Articles

Golomb HM, Braylan R, Polliack A: "Hairy" cell leukaemia (leukaemic reticuloendotheliosis): A scanning electron microscopic study of eight cases. *Br J Haematol* 29:455–460, 1975.

Lossignol D, Bron D, Debusscher L, et al: Basophil leukemia, development of a chronic myeloid leukemia. Apropos of a case and review of the literature. *Nouv Rev Fr Hematol* 29:307–310, 1987.

Torrey E, Simpson K, Wilbur S, et al: Malignant mastocytosis with circulating mast cells. *Am J Hematol* 34:283–286, 1990.

Travis WD, Li CY, Hoagland HC, et al: Mast cell leukemia: Report of a case and review of the literature. *Mayo Clin Proc* 61:957–966, 1986.

Wieselthier JS, Koh HK: Sézary syndrome: Diagnosis, prognosis, and critical review of treatment options. *J Am Acad Dermatol* 22:381–401, 1990.

Winkler CF, Bunn PA Jr.: Cutaneous T-cell lymphoma: A review. *Crit Rev Oncol Hematol* 1:49–92, 1983.

Zucker-Franklin D: In Zucker-Franklin D, Greaves MF, Grossi CE, Marmont AM: *Atlas of Blood Cells: Function and Pathology,* ed 2. Milan, Philadelphia, E. Edi-ermes, Lea & Febiger, 1988, pp 287–320.

CHAPTER 6

Immunophenotype

INTRODUCTION

The hallmark for the diagnosis of the CMLs and related disorders has been morphology, cytochemistry, and cytogenetics. Contrariwise, although morphology, cytochemistry, and cytogenetics may play an important role in the diagnosis of CLL and related disorders, immunophenotyping assumes a much more important role in these disorders. Even though the emphasis has been on immunophenotypic analysis of lymphoid disorders, cell surface analysis has been used to an advantage in blastic crisis of CML. Cell surface marker analysis with monoclonal antibodies has demonstrated that immature cells in blastic transformation heterogeneously express the phenotype of myeloblast, lymphoblast, or, more rarely, megakaryoblast, erythroblast, or mixtures of these blasts. Approximately, one-third of blastic transformations represent early B-cell features that include the expressions of Tdt, CD10-common acute lymphoblastic leukemic–associated antigen (CALLA), HLA-DR, CD19, CD20, and rearrangement in the Ig gene.

The CLLs and related disorders are a heterogeneous group of disorders that are clonal expansions of malignantly transformed cells whose differentiation has been interrupted and arrested early in lymphocyte ontogeny. Since normal lymphocytes share sufficient characteristics with those of lymphocytic and related neoplasms, it is possible to determine both lineage and stage of differentiation of a neoplasm by immunophenotypic analysis and gene rearrangement. Such analysis provides accurate information concerning the lymphoid nature of the leukemia and enables the hematologist and hematopathologist to determine B- or T-cell lineage. This is accomplished by selecting a battery of antibody probes used to identify immunoreactive molecules known to be associated with lineage or differentiation.

Surface markers have been analyzed by various methods (e.g., immunofluorescence microscopy, immunocytochemistry, and flow cytometry). Immunocytochemical staining methods may be used on sections of fresh-frozen tissue, touch preparations, and aspirations of lymphomatous and/or leukemic materials. Both immunofluorescent microscopy and immunocytochemistry have the advantages of direct cell and/or tissue analysis and relatively low budget operation. Also, they allow the hematopathologist to examine the cells in relation to total tissue architecture. Therefore, these techniques are ideally suited for small biopsies and those specimens that are only focally involved with disease. The disadvantages include slow, tedious analysis and some lack of objectivity and reproducibility. Flow cytometry has the following advantages: fast analysis, objectivity, reproducibility, estimation of cell size and granularity, simultaneous measurement of different markers by multicolored analysis fluorescence, sensitivity of small subpopulation detection, accurate quantitation of fluorescence intensity, and good documentation of data. It has these disadvantages: cost of instrumentation and the training of operators, loss of tissue and architecture, and occasional difficulty in sorting and obtaining single-cell suspensions. Furthermore, cytospins need to be evaluated to determine the morphology of the population examined. The parameters of positivity in flow cytometry vary from laboratory to laboratory but depend on the intensity of fluorescence and the number of positive cells observed with a particular monoclonal antibody. Additionally, a caveat associated with any test is that the specimens evaluated must contain the appropriate material for analysis. In general, values <30% positivity within a given cell population (gate) are not considered significant.

MYELOID ONTOGENY

The expression of monoclonal antibody–defined myeloid antigen coincides with the pathways of normal hematopoietic differentiation with the myeloid lineage. A schematic representation of human myeloid differentiations indicating the cell surface marker phenotype (as defined by selected well-characterized monoclonal reagents) of identifiable maturational steps is depicted in Fig. 6.1. Note the hypothesized pluripotent stem cell as the site for leukemogenesis of CML. Since the target cell is a pluripotent stem cell, blast crisis of CML may involve lymphocytic, myelocytic, monocytic, erythrocytic, or megakaryocytic cell lines. Table 6.1 shows the clinically used monoclonal antibodies for myeloid disorders. Although immunophenotyping is not of great importance in the diagnosis of CML and related disorders, it may be helpful in classification of blast crisis cell populations.

LYMPHOCYTE ONTOGENY

Stem cells that develop into B cells arise in the bone marrow and liver. These cells contain nuclear Tdt that disappears as the lymphocyte matures. The B cells acquire surface markers and undergo both heavy and light chain lg gene rearrangement (Fig. 6.2). The progenitors of B lymphocytes (pre-B cells) are found in the bone marrow and fetal liver. The pre-B cells acquire cytoplasmic μ heavy chain (Cμ) (cCD22) and surface markers and undergo gene rearrangement as the lymphocyte matures. However, at this stage they lack intracytoplasmic light chain and surface membrane immunoglobulin (sIg), but may have receptors for the third component of complement (C'_3) and for the Fc portion of IgG. Both Fc and C'_3 receptors are not specific for B-cell lineage and are found on monocytes and on some nonhematopoietic cells. B cells also have these receptors, but, in addition, acquired sIg, the hallmark of a B lymphocyte. Also, Ia or HLA-DR, a histocompatibility-related antigen, is found on the surface of B cells, as well as myeloblasts, immature erythroid elements, the monocytic series, and activated T lymphocytes. Eventually, the lymphocyte may develop into a plasma cell, which is the most mature B cell. Plasma cells lack sIg but contain cytoplasmic immunoglobulin (cIg), which can be released into the bloodstream as a humoral antibody. Spontaneous rosetting using mouse erythrocytes may be employed to demonstrate M-rosettes in B-CLL. Clinically used monoclonal antibodies that identify B-cell-associated antigens are depicted in Table 6.2 with their cell specificity and associated cluster designation (CD). Besides "pan-B" or "pan-T" reagents, which define two main lines of differentiation, some antigens are restricted to certain maturational stages and are useful for subclassification. For example, B lymphocytes of

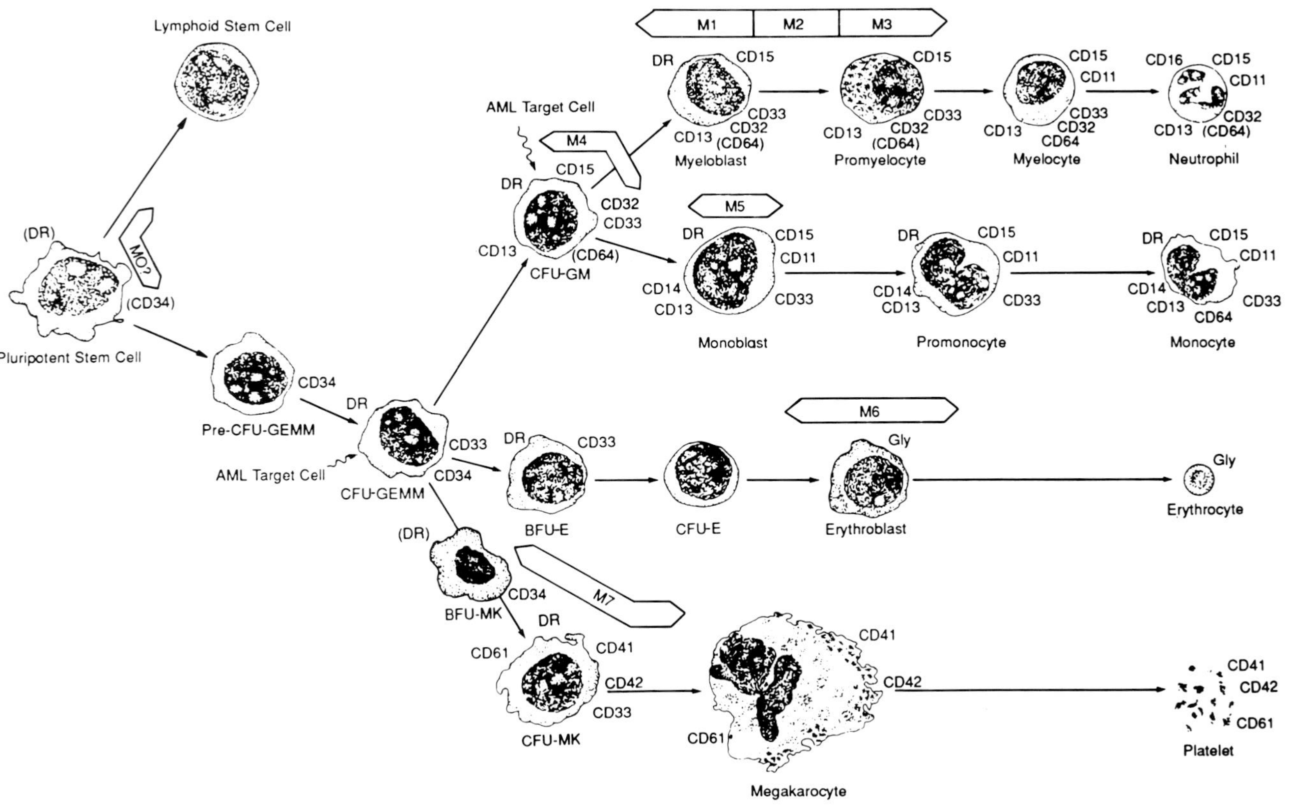

Lymphoid Stem Cell
(DR)
MO?
(CD34)
Pluripotent Stem Cell
CD34
Pre-CFU-GEMM
DR
CD33
CD34
AML Target Cell
CFU-GEMM
AML Target Cell
M4
DR
CD15
CD32
CD33
CD13
(CD64)
CFU-GM
M1
M2
M3
DR
CD15
CD33
CD32
CD13 (CD64)
Myeloblast
CD15
CD33
CD13
CD32
(CD64)
Promyelocyte
CD15
CD11
CD33
CD32
CD13
CD64
Myelocyte
CD16
CD15
CD11
CD32
CD13 (CD64)
Neutrophil
M5
DR
CD15
CD11
CD14
CD13
CD33
Monoblast
DR
CD15
CD11
CD14
CD13
CD33
Promonocyte
DR
CD15
CD11
CD14
CD13
CD64
CD33
Monocyte
DR
CD33
BFU-E
CFU-E
M6
Gly
Erythroblast
Gly
Erythrocyte
(DR)
CD34
BFU-MK
M7
DR
CD61
CD41
CD42
CD33
CFU-MK
CD41
CD42
CD61
Megakarocyte
CD41
CD42
CD61
Platelet

Table 6-1 Clinically Used Myeloid Antibodies

Antibody	*Specificity**	*Cluster Designation*
Mo1, OKM1	N, G, NK	CD11b
M67, 20.2	G, M, Plt	CDw12
My7, MCS-2, 44H	M, G	CD13
Mo2, My4, anti-M3, FMC17, FMC33	M, (G)	CD14
My1, MCS 1, anti-Leu M1, VIM D5, FMC10	G, (M)	CD15
My9, anti-Leu6, L4F3	G, progenitors	CD33
My10, anti-HPCA 1, 12.8, B1-3C5	Progenitors	CD34
My8	G, M	NA
Ep-1	E, BFU-E, CFU-E	NA
LICR, LON, R10	E, glycophorin A	NA
J15, 10E5, PBM 6.4	Plt GP IIb/IIIa, GPIIb	GD41
FMC25, BL-H6, GR-P	Plt GP IX, gp 23	CD42a
AN51, 6D1, PHN 89	Plt GPIb gp 135/25	CD42b
HLe-1, T29/33, T-200	Panleukocyte, leukocyte common antigen	CD45
4D1	Ia (HLA-DR)	NA

*M = monocytes; G = granulocytes; NK = national killer; ( ) = some; E = erythrocytes; N = neutrophils; Plt = platelets; NA = not applicable, no CD assigned.

CLL are characterized by a distinct pattern of reactivity that consists of weak expression of sIg, and of CD5 antigen, high affinity for binding mouse erythrocytes (M-rosettes), and expression of B maturation antigens such as those detected by monoclonal antibodies FMC7 or CD22 in <20% of cases.

T lymphocytes were first identified by their ability to spontaneously bind sheep erythrocytes and form a characteristic E-rosette. T-cell precursors arise in the bone marrow but enter the thymus,

Figure 6-1 Hypothetical myeloid differentiation scheme indicates the cell surface markers—as defined by selected, well-characterized cluster designations (CDs)—that have been detected on cells at the various maturational stages either by immunofluorescence, positive selection (sorting followed by colony forming units (CFU) assay, or negative selection (complement-mediated lysis). Hypothetical target cells in AML are indicated by small, wavy arrows. Major phenotypic manifestations of the FAB subtypes (M0–M7) are in boxes. Parenthesis around a CD marker indicate speculative placement (CD34, DR on pluripotent stem cell), weak expression (CD64 on myeloid precursors), or inducibility (CD64 on mature neutrophil). From Vaickus L, et al: Immune markers in hematologic malignancies. *CRC Crit Rev Oncol Hematol* 11:267–297, 1991.

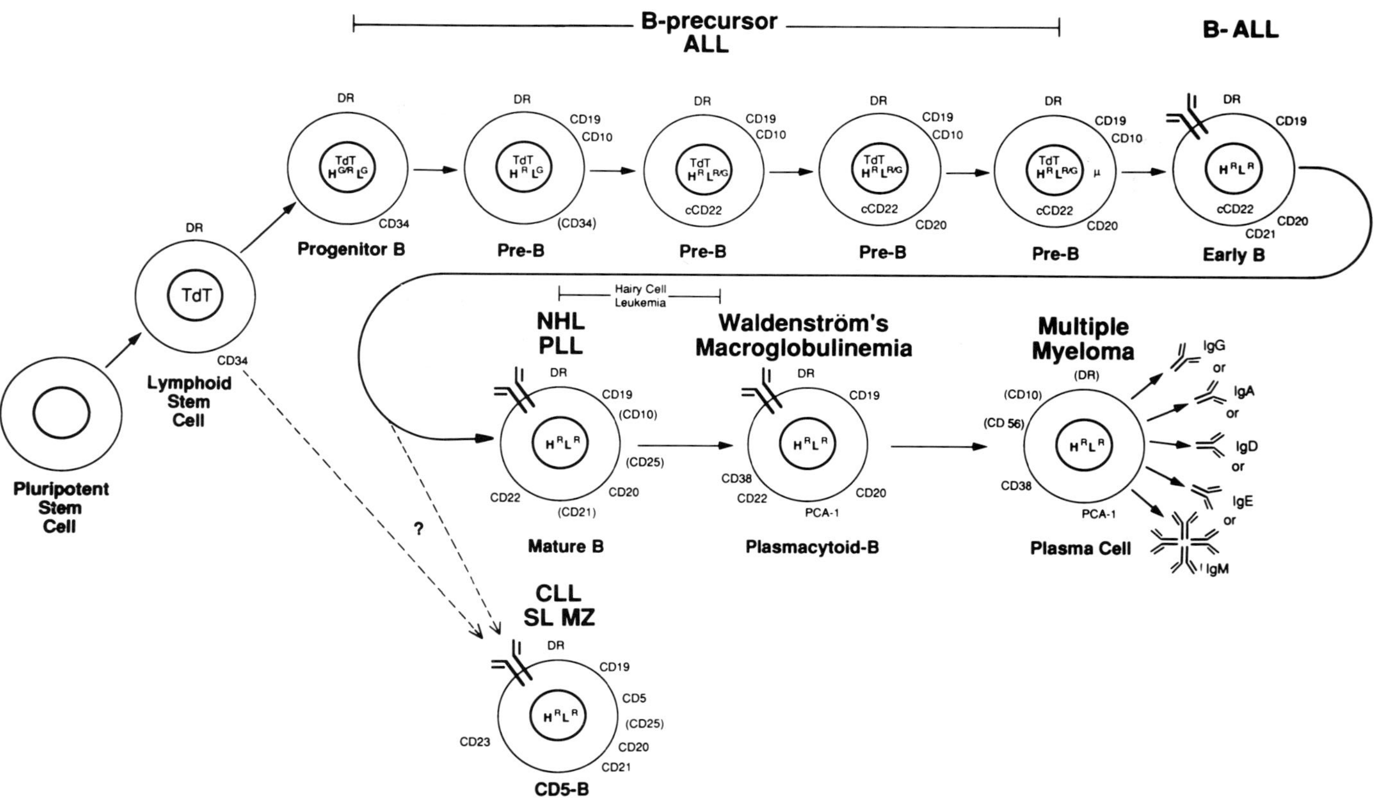

B-precursor ALL
B-ALL
Pluripotent Stem Cell
DR
TdT
CD34
Lymphoid Stem Cell
DR
$TdT\ H^{G/R}L^{G}$
CD34
Progenitor B
DR
CD19
CD10
$TdT\ H^{R}L^{G}$
(CD34)
Pre-B
DR
CD19
CD10
$TdT\ H^{R}L^{R/G}$
cCD22
Pre-B
DR
CD19
CD10
$TdT\ H^{R}L^{R/G}$
cCD22
CD20
Pre-B
DR
CD19
CD10
$TdT\ H^{R}L^{R/G}$
μ
cCD22
CD20
Pre-B
DR
CD19
$H^{R}L^{R}$
cCD22
CD21
CD20
Early B
Hairy Cell Leukemia
NHL
PLL
DR
CD19
(CD10)
$H^{R}L^{R}$
(CD25)
CD22
CD20
(CD21)
Mature B
Waldenström's Macroglobulinemia
DR
CD19
$H^{R}L^{R}$
CD38
CD22
PCA-1
CD20
Plasmacytoid-B
Multiple Myeloma
(DR)
(CD10)
(CD 56)
$H^{R}L^{R}$
CD38
PCA-1
Plasma Cell
IgG
or
IgA
or
IgD
or
IgE
or
IgM
?
CLL
SL MZ
DR
CD19
CD5
$H^{R}L^{R}$
(CD25)
CD23
CD20
CD21
CD5-B

Table 6-2 Clinically Used Lymphoid Antibodies for B-Cell Disorders

Antibody	*Specificity†*	*Cluster Designation*
OKT1, T1, Leu 1, T101, UCHT2	Pan T-LC, Pan Thy, B subset (B-CLL)	CD5
J5, anti-CALLA, BA-3, OK B-CALLA	Common ALL antigen, early B cells, some NHL (follicular lymphomas)	CD10
B4, Leu12	Pan B-LC, LB	CD19
B1, Leu16, RFB7, NU-B2	B-LC, malignant B cells	CD20
B2, Leu CR2, BA-5, RFB6	B-LC, malignant B cells, receptor EBV and C3d	CD21
B3, Leu 14, To15, RFB4, CLB/BLyl	Late B cells, hairy cells	CD22
FMC7*	Late B cells, hairy cells, B prolymphocytes	NA
BA-1	B-LC, malignant B cells	CD24
Anti-Tac, Tac 1, IL-2R1	IL-2 receptor, activated B, T; hairy cells	CD25
Anti-HPCA 1, My10, B1-3C5	Early progenitors (myeloblastic and lymphoblastic leukemia)	CD34
OKT10	Activated T, B; plasma cells	CD38
HLA-DR, OK1a, FMC4	Anti-class II MHC antigens, B-LC up to plasma cells, activated T, hematopoietic precursors	NA
HLe-1, T29/33, T-200	Panleukocyte, leukocyte common antigen	CD45

*FMC7 is probably distinct from CD22, although findings in some of the B-cell leukemias suggest that both appear on the cell membrane at a relatively late stage of B-cell maturation.

†ALL = acute lymphoblastic leukemia; Thy = thymocyte; LB = lymphoblast; LC = lymphocyte; H = helper; I = inducer; M = monocyte; C = cytotoxic; S = suppressor; EBV = Epstein-Barr virus; NA = none assigned; IL = interleukin; NHL = non-Hodgkin's lymphoma; MHC = major histocompatibility complex.

Figure 6-2 Hypothetical B-lineage differentiation scheme with selected stage-associated cell markers and putative phenotypic manifestations of B-lymphoid malignancies. Abbreviations: ALL, acute lymphoblastic leukemia; NHL, non-Hodgkin's lymphoma; PLL, prolymphocytic leukemia; CLL, chronic lymphocytic leukemia; SL, small lymphocytic, NHL; MZ, mantle zone, NHL; Tdt, terminal deoxynucleotidyl transferase; H, Ig heavy chain gene; G, germ line; R, rearranged; L, Ig light chain gene; cCd22, cytoplasmic CD22; μ, cytoplasmic IgM heavy chain (Cμ). Alternate names for Cμ+ B-precursor ALL = pre-B ALL; Cμ- B-precursor ALL = early pre-B-ALL. CD antigens in parentheses indicate tentative assignment to a particular stage, presence of only a percentage of cases (e.g., CD56 found on 80% of multiple myelomas), or presence on transformed cells only (e.g., CD56 not found on normal plasma cells). From Vaickus L, et al: Immune markers in hematologic malignancies. *CRC Crit Rev Oncol Hematol* 11:267–297, 1991.

Table 6-3 Clinically Used Lymphoid Antibodies for T-Cell Disorders

Antibody	*Specificity*	*Cluster Designation*
OKT6, T6, Leu 6, NA 134	Cortical Thy, T-LB	CD1a
OKT11, T11, Leu 5	Pan T-LC, sheep erythrocyte receptor	CD2
OKT3, T3, Leu 4, UCHT1, 41F	Pan T-LC (mitogenic)	CD3
OKT4, T4, Leu 3	T-H/I, M	CD4
OKT1, T1, Leu 1, T101, UCHT2	Pan T-LC, Pan Thy, B subset (B-CLL)	CD5
OKT16, Leu 9, 3A1, WT1, T-55	Pan T-LC, LB	CD7
OKT8, T8, Leu 2, UCHT4	T-C/S	CD8
Anti-Tac, Tac 1, IL-2R1	IL-2 receptor, activated B, T; hairy cells	CD25
Anti-HPCA 1, My10, B1-3C5	Early progenitors (myeloblastic and lymphoblastic leukemia)	CD34
HLe-1, T29/33, T-200	Panleukocyte, leukocyte common antigen	CD45

where they undergo changes that ultimately lead to mature T-cell function. While in the thymus, the T-cell precursors acquire a sequential array of cell surface markers that serve as markers of differentiation (Fig. 6.3). These cell surface markers, similar to those of B cells, are demonstrated by a battery of monoclonal antibodies. The more common T monoclonal antibodies and specific antisera are shown in Table 6.3. The earliest identifiable stages of T-cell differentiation are observed in the thymic cortex, which is depicted as an early thymocyte (Fig. 6.3). Later in development, the cortical thymocyte acquires the cortical thymocyte marker CD1a and is referred to as a common thymocyte (Fig. 6.3). Also, simultaneously during cortical thymic development, the cells express CD4 and CD8, which are associated with

Figure 6-3 Hypothetical T-lineage differentiation scheme with stage-associated cell markers, anatomic localization of normal T cells, and putative phenotypic manifestations of different T-ALL subtypes. Cell markers in parentheses are not always expressed or are speculative (e.g., CD34 on progenitor T cell). Abbreviations: TdT, terminal deoxynucleotidyl transferase; TCR, T-cell receptor β, TCR β-chain gene; α, chain gene; G, germ line; R, rearranged; cCD3, cytoplasmic CD3. From Vaickus L, et al: Immune markers in hematologic malignancies. *CRC Crit Rev Oncol Hematol* 11:267–297, 1991.

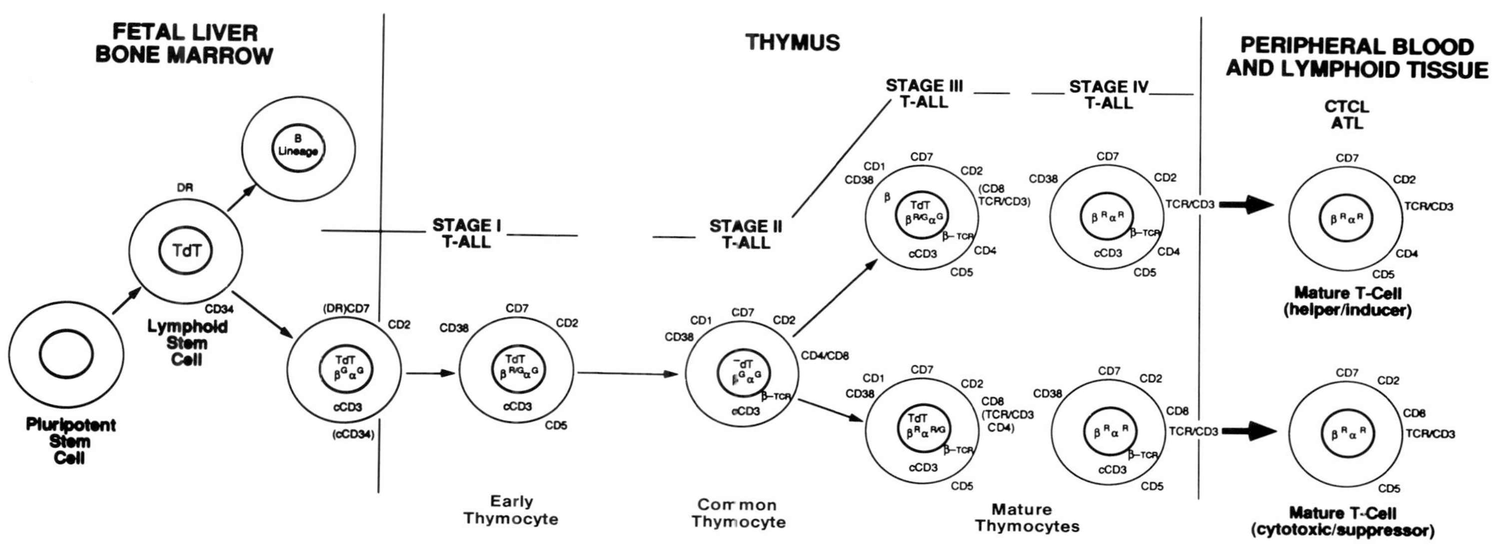

FETAL LIVER
BONE MARROW
THYMUS
PERIPHERAL BLOOD
AND LYMPHOID TISSUE
STAGE I
T-ALL
STAGE II
T-ALL
STAGE III
T-ALL
STAGE IV
T-ALL
CTCL
ATL
Pluripotent
Stem
Cell
DR
TdT
CD34
Lymphoid
Stem
Cell
B
Lineage
(DR)CD7
CD2
TdT
cCD3
(cCD34)
CD38
CD7
CD2
TdT
cCD3
CD5
Early
Thymocyte
CD1
CD38
CD7
CD2
CD4/CD8
cCD3
β-TCR
Common
Thymocyte
CD1
CD38
CD7
CD2
(CD8
TCR/CD3)
β
TdT
β-TCR
cCD3
CD4
CD5
CD1
CD38
CD7
CD2
CD8
(TCR/CD3
CD4)
TdT
β-TCR
cCD3
CD5
Mature
Thymocytes
CD38
CD7
CD2
TCR/CD3
β-TCR
cCD3
CD4
CD5
CD38
CD7
CD2
CD8
TCR/CD3
β-TCR
cCD3
CD5
CD7
CD2
TCR/CD3
CD4
CD5
Mature T-Cell
(helper/inducer)
CD7
CD2
CD8
TCR/CD3
CD5
Mature T-Cell
(cytotoxic/suppressor)

helper and suppressor functions, respectively. The CD1 disappears when the cells enter the thymic medulla and acquire a more mature T-cell phenotype. The CD4 and CD8 are only coexpressed for a brief period of intrathymic differentiation, since they are mutually exclusive in mature T cells. It is the latter cell types that are pathologically involved in the chronic T-cell disorders. Although Tdt is found in all thymocytes, it is not found in the chronic T-cell disorders that develop in cells beyond the thymocyte stage (Fig. 6.3). Furthermore, Tdt is not specific for T-cell lineage since it appears in precursor B cells and occasionally in myeloid leukemias.

CHRONIC MYELOID LEUKEMIA AND RELATED DISORDERS

The use of monoclonal antibodies in the characterization of the chronic myeloid malignancies is limited since the diagnosis of those disorders is usually established with ease utilizing morphology, cytochemistry, and cytogenetics. However, in blastic crisis of these disorders, the blast cells show the same cellular diversity as the increased progenitor cell compartment observed in these disorders, and their differentiation stages seem to be very closely interrelated. Therefore, cell surface marker analysis with monoclonal antibodies has demonstrated that immature cells heterogeneously express the phenotype of myeloblast, lymphoblast, or, more rarely, megakaryoblast, erythroblast, or a mixture of these blasts. In general, approximately one-third of blastic transformations in CML represent early B-cell features that include the expressions of Tdt, CD10, HLA-DR, CD19, CD20 and rearrangement of the Ig gene. The other two-thirds of these blast crises are dominated by expression of myeloid antigens. These myeloid precursors may be detected by CD13 and CD33, which represent broad panmyelomonocytic markers (Fig. 6.1). Also, CD11b, CD11c, My8, and CD15 may be used to detect mixed myeloid and monocytic elements. Finally, CD14 is more specific and may be used to detect monocytic elements. Discordance has been observed between morphology, cytochemistry, and immunophenotyping particularly when poorly differentiated leukemic cells are involved; therefore, caution is emphasized in the interpretation and use of these markers. This becomes of specific importance in blast crisis of CML, the cells of which arise from a pluripotential precursor.

Therefore, the concept of lineage specificity has been challenged by an increasing number of reports that indicate that phenotypic and genotypic markers of different lineages have been coexpressed in individual cells. These findings of lineage infidelity or promiscuity have been further clarified by the use of flow cytometric two-color immunofluorescent analysis. Furthermore, a consistent pattern of reactivity with monoclonal antibodies is found in all patients exhibiting blast crisis, showing that the blast cells are heterogeneous. Minor components of the blast cells react with platelet antibodies, most of them being labeled with monoclonal antibodies J15 (CD41) to platelet glycoproteins IIb/IIIa. Monoclonal antibodies AN51 (CD42b) to glycoprotein 1b detected fewer megakaryocytic blast cells, suggesting that these markers detect more mature cells in the megakaryocytic series.

Besides myelomonoblastic, lymphoblastic, and megakaryoblastic cells in this heterogeneous array, early erythroid components may be detected. Monoclonal antibodies to glycophorin, the transferrin receptor CD71, CD45, and erythropoietin (Ep-1) have been useful in detecting erythroid lineage. CD45 is expressed on the earliest identifiable erythroid cells and is progressively lost as cells undergo maturation. Ep-1 and CD71 will detect erythrocyte burst-forming units (BFUs-E) and erythroid colony-forming units (CFUs-E), whereas glycophorin is first observed on morphologically recognizable erythroblasts just after the CFU-E stage. Loken et al. (1987) have utilized the above markers effectively in analyzing erythroid ontogeny.

Recent studies using peroxidase-antiperoxidase and avidin-biotin peroxidase techniques on juvenile chronic myeloid leukemia (JCML) (Ph^1-absent) have revealed immunophenotypes with EMB11+, KiM1+, KiM6+, KiM8+, CD4+, HLA-DR+, and S-100 protein +. The first four antibodies mark monocytes-histiocytes. KiM1 also detects interdigitating reticulum cells. Furthermore, these cells express S-100 protein, which occurs in antigen-presenting cells including indeterminate cells, interdigitating reticulum cells, Langerhans' cells, and veiled cells. S-100 protein has also been detected in a population of CD2+, CD3+, CD8+ T lymphocytes and rare examples of T-cell lymphoma and HCL. Considerable overlap in immunophenotypic characteristics has been noted in dendritic and phagocytic histiocytes. Therefore, JCML may be derived from a common stem cell of dendritic cells and phagocytic histiocytes. Alternatively, JCML may be the malignant counterpart of dendritic cells exhibiting some immunophenotypic features of phagocytic histiocytes.

CHRONIC LYMPHOCYTIC LEUKEMIA AND RELATED DISORDERS (B-CELL)

The B-cell lymphoid leukemias and related disorders are in general characterized by clinical, morphologic, and histologic features. The

Table 6-4 Markers for Chronic B-Cell Leukemias and Related Entities*

				NHL†			
Marker	*CLL*	*PLL*	*HCL*	*Follicular lymphoma*	*Intermediate*	*SLVL*	*Plasma Cell Tumors‡*
sIg	Weak	Strong	Strong	Strong	Moderate	Strong	Negative
cIg	+	+	+	–	–	–/+	+ +
M-rosettes	+ +	–	–/+	–/+	–/+	–	–
CD5	+ +	–/+	+ –	–	+ + (MZL)	–	–
CD19/20/24	+ +	+ +	+ +	+ +	+ +	+ +	–
Anti-class II	+ +	+ +	+ +	+ +	+ +	+ +	–
FMC7/CD22	–/+	+ +	+ +	+	+	+ +	–
CD10	–	–/+	–	–/+	–/+	–	–/+
CD25	–	–	+ +	–	–	–/+	–
CD38	–	–	–/+	–/+	–	–/+	+ +

Source: Bennett JM, et al: Proposals for the classification of chronic (mature) B and T lymphoid leukemias. *J Clin Pathol* 42:567–584, 1989.

*A plus sign indicates incidence at which a marker is positive in >30% of cells in a particular B-cell tumor (+ + = 80–100%; + = 40–80%; –/+ = 10–40%; – = 0–9% of cases).

†NHL with a high incidence of peripheral blood or bone marrow disease. Mantle zone lymphoma (MZL).

‡Myelomatosis and plasma cell leukemia: WM cells show a similar phenotype except for sharing some features with PLL, HCL, and NHL (expression of FMC7, CD22, and some other B-cell antigens).

defining criterion for diagnosis is the presence of a monoclonal population of B cells, demonstrating B lineage differentiation as shown by one or more specific monoclonal antibodies such as CD19, CD20, and CD24, and gene rearrangement. The markers for the chronic B-cell leukemias and related disorders used in the diagnosis of these entities are depicted in Tables 6.2 and 6.4.

CLL results from the malignant transformation of a B lymphocyte, and T-CLL was originally believed to account for approximately 5% of CLL cases, but recently some authors question the existence of this disorder. They suggest that T-CLLs most likely represent misdiagnosed cases of other chronic T-lymphoid leukemias. The B lymphocytes of CLL are characterized by a distinct pattern of reactivity that includes expression of sIg (weak) typically mμ or mμ and delta chain, less commonly gamma, alpha, or no heavy chain; CD5 antigen, high affinity for binding mouse erythrocytes (M-rosettes); and in <20% cases, expression of B maturation antigens such as FMC7 and CD22. Besides CLL, some NHLs (intermediate or diffuse small cleaved) express CD5 and weak sIg, which is not observed in other NHLs and B-cell PLLs. CD5 expression on CLL cells is unexpected since this 65–69 kd glycoprotein antigen was previously thought to be restricted to T lymphocytes. The exact meaning of this finding is not clear.

However, a normal B-cell counterpart that expresses CD5 is identified in 5–10% of normal B cells. Interestingly, phorbol myristate acetate induces expression of this antigen on normal peripheral blood B lymphocytes.

The immunophenotype of a chronic B-cell leukemia is immunologically mature and should be distinguished from that of early B lineage ALL that are immunologically immature and Tdt-positive. Contrariwise, more maturation beyond the CLL lymphocyte ultimately forms plasma cells that are associated with loss of B-cell antigens and class II molecules. However, new antigens such as those detected by CD38 and other monoclonal antibodies such as PCA-1 or BU-11 make their appearance.

Deviation from the typical CLL phenotype is observed in cases with an increased proportion of prolymphocytes, or CLL/PLL in which marker characteristics intermediate between CLL and PLL may be perceived (e.g., strong expression of sIg and reactivity with FMC7). If the following four criteria for B-cell CLL are utilized—weak sIg, >30% M-rosettes, >50% CD5+ cells, and <30% FMC7+ cells—a combination of three or four of these markers is seen in 80% of typical CLLs, in 65% of CLL/PLL cases, and in none of those with a diagnosis of B-PLL.

Recently, a unique subset of a B-cell chronic lymphoproliferative disorder with features of both CLL and HCL was reported. Morphologically, the cases appeared to be cases of CLL with abundant cytoplasm. They had no morphologic features of hairy cells, did not express TRAP, but did express CD11c, a hairy cell immunophenotypic marker. This unique group of leukemias appears to represent the malignant transformation of lymphocytes arising from a stage of lymphocyte differentiation between cases of typical CLL and HCL. The CD11c is known to have important function in cellular adhesion and may be important in determining the pattern of lymphocyte tissue distribution found in this group of patients.

B-PLL cells resemble activated lymphocytes. They express strong sIg staining with either kappa or lambda light chain, HLA-DR, CD10, CD20, CD21, and FMC7/CD22. The cells exhibit heavy and light chain Ig gene rearrangements. PLL cells do not exhibit Tdt positivity, and the PAS reaction is typically positive. In approximately two-thirds of B-PLLs, the phenotype is strikingly different from that of CLL.

The immunophenotype of HCL is most compatible with clonal proliferation of B lymphocytes. B-cell-associated antigens including CD19, CD20, CD21, FMC7/CD22, and sometimes CD23 and CD24 are also observed. The PCA-1 antigen typical of plasma cells may be present on some hairy cells. Such findings suggest that hairy cells may be pre-plasma cells. Analysis of Ig gene rearrangement reveals clonal rearrangement of heavy chain Ig (IgH) genes and at least one light chain Ig (IgL) gene. Most cases of HCL demonstrate the CD25 antigen (IL-2 receptor) typically identified on malignant and activated T cells. Several antigens appear to be restricted to HCL cells. One such antigen, designated the cCLL antigen, is restricted to CLL and hairy cells. Other reagents that react with hairy cells include anti-HC2 and CD11c. Since CD11c reacts with monocytes, its value for detecting hairy cells must depend on the simultaneous demonstration of a B-cell antigen such as CD20 and CD24. Some HCL cell lines express alpha S-HCL1 and alpha S-HCL3, which expressed alone are nonspecific, however, when coexpressed are characteristic of hairy cells.

HCL-v cells differ from typical hairy cells by not reacting with CD25 and HC2; but some cases are CD11c-positive. Membrane IgG is often found on the cell membrane, and in some cases sIg cannot be demonstrated. Therefore, the membrane phenotype of HCL-v is close to that of B-PLL.

Cawley et al. (1980) described an aggressive variant characterized by higher tumor load, high blood leukocyte count, and minimal marrow fibrosis (so that the aspiration is easy). Another aggressive form, called the blastic variant, is characterized by massive splenomegaly, pancytopenia, minimal marrow fibrosis blastlike hairy cells with immature nuclear chromatin, and deep-blue, granulated cytoplasm. The Japanese variant has a somewhat different immunophenotype: CD10+, CD5+, HC1−, HC2−.

Some NHLs may manifest themselves as a CLL involving both peripheral blood and bone marrow. These include follicular or nodular lymphomas and intermediate differentiated lymphocytic (mantle zone) lymphomas. The former include both nodular (follicular, small cleaved cells) and diffuse (diffuse, small cleaved cells) poorly differentiated lymphocytic lymphoma by the Rappaport classification. Follicular lymphoma cells (buttock cells) circulating in the peripheral blood were formerly referred to as lymphosarcoma leukemia cells. These cells differ from CLL cells, as they may express CD10, are CD5-negative, and generally have a low percentage of mouse erythrocyte rosette formation. In addition, they routinely express HLA-DR, CD19, and CD20 antigens and frequently demonstrate the CD21 antigen. Unlike the follicular lymphoma cells, the diffuse small cleaved cells do not express CD10.

The intermediate differentiated lymphocytic lymphoma show surface B-cell antigenic characteristics intermediate between those of follicular center cell lymphomas and medullary small lymphocytic lymphomas. These cells show SIg, usually IgM and sometimes IgM and IgD with intermediate amounts of surface Ig, CD24, CD20, CD5, CD9 molecules. Sometimes they express CD10 and HLA-DR. Lymph node immunoperoxidase techniques have revealed that intermediate lymphocytic lymphomas mark with LN-2 but not LN-1 antibodies. Okan et al. (1985) have shown that LN-1 antibody selectively reacts with lymphoid cells of the follicular center, whereas LN-2 stains a wider spectrum of lymphoid cells, including mantle zone lymphocytes, hence the term *mantle zone lymphoma*.

SLVL cases are similar to those of B-PLL. Unlike HCL cells, these villous lymphocytes do not react with HC2, CD25, CD11c or cytochemically with the TRAP reaction. The differential diagnoses to be considered are CLL, B-PLL, HCL, and HCL-v. The histologic appearances of the spleen show white pulp disease (lymphoma) in contrast to HCL and HCL-v with or without clinically important red pulp infiltration.

The malignant B cells of WM, heavy chain disease, and multiple myeloma represent a further step in the maturation of medullary and B cells. Like CLL cells, WM cells express SIg, HLA-DR, CD19, and CD20 antigens; however, unlike CLL cells, the WM cells express PCA-1 antigen and do not express CD21 antigen, nor rosette with mouse erythrocytes.

The plasma cell and its malignant counterpart, the myeloma cell, represent the most differentiated B lymphocytes. These cells synthesize large quantities of lg and have CIg. Both plasma cells and myeloma cells stain intensely with CD38 monoclonal antibody as well as anti-PCA 1 and anti-PC 1 antibodies. However, they usually lack SIg, HLA-DR, CD19, CD20, and CD21 antigens. Although CD10 is usually absent on myeloma cells, rare cases of CD10–positive myeloma with an aggressive course and poor prognosis have been reported.

CHRONIC LYMPHOCYTIC LEUKEMIA AND RELATED DISORDERS (T-CELL)

There is considerable heterogeneity in this group of disorders because of the existence of many functional subsets and stages of maturation of T lymphocytes from which the leukemias originate. The monoclonal antibodies used in the diagnosis of T-cell leukemias are shown in Table 6.3, and the markers in various chronic (mature) T-cell leukemias in Table 6.5.

Table 6-5 Markers in Chronic (Mature) T-Cell Leukemias*

Marker	*T-CLL†*	*T-PLL*	*ATLL*	*SS*
Tdt	−	−	−	−
CD1a	−	−	−	−
CD2	+ +	+ +	+ +	+ +
CD3	−	+	+ +	+ +
CD4	−	+	+ +	+ +
CD5	−	+ +	+ +	+ +
CD7	−	+ +	−	−
CD8	+ +	−/+	−	
CD25	−	−	+ +	−
CD38	−	−	−	−

Source: Bennett JM, et al: Proposals for the classification of chronic (mature) B and T lymphoid leukemias. *J Clin Pathol* 42:567–584, 1989.

*A plus sign indicates rate at which a marker is positive in >30% of cells in particular T-cell leukemias (+ + = 80–100%; −/+ = 10–40%; − = 0–9% of cases).

†Some authors question the existence of T-CLL.

The immature T-cell or thymic-derived disorders constitute acute T-lymphoblastic lymphoma and are recognized by Tdt and CD1a positivity. Contrariwise, the mature or postthymic T-cell disorders do not express CD1a or Tdt, but demonstrate pan-T markers such as CD2 (E-rosettes) and CD3. The pan-T-monoclonal antibodies CD5 and CD7 are more consistently positive in thymic rather than in postthymic T-cell malignancies.

Although previous reviews indicated that approximately 5% of CLL cases involve T cells, some authors consider these findings incorrect. If such cases are carefully examined, they can be reclassified as T-gamma lymphoproliferative disease (TGLD), adult T-cell leukemia-lymphoma (ATLL), T-prolymphocytic leukemia (T-PLL), or the leukemic phase of NHL. In TGLDs the majority of the cases demonstrate LGLs. These lymphocytes have receptors for the Fc portion of IgG, natural killer (NK)-associated antigens CD56, CD57, and CD16.

Two general forms of TGLD exist exhibiting the above surface markers, which were formerly believed to be T-CLL. One (large granular lymphocytic leukemia or TGLD shows a benign clinical course, gradually increasing lymphocytosis (WBC rarely $>20 \times 10^9$/L), neutropenia, and recurrent infections. Most with this chronic course have a CD3+, CD8+, CD4− membrane phenotype. Contrariwise, the more aggressive form shows more bulky disease of liver and spleen and a progressive course with rising WBCs. These are associated with a CD4+, CD16+, CD8+, CD11b+ membrane phenotype. They also express receptors for the Fc portion of IgG and NK-associated HNK-1.

Some of these cases are probably best diagnosed as ATLL. Finally, some cases of T-cell lymphocytosis may be benign, although they have similar immunophenotypic findings. However, the reactive lymphocytosis is self-limiting, rarely above 5 × 10^9/L, and lacks both T-cell antigen receptor (TCR) rearrangement and cytogenetic abnormalities.

Recent investigation has proposed that TGLD be divided into two groups with subgroups. The first group is composed of two subgroups of natural killer cells (CD2+, CD3−, CD16+, CD57+) and (CD2+, CD3−, CD16+, CD57−). Apparently the CD57− may have a poorer prognosis. The second group (CD2+, CD3+, CD8+, CD57+) is subdivided on the basis of CD16. The CD16+ demonstrates TCR_B rearrangement, whereas CD16− show a germline configuration suggesting a reactive rather than a neoplastic process. Although much progress has been made concerning TGLD, important aspects of the biology and clinical nature of this disorder have not been satisfactorily addressed. Foremost among these are the malignant and benign nature of TGLD. Whatever the outcome it appears fairly clear that TGLD is a heterogeneous disorder that will require detailed investigation and lucid thinking. Because of this heterogeneous group of disorders, some authors prefer use of the term lymphoproliferative disorder of granular lymphocytes.

Approximately 20% of patients who present with clinical and morphologic features of PLL have a T-cell malignancy. As in B-PLL, the WBC is usually >100 × 10^9/L at onset, but in contrast, lymphadenopathy, skin lesions, serous effusions, and splenomegaly dominate an aggressive course. T-PLL cells may resemble B-PLL cells, or may demonstrate a higher nuclear cytoplasmic ratio, irregular nuclear outline, or small nuclei with indistinct nucleoli. Because of this morphologic heterogeneity, some cases have been described as T-CLL, as alluded to above. Membrane markers of most T-PLL are CD4+, CD8−; a minority coexpress CD4 and CD8, and a few are CD4−, CD8+. Unlike other mature T-cell leukemias, in particular those with a CD4+ phenotype, T-PLL cells strongly express the CD7 antigen.

ATLL is associated with HTLV-I. Virtually all patients have antibodies to HTLV-I. Patients with this disease have been identified primarily in Japan, southern United States, and the Caribbean. There is a spectrum of clinical syndromes in ATLL including acute (high WBC, hypercalcemia, <1-year survival), chronic, and smoldering types. Chronic ATLL patients have lower WBCs, fewer circulating abnormal cells, and >1-year survival. The smoldering variant demonstrates normal WBCs, few nonspecific symptoms, and a low proportion of abnormal T lymphocytes in the peripheral blood. These cells with markedly irregular nuclear contour (propeller cells) express the phenotype of helper-inducer T lymphocytes CD4 and CD25 that identifies the IL-2 receptor. Variability in the expression of CD2 and CD3 has been observed. The ATLL cells suppress B-cell Ig secretion by a complex mechanism involving induction of suppressor cells following activation of normal suppressor cell precursors.

SS is characterized by generalized exfoliative erythroderma, an epidermal infiltrate of atypical mononuclear cells, and increased numbers of circulating Sézary cells in the peripheral blood. The nucleus of these cells demonstrates a marked convoluted-cerebriform appearance and small rarely visible nucleoli. Small (more common) and large cell variants have been reported. Sézary and mycosis cells form E-rosettes, react with T antisera and anti-T monoclonal antibodies, and have clonal rearrangement of the TCR_B receptors. In most cases the cells express the phenotype associated with normal helper-inducer T lymphocytes CD5, CD3, CD4 and function as helper T lymphocytes in in vitro assays. A complete list of the cluster designation antigens is shown in Table 6.6.

Table 6.6 CD Antigens*

CD Design	*Selection of Assigned Monoclonal Antibodies*	*Main Cellular Reactivity*	*Recognized Membrane Component†*	*Sequence/ CH-Structure Analyzed‡*
CD1a	NA 1/34; T6; VIT6; Leu6	Thy, DC, B subset	gp49	Y
CD1b	WM-25; 4A76; NUT2	Thy, DC, B subset	gp45	Y
CD1c	L161; M241; 7C6; PHM3	Thy, DC, B subset	gp43	Y
CD2	9.6; T11; 35.1	T	CD58 (LFA-3) receptor, gp50	Y
CD2R	T11.3; VIT 13; D66	Activated T	CD2 epitopes restr. to activ. T	Y
CD3	T3; UCHT1; 38.1; Leu4	T	CD3-complex (5 chains), gp/p 26,20,16	Y
CD4	T4; Leu3a; 91.D6	T subset	Class II/HIV receptor, gp59	Y
CD5	T1; UCHT2; T101; HH9; AMG4	T, B subset	gp67	Y
CD6	T12; T411	T, B subset	gp100	—
CD7	3A1; 4A; CL1.3; G3-7	T	gp40	Y
CD8	α chain: T8; Leu2a; M236; UCHT4; T811 β chain: T8/2T8-5H7	T subset	Class I receptor, gp 32α, / or / β dimer	Y
CD9	CLB-thromb/8; PHN200; FMC56	Pre-B, M, Plt	p24	—
CD10	J5, VILA1, BA-3	Lymph. Prog., cALL, Germ. Ctr. B, G	Neutral endopeptidase, gp100, CALLA	Y
CD11a	MHM24; 2F12; CRIS-3	Leukocytes	LFA-1, gp180/95	Y

Table 6.6 CD antigens* *(continued)*

CD Design	*Selection of Assigned Monoclonal Antibodies*	*Main Cellular Reactivity*	*Recognized Membrane Component†*	*Sequence/ CH-Structure Analyzed‡*
CD11b	Mo1; 5A4.C5; LPM19C	M, G, NK	C3bi receptor, gp155/95	—
CD11c	B-LY6; L29; BL-4H4	M, G, NK, B sub	gp150/95	—
CDw12	M67	M, G, Plt	(p90-120)	—
CD13	MY7, MCS-2, TÜK1, MOU28	M, G	Aminopeptidase N, gp150	Y
CD14	Mo2, UCHM1, VIM13, MoP15	M, (G), LHC	gp55	Y
CD15	My1, VIM-D5	G, (M)	3-FAL, X-Hapten	Y
CD16	BW209/2; HUNK2; VEP13; 3G8	NK, G, Mac	FcRIII, gp50-65	Y
CDw17	GO35, Huly-m 13	G, M, Plt	Lactosylcaramide	—
CD18	MHM23; M232; 11H6; GLB54	Leukocytes	β chain to CD11a,b,c	Y
CD19	B4; HD37	B	gp95	Y
CD20	B1; 1F5	B	p37/32, ion channel?	Y
CD21	B2; HB5	B subset	C3d/EBV-Rec. (CR2), p140	Y
CD22	HD39; S-HCL1; To15	Cytopl. B/surface B subset	gp135, homology to myelin assoc. gp (MAG)	Y
CD23	Blast-2, MHM6	B subset, act. M, Eo	FceRII, gp45-50	Y
cd24	VIBE3; BA-1	B, G	gp41/38?	—
CD25	TAC; 7G7/B6; 2A3	Activated T, B, M	IL-2R βchain, gp55	Y
CD26	134-2C2; TS145	Activated T	Dipeptidylpeptidase IV, gp120	Y
CD27	VIT14; S152; OKT18A; CLB-9F4	T subset	p55 (dimer)	—
CD28	9.3; KOLT2	T subset	gp44	Y
CD29	K20; A-1A5	Broad	VLA β-, integrin β1-chain, Plt GPIIa	Y
CD30	Ki-1; Ber-H2; HSR4	Activated T, B; Sternberg-Reed	gp120, Ki-1	—
CD31	SG134; TM3; HEC-75; ES12F11	Plt, M, G, B, (T)	gp140, Plt GPIIa	—
CDw32	CIKM5; 41H16; IV.3; 2E1; KB61	M, G, B, Plt	FcRII, gp40	Y
CD33	My9; H153; L4F3	M, Prog., AML	gp67	Y
CD34	My10, Bl-3C5, ICH-3	Prog.	gp105-120	Y
CD35	TO5, CB04, J3D3	G, M, B	CR1	Y
CD36	5F1, CIMeg1; ESIVC7	M, Plt, (B)	gp90, Plt GPIV	—
CD37	HD28; HH1; G28-1	B, (T, M)	gp40-52	Y
CD38	HB7; T16	Lymph. Prog., PC, Act. T	p45	Y
CD39	AC2; G28-2	B subset, (M)	gp70-100	—
CD40	G28-5	B, carcinomas	gp50, homology to NGF-receptor	Y
CD41	PBM 6.4; CLB-thromb/7; PL273	Plt	Plt GPIIb/IIIa complex and GPIIb	Y
CD42a	FMC25; BL-H6; GR-P	Plt	Plt GPIX, gp23	Y
CD42b	PHN89; AN51; GN287	Plt	Plt GPIb, gp135/25	Y

Table 6.6 CD antigens* *(continued)*

CD Design	*Selection of Assigned Monoclonal Antibodies*	*Main Cellular Reactivity*	*Recognized Membrane Component†*	*Sequence/ CH-Structure Analyzed‡*
CD43	OTH 71C5; G19-1; MEM-59	T, G, M, brain	Leukosialin, gp95	Y
CD44	GRHL 1; F10-44-2; 33-3B3; BRIC35	T, G, M, brain, RBC	Pgp-1, gp80-95	Y
CD45	T29/33; BMAC 1; AB187	Leukocytes	LCA, T200	Y
CD45RA	G1-15; F8-11-13; 73.5	T subset, B, G, M	Restricted T200, gp220	Y
CD45RB	PTD/26/16	T subset, B, G, M	Restricted T200	Y
CD45RO	UCHL 1	T subset, B, G, M	Restricted T200, gp180	Y
CD46	HULYM5; 122-2; J4B	Leukocytes	Membrane cofactor protein (MCP), gp66/56	Y
CD47	BRIC 126; CIKM1; BRIC 125	Broad	gp47-52, *N*-linked glycan	—
CD48	WM68; LO-MN25; J4-57	Leukocytes	gp41, PI-linked	—
CDw49b	CLB-thromb/4; Gi14	Plt, cultured T	VLA-alpha2-chain, Plt GPIa	Y
CDw49d	B5G10; HP2/1; HP1/3	M, T, B, (LHC), Thy	VLA-alpha4-chain, gp150	—
CDw49f	GoH3	Plt, (T)	VLA-alpha6-chain, Plt GPIc	—
CDw50	101-1D2; 140-11	Leukocytes	gp148/108, PI-linked	—
CD51	13C2; 23C6; NKI-M7; NKI-M9	(Plt)(B)	VNR α chain	Y
CDw52	097; YTH66.9; Campath-1	Leukocytes	Campath-1, gp21-28	—
CD53	MEM-53; HI29; HI36; HD77	Leukocytes	gp32-40	—
CD54	RR7/7F7; WEHI--CAMI	Broad, Activ.	ICAM-1	Y
CD55	143-30; BRIC 110:BRIC 128; F2B-7.2	Broad	DAF (decay accelerating factor), PI-linked	Y
CD56	Leu19; NKH1; FP2-11.14, L185	NK, activ. lymphocytes	gp220/135, NKH1, isoform of N-CAM	Y
CD57	Leu7; L183; L186	NK, T, B sub, brain	gp110, HNK1	—
CD58	TS2/9; G26; BRIC 5	Leukocytes, Epithel	LFA-3, gp40-65, PI-linked	Y
CD59	YTH53.1; MEM-43	Broad	gp18-20, PI-linked	—
CDw60	M-T32; M-T21; M-T41; UM4D4	T sub	NeuAc-NeuAc-Gal-	Y
CD61	Y2/51; CLB-thromb/1; VI-PL2; BL-E6	Plt	Integrin β3-, VNR β-chain, Plt GPIIIa	Y
CD62	CLB-thromb/6; CLB-thromb/5; RUU-SP1.18.1	Plt activ.	CMP-140 (PADGEM), gp140	Y
CD63	RUU-SP2.28; CLB-gran/12	Plt activ., M, (G, T, B)	gp53	—
CD64	Mab32.2; Mab22	M	FcRI, gp75	Y

Table 6.6 CD antigens* *(continued)*

CD Design	*Selection of Assigned Monoclonal Antibodies*	*Main Cellular Reactivity*	*Recognized Membrane Component*†	*Sequence/ CH-Structure Analyzed*‡
CDw65	VIM2; HE10; CF4; VIM8	G, M	Ceramide-dodecasaccharide 4c	Y
CD66	CLB gran/10; YTH71.3	G	Phosphoprotein pp 180-200	—
CD67	B13.9; G10F5; JML-H16	G	p100, PI-linked	—
CD68	EBM11; Y2/131; Y-1/82A; Ki-M7; Ki-M6	Macrophages	gp110	—
CD69	MLR3; L78; BL-Ac/p26; FN50	Activated B, T	gp32/28, AIM	—
CDw70	Ki-24; HNE 51; HNC 142	Activated B, T, Sternberg-Reed cells	Ki-24	—
CD71	138-18; 120-2A3; MEM-75; VIP-1; Nu-TfR2	Proliferating cells, Mac.	Transferrin receptor	Y
CD72	S-HCL2; J3-109; BU-40; BU-41	B	gp43/39	—
CD73	1E9.28.1; 7G2.2.11; AD2	B subset, T subset	ecto-5′-nucleotidase, p69	—
CD74	LN2; BU-43; BU-45	B, M	Class II assoc. invariant chain, gp41/35/33	—
CDw75	LN1; HH2; EBU-141	Mature B, (T subset)	p53?	—
CD76	HD66; CRIS-4	Mature B, T subset	gp85/67	—
CD77	38.13(BLA); 424/4A11; 424/3D9	Restr. B	Globotriaosylceramide (Gb3)	—
CDw78	Anti Ba; LO-panB-a; 1588	B, (M)	?	

Source: W. Knapp and Grune & Stratton.

*Members of the Nomenclature Committee of the Fourth International Workshop on Human Leukocyte Differentiation Antigens: *Workshop Council:* A. Bernard, P. Beverley, L. Bournsell, T. Kishimoto, W. Knapp, A. McMichael, C. Milstein, S.F. Schlossman, E. Reinherz, G. Riethmüller, T.A. Springer, R. Winchester. *Workshop Organizers: T-Cell Section:* P. Rieber, R. Kurrle, S. Meuer. *B-Cell Section:* B. Dörken, G. Moldenhauer, P. Möller, A. Pezzutto, R. Schwartz-Albiez. *Myeloid Antigen Section:* W. Knapp, P. Bettelheim, S. Gadd, U. Köller, O. Majdic, C. Peschel, T. Radaszkiewicz, H. Stockinger, P.A.T. Tetteroo, C. E.v. d. Schoot. *NK-/NL-Section:* R.E. Schmidt, A.C. Feller, M.R. Hadam, J. Johnson, J. Schubert, R. Schwinzer, M. Stoll, P. Uciechowski, K. Wonigeit. *Activation Antigen Section:* H. Stein, R. Schwarting. *Platelet Section:* A.E.G.Kr.v.d. Borne, L.G. de Bruijne-Admiraal, P.W. Modderman, H.K. Nieuwenhuis. *Statistics Section:* W.R. Gilks, L. Oldfield, A. Rutherford.

†Abbreviations: Thy, thymocytes; DC, dendritic cells; B, B cells; T, T cells; M, monocytes; G, granulocytes; Plt, platelets; Prog., progenitor cells; Germ.Ctr. B, germinal center B cells; NK, NK cells; Mac, macrophages; cytopl., cytoplasmic; LHC, epidermal Langerhans cells.

‡Y, for protein antigens: sequence data available; for carbohydrate antigens: reactive oligosaccharide structure known.

BIBLIOGRAPHY

Articles

Abramson CS, Kersey JH, LeBien TW: A monoclonal antibody (BA-1) reactive with cells of human B lymphocyte lineage. *J Immunol* 126:83–88, 1981.

Adachi K, Okumura M, Tanimoto M, et al: Analysis of immunophenotype, genotype, and lineage fidelity in blastic transformation of chronic myelogenous leukemia: A study of 20 cases. *J Lab Clin Med* 111:125–132, 1988.

Almasri NM, Iturraspe JA, Benson NA, et al: Flow cytometric analysis of terminal deoxynucleotidyl transferase. *Am J Clin Pathol* 95:376–380, 1991.

Anderson KC, Boyd AW, Fisher DC, et al: Hairy cell leukemia: A tumor of pre-plasma cells. *Blood* 65:620–629, 1985.

Bakhshi A, Minowada J, Arnold A, et al: Lymphoid blast crises of chronic myelogenous leukemia represent stages in the development of B cell precursors. *N Engl J Med* 309:826–831, 1983.

Cawley JC, Burns GF, Hayho FGJ: A chronic lymphoproliferative disorder with distinctive features. A variant of hairy cell leukemia. *Leuk Res* 4:547–549, 1980.

Chan WC, Zaatari G: Lymph node interdigitating retriculum cell sarcoma. *Am J Clin Pathol* 85:739–744, 1986.

Dietz ML, Li CY, Banks PM: Blastic variant of hairy cell leukemia. *Am J Clin Pathol* 87:576–583, 1987.

Durie BG, Grogan TM: CALLA-positive myeloma: An aggressive subtype with poor survival. *Blood* 66:229–232, 1985.

Faguet GB, Agee JF: Monoclonal antibodies against the chronic lymphatic leukemia antigen cCLLa: Characterization and reactivity. *Blood* 70:437–443, 1987.

Faguet CB, Satya-Prakash KL, Agee JF: Cytochemical, cytogenetic, immunophenotypic and tumorigenic characterization of two hairy cell lines. *Blood* 71:422–429, 1988.

Gadol N, Ault KA: Phenotypic and functional characterization of human Leu1 (CD5) B cells. *Immunol Rev* 93:23–34, 1986.

Greaves MF, Chan LC, Furley AJ, et al: Lineage promiscuity in hemopoietic differentiation and leukemia. *Blood* 67:1–11, 1986.

Griffin JD, Todd RF III, Ritz J, et al: Differentiation patterns in the blastic phase of chronic myeloid leukemia. *Blood* 61:85–91, 1983.

Hanson CA, Gribbin TE, Schnitzer B, et al: CD11c(Leu-M5) expression characterizes a B-cell chronic lymphoproliferative disorder with features of both chronic lymphocytic leukemia and hairy cell leukemia. *Blood* 76:2360–2367, 1990.

Janossy G, Greaves MF, Revesz T, et al: Blast crisis of chronic myeloid leukaemia (CML): II. Cell surface marker analysis of "lymphoid" and myeloid cases. *Br J Haematol* 34:179–192, 1976.

Kabral A, Bradstock KF, Grimsley P, et al: Immunophenotype of clonogenic cells in myeloid leukaemia. *Leuk Res* 12:51–59, 1988.

Katayama I, Hirashima K, Maruyama K: Hairy cell in Japanese patients: A study with monoclonal antibodies. *Leukemia* 1:301–304, 1987.

Kung PC, Berger CL, Goldstein G, et al: Cutaneous T cell lymphoma: Characterization by monoclonal antibodies. *Blood* 57:261–266, 1981.

Loken MR, Shah VO, Dattilio KL, et al: Flow cytometric analysis of human bone marrow: I Normal erythroid development. *Blood* 69:255–263, 1987.

Loughran TP Jr, Kadin ME, Starkebaum G, et al: Leukemia of large granular lymphocytes: Association with clonal chromosomal abnormalities and autoimmune neutropenia, thrombocytopenia, and hemolytic anemia. *Ann Intern Med* 102:169–175, 1985.

Nadler LM, Korsmeyer SJ, Anderson KC, et al: B cell origin of non-T cell acute lymphoblastic leukemia. A model for discrete stages of neoplastic and normal pre-B cell differentiation. *J Clin Invest* 74:332–340, 1984.

McCulloch EA: Stem cells in normal and leukemic hemopoiesis. (Henry Stratton Lecture, 1982). *Blood* 62:1–13, 1983.

McDaniel HL, MacPherson BR, Tindle BH, et al: Lymphoproliferative disorder of granular lymphocytes: A heterogeneous disease. *Arch Pathol Lab Med* 116:242–248, 1992.

McKenna RW: Lymphoproliferative disorder of granular lymphocytes: More questions than answers. *Arch Pathol Lab Med* 116:235–237, 1992.

Miller RA, Gralow J: The induction of Leu-1 antigen expression in human malignant and normal B cells by phorbol myristic acetate (PMA). *J Immunol* 133:3408–3414, 1984.

Morimoto C, Matsuyama T, Oshige C, et al: Functional and phenotypic studies of Japanese adult T cell leukemia cells. *J Clin Invest* 75:836–843, 1985.

Ng CS, Lam TK, Chan JK, et al: Juvenile chronic myeloid leukemia. A malignancy of S-100 protein-positive histiocytes. *Am J Clin Pathol* 90:575–582, 1988.

Okon E, Felder B, Epstein A, et al: Monoclonal antibodies reactive with B-lymphocytes and histiocytes in paraffin sections. *Cancer* 56:95–104, 1985.

Uchiyama T, Sagawa K, Takatsuki K, et al: Effect of adult T-cell leukemia cells on pokeweed mitogen–induced normal B-cell differentiation. *Clin Immunol Immunopathol* 10:24–34, 1978.

Valiron O, Clemancey-Marcille G, Troesch A, et al: Immunophenotype of blast cells in chronic myeloid leukemia. *Leuk Res* 12:861–872, 1988.

Witzig TE, Banks PM, Stenson MJ, et al: Rapid immunotyping of B-cell non-Hodgkin's lymphomas by flow cytometry. A comparison with the standard frozen-section method. *Am J Clin Pathol* 94:280–286, 1990.

Review Articles

Bennett JM, Catovsky D, Daniel MT, et al: Proposals for the classification of chronic (mature) B and T lymphoid leukaemias. French-American-British (FAB) Cooperative Group. *J Clin Pathol* 42:567–584, 1989.

Caligaris-Cappio F, Janossy G: Surface markers in chronic lymphoid leukemias of B cell type. *Semin Hematol* 22:1–12, 1985.

Chang KL, Stroup R, Weiss L: Hairy cell leukemia: Current status. *Am J Clin Path* 97:719–738, 1992.

Dalal BI, Fitzpatrick LA: Hairy cell leukemia: An update. *Lab Med* 22:31–36, 1991.

Dighiero G, Travade P, Chevrets, et al: B-cell chronic lymphocytic leukemia: Present status and future directions. French Cooperative Group on CLL. *Blood* 78:1901–1914, 1991.

Foon KA, Gale RP: Immunologic classification of lymphoma and lymphoid leukemia. *Blood Rev* 1:77–88, 1987.

Foon KA, Gale RP: Chronic lymphoid leukemias. In Handin RI, Lux SE, Stassel TP: *Blood:* Principles and Practice of Hematology. Philadelphia, JB Lippincott, 1989.

Foon KA, Todd RF III: Immunologic classification of leukemia and lymphoma. *Blood* 68:1–31, 1986.

Foon KA, Schroff RW, Gale RP: Surface markers on leukemia and lymphoma cells: Recent advances. *Blood* 60:1–19, 1982.

Foon KA, Rai KR, Gale RP: Chronic lymphocytic leukemia: New insights into biology and therapy. *Ann Intern Med* 113:525–539, 1990.

Mayer R, Stone K, Han A, et al: Malignant CD5 B cells-biased immunoglobulin variable gene usage and autoantibody production. *Int Rev Immunol* 7:189–203, 1991.

Miller ML: Immunologic characterization of lymphocytic leukemias. Methodologic and immunophenotypic considerations. *Cleve Clin J Med* 56:722–739, 1989.

Ryan DH, Fallon MA, Horan PK: Flow cytometry in the clinical laboratory. *Clin Chim Acta* 171:125–173, 1988.

Turner RR, Wood GS, Backstead JH, et al: Histiocytic malignancies. Morphologic, immunologic, and enzymatic heterogeneity. *Am J Surg Pathol* 8:485–500, 1984.

CHAPTER 7

Cytogenetics

INTRODUCTION

Disturbances in the mitotic activity of tumor cells were recognized as early as the late nineteenth century. It was suggested early on that the disordered growth of tumors is based on mitotic irregularities; and Boveri proposed the hypothesis that mitotic errors are directly responsible for the origin of neoplasia. The foundations for proof of this hypothesis were established by Tjio and Levan, who applied cytogenetics techniques that clearly established the diploid chromosome number of 46 for human cells.

The next great discovery, a historic landmark, was made in 1960 by Nowell and Hungerford, who identified Ph^1 in leukemic cells from patients with CML. The Ph^1 has proved to be an exemplary model for studying the role of the genome in etiology and pathogenesis of malignancy. Also, its discovery became extremely important in the diagnosis of CML and myeloproliferative and associated disorders. However, further advancement in cytogenetics was limited at this time by lack of sophisticated banding techniques, and only gross structural abnormalities were identified in leukemic cells.

The next era began in the 1970s, when banding techniques (Caspersson et al, Seabright) were developed that allowed better detection and definition of specific structural abnormalities, many of which were not previously recognized. These techniques clearly showed that gains and losses, deletions, translocations, and inversions of chromosomes in the leukemias and lymphomas are nonrandom events. However, perhaps of even more importance was the discovery of chromsomal translocations that pioneered the concept of activation of cellular oncogenes. This hypothesis has been strongly implicated in the pathogenesis of hematopoietic tumors. The quintessential example of this occurs in CML, in which the Ph[1] is a shortened chromosome 22 that arises from a reciprocal translocation, t(9;22)(q34;q11).

In the late 1970s cell synchronization and high-resolution banding techniques were developed. Some laboratories have observed an increase in the quality of their analyses using these methods, but others have not. Most laboratories have noted improvements in quality during the last decade, because of a gain in experience. The major change in processing methods in the past 10 years is the new use of DNA-binding agents such as ethidium bromide to elongate the chromosome. In earlier studies, chromosomes were contracted and fuzzy and demonstrated poor banding patterns. The underlying cause for fuzzy chromosomes in the leukemias is unknown but may be intimately related to the leukemic process. In the past, metaphases with such fuzzy chromosomes were overlooked, resulting in a false-negative report (e.g., only normal cells examined) or claim of technical failure as the responsible culprit. Improvements in cell techniques have permitted the precise identification of recurring abnormalities, including specific breakpoints involved in structurally altered chromosomes. These technical advances have increased the observed incidence of chromosomal abnormalities from 50% to 70–90% in AML (Yunis, Bloomfield, Ensrud). Indeed, increased meticulous chromosomal analyses and oncogene studies in the chronic leukemias have identified additional subgroups in the CMLs and CLLs and related entities, which demonstrate independent clinical relevance. Although the great impact of cytogenetics in the chronic leukemias has been almost entirely in the domain of CML, recent studies of CLL have demonstrated differences in survival based upon single and multiple chromosomal abnormalities. Therefore, it is imperative that cytogenetic studies be performed on leukemias to expedite diagnosis, prognosis, and treatment and provide information vital to our understanding of the leukemic process.

CHRONIC MYELOGENOUS LEUKEMIA AND RELATED DISORDERS

CML is a clonal cancer arising from neoplastic transformation of the hematopoietic stem cell. Approximately 95–99% of cases demonstrate

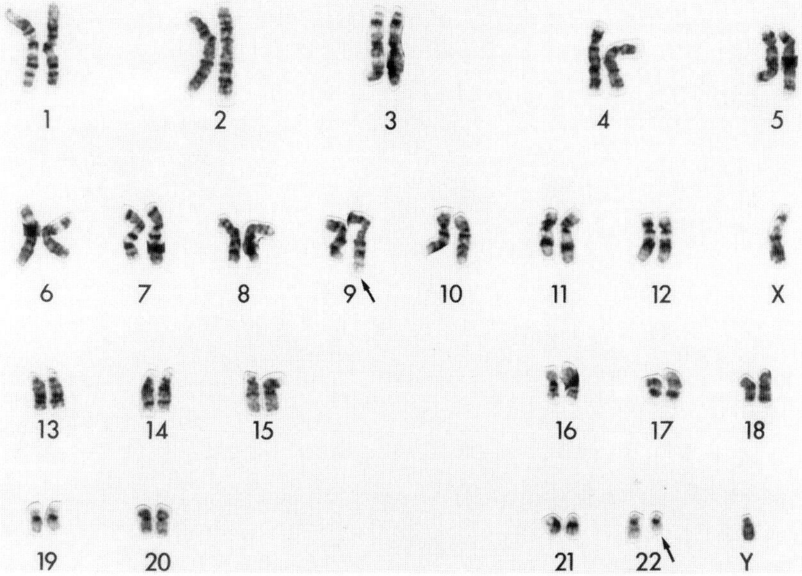

Figure 7-1 Trypsin-Giemsa banded metaphase cell from a bone marrow aspirate of a patient with CML, illustrating the 9;22 translocation. The karyotype is 46,XY,t(9;22)(q34;q11). The rearranged chromosome 9 and 22 homologues are identified with arrows. Courtesy of Michelle M. LeBeau.

a truncated chromosome 22, which was designated Ph^1 by Nowell and Hungerford. This karyotypic anomaly is generally detected in 100% of bone marrow metaphases observed in patients with CML who are Ph^1-positive (Fig. 7.1). Initially this chromosome was identified as a deleted chromosome; however, Rowley, in an important landmark discovery in 1973, showed that the Ph^1 abnormality is not a deletion but a translocation of the distal segment of 22q to the distal portion of 9q, [t(9;22)(q34;q11)]. Although this rearrangement was presumed to be reciprocal and balanced, the transposition of material from 9q to 22q was not microscopically visible by standard cytogenetic techniques. The reciprocal nature of the t(9;22) was confirmed 10 years later by molecular techniques, when it was demonstrated that the cellular protooncogene *ABL* is transposed from its normal location on 9q34 to 22q11 in Ph^1-positive CML.

The *ABL* protooncogene resides on the long arm of chromosome 9 (band 34) (Fig. 7.2). This DNA region is highly conserved in evolution and suggests that the normal *ABL* gene has an important role in

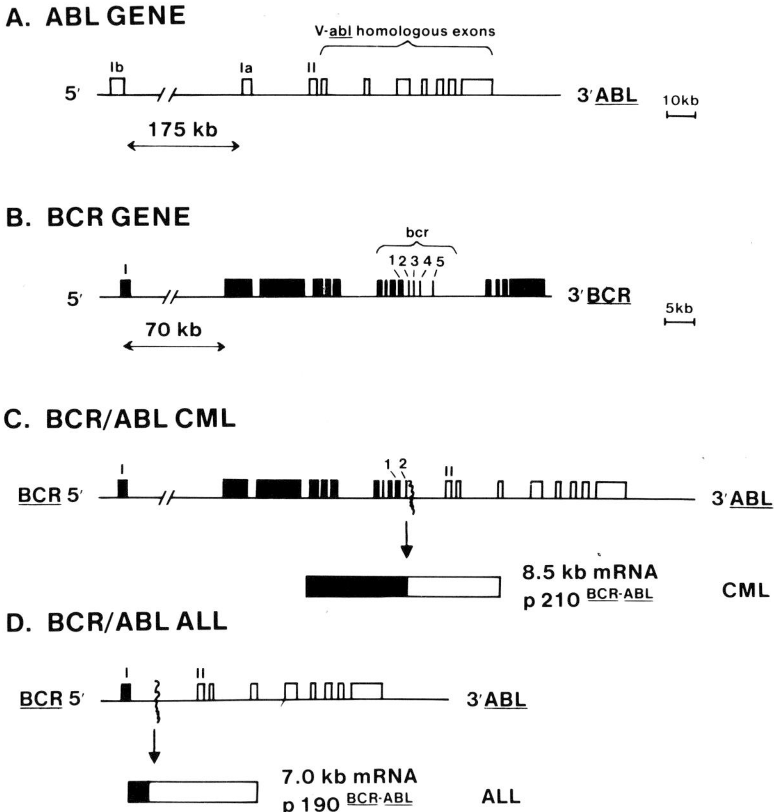

Figure 7-2 Schematic diagram of the molecular structure of the normal *ABL* and *BCR* genes, and the *BCR-ABL* fusion genes characteristic of Ph[1]-positive CML and ALL. **(a)** Structure of the normal *ABL* gene on chromosome 9, band q34. **(b)** Structure of the normal *BCR* gene on chromosome 22, band q11. **(c)** Structure of the *BCR-ABL* fusion gene on the Ph[1] in CML. In this disease, the break in the *BCR* gene occurs within the 5.8-kb bcr. An 8.5-kb fusion mRNA is transcribed from this fusion gene, resulting in the production of a 210-kd fusion protein ($p210^{BCR\text{-}ABL}$). **(d)** Structure of the *BCR-ABL* fusion gene on the Ph[1] in ALL. In Ph[1]-positive ALL, the break on chromosome 22 occurs within the first intron of the *BCR* gene, resulting in the transcription of a 7.0-kb *BCR-ABL* fusion mRNA, and the production of a smaller fusion protein ($p190^{BCR\text{-}ABL}$). Courtesy of Michelle M. LeBeau.

human ontogeny. The *ABL* gene spans approximately 230 kb and contains two alternative 5′ exons (Ia and Ib) spliced to a common set of 10 3′ exons, to yield the two major RNA transcripts of 6 and 7 kb (Fig. 7.2). The alternative first exons are separated from each other by an extremely long intron of approximately 175 kb. The introns immediately 5′ to the first alternative exons lack TATA and CAAT initiation sequences, are GC-rich regions, and contain multiple GGGCGG repeats. This repeat was previously identified as the core within the consensus binding site of SPL factor, which regulates transcription in vitro. The *ABL* gene encodes a p145 protein with tyrosine kinase activity. Breaks in chromosome 9 occur at variable sites, usually 5′ to *ABL* exon II and typically in the long intron between exons Ia and Ib. Rarely breaks occur 5′ of exon Ib. The result of these breaks in most instances is that the 10 3′ exons of *ABL* are translocated from chromosome 9 to chromosome 22. In addition, exon Ia may be included in the translocated segment (Fig. 7.2).

In 1984, Groffen et al. reported that the breakpoints on chromosome 22 in patients with Ph^1-positive CML are clustered within a 5.8 kb DNA segment designated the bcr. Shortly thereafter, Heisterkamp et al. showed that the 5.8 kb bcr is actually a part of a gene that spans 90-kbp of DNA and is composed of approximately 20 exons encoding 1271 amino acids. This gene was named the *BCR* gene (Fig. 7.2). The DNA segment upstream of the open reading frame contains many GC nucleotides and an inverted repeat of 18 nucleotides at positions −113 to −130 and −376 to −393. Since this repeat may form a stem and loop structure, it could play a role in regulation of *BCR* transcription. The sequences upstream of the presumed transcriptional initiation point show no TATA or CAAT boxes, but rather CCGCC sequences at positions −545 and −563 and the inverted sequence at position −351. Similar motifs are present within the promoter regions of a number of genes including *ABL*. A number of genes with homology to the *BCR* gene have been identified; whether the *BCR*-related genes are functional genes or pseudogenes is not clear. Current evidence is conflicting. The protein product of *BCR* is a 160-kd protein (p160). The protein does not appear to be a membrane receptor, and it can be phosphorylated on serine or threonine, but whether the phosphokinase enzymatic activity associated with this protein is intrinsic to this molecule or is only coprecipitated with it is unclear. Unfortunately, the role of this 160-kd protein in normal hematopoietic processes is unknown. The genetic consequence of the t(9;22) is the juxtaposition of coding sequences of the *ABL* gene on chromosome 9 with those of the *BCR* gene on chromosome 22. The product of the *BCR-ABL* fusion gene is a 210-kd fusion protein; the amino-terminal portion of the protein is encoded by the *BCR* gene; the carboxy-terminal region is encoded by the *ABL* gene and contains the *ABL* tyrosine kinase domain (Fig. 7.2). In CML, it is hypothesized that the abnormal fusion protein product $p210^{BCR\text{-}ABL}$ expressed by the *BCR-ABL* fusion gene causes malignant transformation because of the abnormally regulated phosphorylating activity of the chimeric

Table 7-1 Patterns of *BCR-ABL* Rearrangements in Ph[1] + Leukemias

Disorder	BCR-ABL *Genomic Rearrangements*	BCR-ABL *Transcripts*	*Proteins*
Normal cells	None	6.0,7.0-kb ABL 4.5,6.7-kb BCR	145-kd ABL 160-kd BCR
CML	*BCR* 5.8-kb bcr *ABL*-5′ common exon II	8.5-kb BCR-ABL Fusion mRNA	210-kd BCR-ABL
CML/blast crisis	*BCR* 5.8-kb bcr *ABL*-5′ common exon II	8.5-kb BCR-ABL Fusion mRNA	210-kd BCR-ABL
Ph[1]+ de novo AML	*BCR* intron 1 *ABL*-5′ common exon II	7.0-kb BCR-ABL Fusion mRNA	185–190 kd BCR-ABL
Ph[1]+ ALL Adults	25%: *BCR* 5.8-kb bcr *ABL*-5′ common exon II	8.5-kb BCR-ABL Fusion mRNA	210-kd BCR-ABL
	75%: BCR intron 1 *ABL*-5′ common exon II	7.0-kb BCR-ABL Fusion mRNA	185–190 kd BCR-ABL
Children	100%: BCR intron 1 *ABL*-5′ common exon II	7.0-kb BCR-ABL Fusion mRNA	185–190 kd BCR-ABL

Source: Willman C: *Molecular Diagnostics in Pathology*. Baltimore, Williams & Wilkins, 1991, p. 121.

tyrosine kinase protein. Transplantation of bone marrow cells containing the *BCR-ABL* fusion gene in a retroviral vector into lethally irradiated mice results in the development of myeloid leukemias, providing direct evidence that the fusion of *ABL* and *BCR* is involved in the pathogenesis of CML. A summary of the patterns of *BCR-ABL* rearrangements is shown in Table 7.1.

Approximately 1–5% of patients do not have the Ph[1]. Some of these patients have all the classic features of Ph[1]-positive CML but others, who are either younger (juvenile type) or older than the average patient with Ph[1]-positive CML, show clinical and hematologic differences distinguishing them from those with Ph[1]-positive CML. The most important difference is a significantly lower median survival in the Ph[1]-negative group: 8–20 months versus 30–55 months in various adult series. Ph[1]-negative CML is characterized by (1) hypercellular marrow with granulocytic hyperplasia, (2) peripheral granulocytic leukocytosis with left maturation shift and a WBC greater than 20 × 10^9/L on two occasions, and (3) absence of the Ph[1] by cytogenetic analysis. Therefore, the morphologic picture is similar to that of Ph[1]-positive CML except for the absence of Ph[1] or Ph[1] variant abnormalities. Approximately 30–50% of the patients with these so-called Ph[1]-negative CMLs do show the *BCR-ABL* rearrangement resulting in the $p210^{BCR\text{-}ABL}$ fusion protein. In addition to its occurrence in CML, the Ph[1] chromosome is also observed in de novo ALL (5% of children, 20–30% of adults) (Fig. 7.2) and in rare cases of AML (<2% of cases). In approximately one-quarter of these patients, the *BCR-ABL* rearrangement is similar to the CML-type rearrangement; however, in the majority of Ph^1-positive ALL cases, the *ABL* common exons are translocated into the first intron of the *BCR* gene resulting in the production of a 185–190 $kd^{BCR\text{-}ABL}$ fusion protein containing only the first *BCR* exon fused to *ABL* (Fig. 7.2). Interestingly, replacement of the amino-terminal domain of *ABL* with *BCR* sequences in the *BCR-ABL* fusion proteins produced from the t(9;22) in CML and de novo acute leukemias leads to an increase in the tyrosine kinase activity of the protein. Presumably this translocation creates an altered *BCR-ABL* tyrosine kinase protein that phosphorylates the wrong target proteins, or the same target proteins at an inappropriate stage, leading to cellular transformation. These alterations in *ABL* most likely contribute to the transformation of hematopoietic cells in leukemias. Intriguingly, the $p185\text{–}190^{BCR\text{-}ABL}$ fusion protein has a more potent transforming potential for more aggressive leukemia than does the $p210^{BCR\text{-}ABL}$ fusion protein.

In addition to the classic t(9;22), variant 9;22 translocations have been reported in well over 300 patients (Fig. 7.3) (Fig. 7.4). All chromosomes, apart from the Y, have been involved in variant translocations with 22q11. These variants were classified as simple if the involved segment of 22q was translocated to a chromosome other than 9, or complex if three or more chromosomes, one of them 22q and usually chromosome 9, were interchanged. Rarely, the Ph^1 is not recognizable in these complex exchanges, resulting in a "masked" Ph^1 (Fig. 7.3). Since all chromosomes apart from Y have been involved in simple variant translocations with 22q11, it was initially postulated that the critical factor in the pathogenesis of CML is the deletion and transposition of genes from the donor chromosome 22, rather than the specificity of material from chromosome 9 relocating to chromosome 22. However, in 1980, Rowley proposed that the translocation of 9q to 22q is the critical event! Later, this hypothesis was confirmed by molecular analysis as well as high-resolution R banding and telomeric (T) banding that demonstrated 9q34 → qter on the Ph^1 in some ostensibly simple variants, and in situ hybridization confirmed that *ABL* is translocated to 22q11 in both simple and complex variants. Transposition of *ABL* and rearrangements of the bcr on 22q11 have also been demonstrated in masked Ph^1 abnormalities. Although the Ph^1 translocation may not be the first step in the leukemogenesis of CML, one of the crucial molecular events in the pathogenesis of CML appears to be the juxtaposition of *ABL* (transposed from 9q34) and the *BCR* sequence on 22q11 to form a new fusion gene with a novel RNA transcript.

A. SIMPLE 9;22 TRANSLOCATION

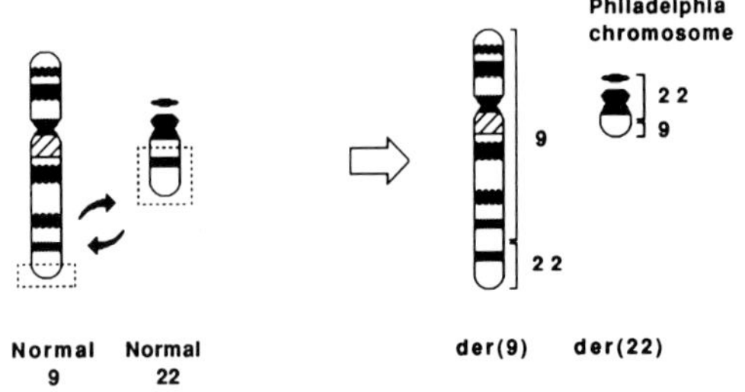

B. COMPLEX 9;22 TRANSLOCATION

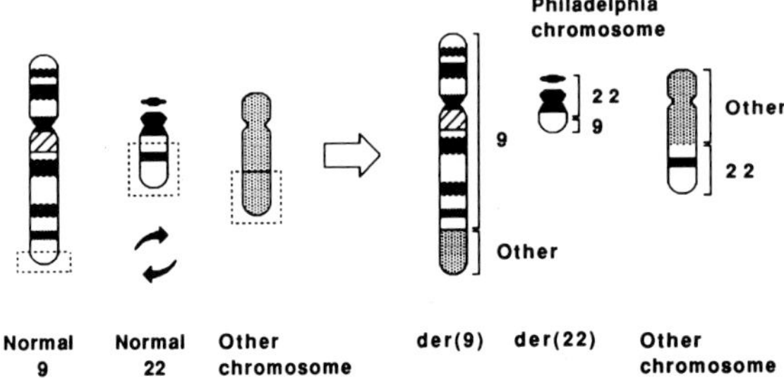

C. MASKED 9;22 TRANSLOCATION

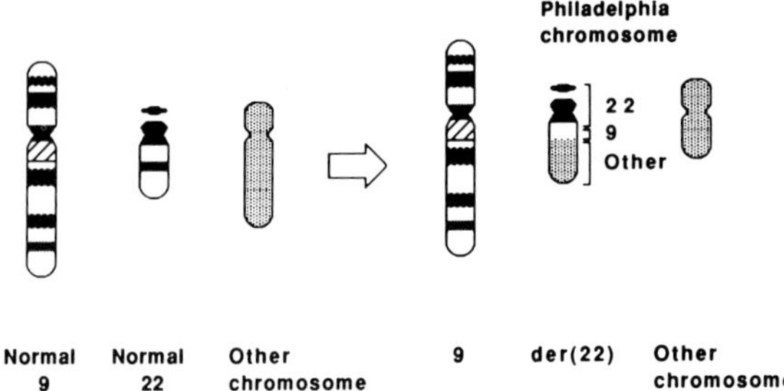

Figure 7-3 Schematic diagram of simple and variant 9;22 translocations characteristic of CML. **(a)** Simple t(9;22). Chromosome breaks occur in chromosomes 9 (band q34) and 22 (band q11), followed by a reciprocal exchange of chromosomal material. **(b)** Complex 9;22 translocation. Chromosome breaks occur in chromosomes 9 (band q34) and 22 (band q11), and in a third chromosome, followed by an exchange of chromosomal material. In variant 9;22 translocations, material from chromosome 9 containing the *ABL* oncogene is translocated to chromosome 22. **(c)** Masked 9;22 translocation. In masked translocations, a complex rearrangement results in the relocation of chromosomal material from chromosome 9, and from another chromosome to chromosome 22, masking the typical Ph^1. In each panel, the origin of the chromosomal segments in each of the rearranged chromsomes is indicated by a bracket on the side of the chromosome. Courtesy of Michelle M. LeBeau.

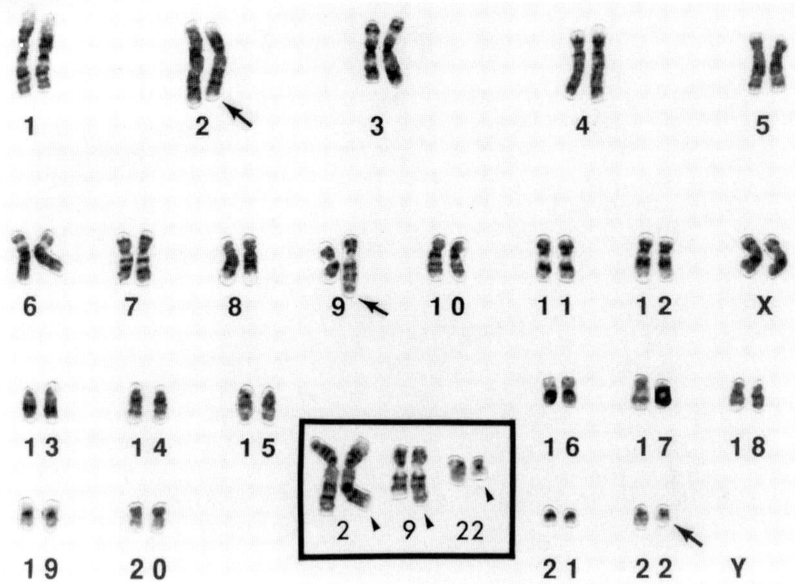

Figure 7-4 Trypsin-Giemsa banded metaphase cell from a bone marrow aspirate illustrating a variant, complex 9;22 translocation. In this rearrangement, chromosome breaks occurred in chromosomes 2 (band p23), 9 (band q34), and 22 (band q11). Chromosomal material from 2p is translocated to 9q, material from 9q is translocated to 22q, and material from 22q is translocated to 2p [t(2;9;22)(p23;q34;q11)]. The rearranged homologues are identified with arrows. The inset illustrates a partial karyotype of the normal and rearranged chromosomes 2, 9, and 22 homologues from another metaphase cell. Courtesy of Michelle M. LeBeau.

CNL has been associated with occasional abnormalities of chromosomes. The Ph^1 and bcr rearrangements have not been observed in the cases examined for cytogenetic abnormalities. Some cases have shown normal karyotypes, others, mosaic karyotypes of 46,XY/46,XY,t(7;16)(q22;q24); trisomy of chromosome 9, and partial deletion of the long arm of chromosome 20; multiple chromosomal aberrations such as breaks and gaps, and deletions of 7q. Of these, +9, and deletions of 20q and 7q, are recurring abnormalities in myeloid neoplasms.

CMoL is an extremely rare disorder, and karyotypic abnormalities must be interpreted with caution since these cases are frequently misdiagnosed. In an evaluation of 28 cases of CMoL from the literature, Bearman et al. (1981) considered only two cases that had the characteristics of CMoL. The remainder represented a variety of he-

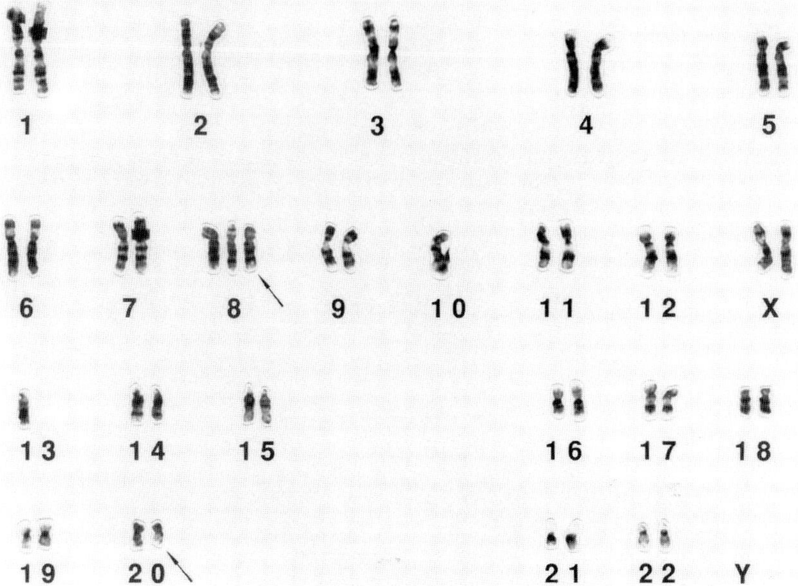

Figure 7-5 Trypsin-Giemsa banded metaphase cell from a bone marrow aspirate of a patient with CMML, illustrating two recurring abnormalities in the MDSs, a gain of chromosome 8, and a deletion of the long arm of chromosome 20. The karyotype was 47,XX, +8, del(20)(q13.1q13.3). The additional and rearranged chromosomes are identified with arrows. Loss of chromosomes 10 and 13 observed in this cell represents the random (artifactual) loss of chromosomes due to processing techniques. Courtesy of Michelle M. LeBeau.

matologic disorders including CMML, acute leukemia, histiomonocytic proliferations that could not be subclassified, and cases in which the data were insufficient for analysis. However, Sherman et al. (1979) evaluated by karyotypic analysis 20 patients whom they classified as CMoL. Although no distinct chromosomal abnormality was detected, random numerical and structural chromosome abnormalities were observed.

In contrast to studies in CMoL, cytogenetic studies have been performed in many cases of CMML which is much more common. Karyotypic abnormalities have been observed in 30–50% of patients evaluated (Fig. 7.5). Common chromosomal abnormalities include trisomy 8; abnormalities involving the long arms of chromosome 11 [del(11)(q23)]; or loss or deletion of chromosomes 5 or 7 [−5, −7], [del(5q), del(7q)]; or loss of the Y chromosome. Some chromosomal abnormalities, such as del(11)(q23), are more common in monocytic disorders, while others, such as the del(5q) or +8, are found in all myeloid disorders, pointing to the association of cytogenetic and molecular aberrations with lineage-specific transformation.

Although molecular studies have demonstrated the presence of bcr rearrangements in 30–50% of patients with Ph[1]-negative CML, patients with CMML have not demonstrated such a change. However, *RAS* gene mutations occur in 30–50% of patients with CMML, but are unusual in Ph[1]-positive and Ph[1]-negative CML.

Even though there has been ongoing discussion concerning the existence of EL, there seems to be no good reason why this cell cannot develop neoplastic transformation. The difficulty is to separate EL from the hypereosinophilic syndromes, which may be secondary to chronic hypersensitivity of undetermined etiology. Some cases of EL may represent a variant of CML since they demonstrate a Ph[1] chromosome. Others may represent the eosinophilic variant of AMML associated with an inversion of chromosome 16 [inv(16)(p13q22) or translocation t(16;16)(p13;q22)]. Finally, some cases are neither of the above and may show trisomy 8 or monosomy 7. Although cytogenetic studies may help, such abnormalities may not be present, and, therefore, there is no easy way of differentiating hypereosinophilic syndrome from EL. Indeed, some authors have reported a case of "hypereosinophilic syndrome" that was characterized by a chronic indolent course and evolved into an EL. This case developed a granulocytic sarcoma (chloroma) with a hyperdiploid karyotype (49,XY,+10,+10,+15,3q−). An alternative explanation suggested by the authors was that the case might represent a variant Ph[1]-negative CML with EL. In conclusion, EL, despite cytogenetic investigation, continues to remain an elusive diagnostic dilemma probably because of its heterogeneous origin and associated benign mimicry.

Extreme basophilia may occur in the chronic phase of Ph[1]-positive CML or as a manifestation of the accelerated phase of CML. Most cases of BL so far studied cytogenetically demonstrate the Ph[1], and since the Ph[1] is absent in the majority of ELs, some authors believe it more appropriate to call BL *basophilic CML.* However, although rare, Ph[1]-negative LAP-positive BL does occur. It is typically very aggressive, complicated by histamine excess, asthma, and DIC in spite of therapy. Besides so-called chronic forms, acute BL can occur de novo; marrow basophilia can be quite pronounced in AML with t(6;9) or inv(16). In addition, acute promyelocytic leukemia with the t(15;17) may demonstrate some basophilic maturation. Patients with basophilic excess may occasionally manifest flushing, pruritus, and hypotension secondary to release of mediators (especially histamine).

Mast cells are connective tissue cells that most likely arise from marrow progenitors. They have no ancestral relationship to the blood basophil or its antecedents. Unlike the blood basophil, they are capable of mitotic activity. Chromosome analysis of bone marrow mast cells from one patient with malignant mastocytosis revealed near-haploid (59%), near-diploid (36%), and polyploid (5%) cells. Near-haploid cells had a mode of 25 chromosomes with variable disomy and nullisomy, particularly of chromosomes 19 and 20. A 17p+ marker was observed in all cells. Other structural chromosomal changes included dicentrics, ring chromosomes, translocations, and double minutes. The modal number in near-diploid cells was 46 with a range of 41–52. The majority of cells with 46 chromosomes were pseudodiploid, and only a few had a normal karyotype. The presence of the 17p+ marker in occasional cells suggested a relationship between the two tumor cell populations. Strikingly, chromosome numbers in polyploid cells ranged from 70 to about 600.

CHRONIC LYMPHOCYTIC LEUKEMIA AND RELATED DISORDERS

Until recently, chromosomal analysis of CLL was most difficult and frequently did not yield sufficient numbers of metaphases. However, with the advent of B-cell mitogens such as lipopolysaccharides and Epstein-Barr virus, adequate numbers of metaphases can be obtained in nearly 90% of cases; however, these agents induce mitosis of all B cells, rather than selective stimulation of the leukemia cells. When G and/or Q banding techniques are used, approximately 50% of patients with CLL are found to have chromosomal abnormalities, which commonly involve chromosomes 12, 13, or 14. Structural abnormalities frequently involve 14q32. Rarely, other chromosomal changes such as −8, i(7p), i(2p), t(13;21), trisomy 18, del(6q), del(14q), or −X have been found. Karyotypic abnormalities increase from 20% in early-stage disease to over 70% in patients with advanced disease.

Trisomy 12, the most common chromosomal anomaly, occurs alone in 15–20% or in association with other abnormalities in another 10% of patients with abnormal karyotypes (Fig. 7.6). It has been proposed that trisomy 12 represents the primary chromosomal abnormality, and that the more complex anomalies exemplify clonal evolution with associated poorer prognosis. Trisomy 12 may also be observed in WM, HCL, PLL, and small lymphocytic lymphoma. Chromsome 12 contains the Kirsten *RAS* protooncogene, which en-

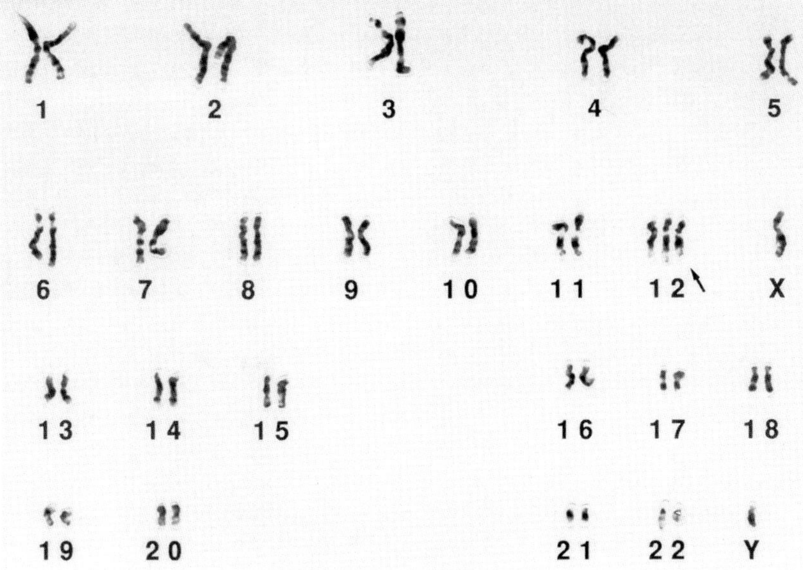

Figure 7-6 Trypsin-Giemsa banded karyotype from a bone marrow aspirate of a patient who has CLL illustrating a gain of chromosome 12 (trisomy 12), a recurring numerical abnormality in this disease. The karyotype of this cell is 47,XY, +12. The additional chromsome 12 is identified with an arrow. Courtesy of Michelle M. LeBeau.

codes a GTP-binding protein that is similar to the G proteins that are vital in signal transduction.

Structural abnormalities of chromosome 13 occur in about 13% of all patients evaluated, most involving the site of the retinoblastoma gene 13q14. CLL patients with 13q14 abnormalities have a survival similar to that of patients with normal karyotypes, who have a median overall survival of more than 15 years, in contrast to 7.7 years for patients with other clonal changes.

Chromosome 14 changes include translocations such as the t(14;19) and t(11;14), deletions (14q−), and inversions. The presence of a translocation involving 14q32 is associated with high WBCs, poor response to therapy, and increased risk for prolymphocytic transformation. Chromosome 14 contains the genes for the IgH (14q32) and for the alpha and delta chains of the human T receptor at band 14q11.2. In CLL cases with translocations involving 14q32, such as the t(11;14), the breakpoint on chromosome 14 is within the J segment of the heavy chain locus. The chromosome 11 segment translocated to this site contains a putative oncogene; however, no mRNA transcript has been identified in over 100-kb of DNA surrounding this locus. This translocation has also been found in patients with PLL and large cell lymphoma and can be used in a polymerase chain reaction to detect minimal residual disease. Patients with structural abnormalities of the long arm of chromosome 14 seem to have the worst prognosis of all of the patients with cytogenetic subsets of CLL. However, complex karyotypes add additional shortened survival. Cytogenetic analysis of cases of T-cell CLL reported in the literature may be difficult to interpret since this disorder may actually be a group of diseases including TGLD, chronic ATLL, T-PLL, or the leukemic phase of a T-cell NHL.

Development of Richter's syndrome, immunoblastic lymphoma, was observed more frequently in those CLL patients with complex karyotypic changes with or without trisomy 12. Richter's transformation, which occurs with comparable frequency in patients with small lymphocytic lymphoma and WM, occurs in about 10% of CLL patients and thus is much better established as an evolutionary end phase of CLL than lymphoblastic crisis. Richter's immunoblastic cells usually synthesize the same monoclonal Ig, suggesting that they represent clonal evolution of the previous neoplastic process; however, independent clones have been sometimes observed. Such chromosomal analysis has been found to offer prognostic information about overall survival in addition to that supplied by clinical data in patients with CLL.

B-PLLs demonstrate abnormalities of chromosome 14, which occur in nearly 80% of B-PLL, but not in T-PLL. These abnormalities, which involve 14q32, are usually seen in most of the metaphase cells in B-PLL. A number of translocations involving 14q32 have been identified in B-PLL. This phenomenon is similar to that observed in NHL; however, the t(8;14) rearrangement characteristic of Burkitt's lymphoma is not observed in B-PLL. In most cases, the donor chromosome responsible for the marker 14q+ is unknown; however, in some instances a t(11;14) may be responsible, as also observed in B-CLL and other B-cell growth disorders. Besides 14q+ and t(11;14), del(6q) and rearrangements affecting chromosomes 1 and 12 are overrepresented and account for one-third of the primary chromsome abnormalities in B-PLL.

A rare case of aggressive B-PLL involving activation of the *MYC* oncogene in a masked t(8;17) has been reported. The abnormal karyotype included a t(14;18) and a 17q+ chromosome. Molecular analysis showed that *BCL2* was rearranged in the major bcr and had joined into the IgH gene as in follicular lymphoma. Cloning and sequencing of the rearranged *MYC* gene revealed that it was truncated at the end of the first exon and had joined into the regulatory elements of *BCL5* (B-cell leukemia-lymphoma, gene 3, formerly called *BCL3*). The *BCL5* locus is mapped to chromosome 17 band 22. The truncated *MYC* gene was highly expressed under the influence of *BCL5* regulatory elements leading to an aggressive B-cell leukemia that presumably had been derived from an indolent lymphoma carrying a rearranged *BCL2* gene.

Besides involvement of *BCL1* sequences, *BCL2*, and *BCL5* in B-PLL, some cases showing del(3)(p13) with possible association with the *RAS* oncogene have been described. In B-cell PLL, as in other B-lymphocytic leukemias-lymphomas, the karyotype often involves chromosomes 3, 6, 11, and 12; several of these chromosomes (6,11,12) contain *RAS* genes or *RAS*-related genes. Although B-PLL undoubtedly has unique karyotypic subsets, aberrant forms exist with unique molecular pathogenetic mechanisms. Trisomy 12, the most frequent and foreboding chromosomal abnormality in B-CLL, is quite rare in B-PLL.

Cytogenetic analysis in HCL has not demonstrated unique or specific changes. Several cases have been reported in which 14q+, del(6q), +3, +Y, +12, +18 anomalies have been reported. HCL patients with clonal abnormalities and nonclonal structural abnormalities do not fare well. However, those with nonclonal numerical abnormalities and normal karyotypes seem to do much better. Apparently, structural chromosome abnormalities in HCL portend a poor prognosis.

Overall 60–70% of all B-cell NHLs have a translocation involving 14q32.3. Lymphomas that may develop a chronic leukemia phase include small lymphocytic lymphoma (well-differentiated lymphocytic), intermediate differentiated lymphoma (mantle zone lymphoma), and follicular and diffuse, small cleaved lymphoma (nodular and diffuse, poorly differentiated lymphocytes). Small lymphocytic lymphoma in the leukemic phase is believed by many pathologists to be CLL. This disorder, intermediate differentiated lymphoma, and CLL are associated with a translocation involving the IgH locus t(11;14)(q13;q32.3) and the *BCL1* sequences (Fig. 7.7). Trisomy 12 and deletions of 11q in the same region have been observed in small lymphocytic lymphoma similar to CLL.

Follicular lymphomas in the leukemic phase are characterized by small cleaved cells (buttock cells) in the peripheral smear. The most common specific karyotypic abnormality is the t(14;18)(q32.3;q21.3) present in 80–90% of these lymphomas (Fig. 7.8). The *BCL2* protooncogene is translocated from chromosome 18 to the IgH locus (chromosome 14) with resultant overproduction of the BCL2 protein. The

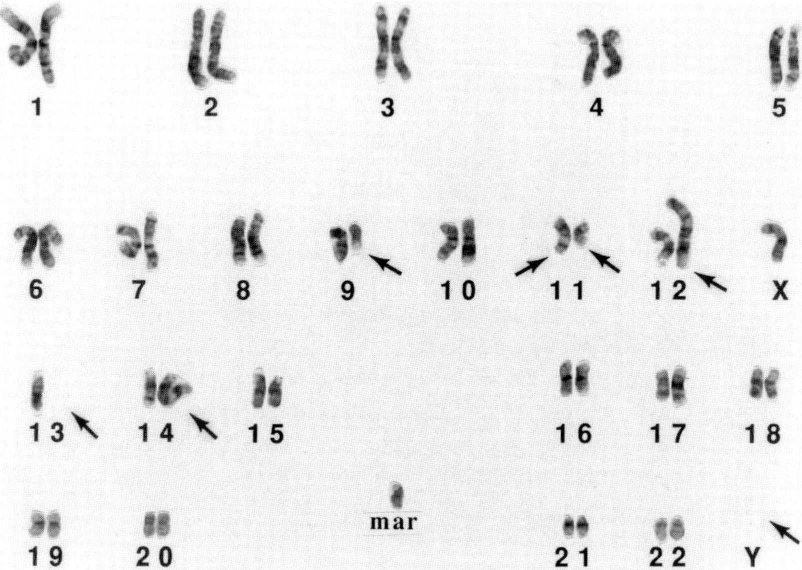

Figure 7-7 Trypsin-Giemsa banded metaphase cell from a lymph node biopsy of a patient with an NHL (mantle zone lymphoma) illustrating the t(11;14)(q13;q32) characteristic of mantle zone lymphoma, and other lymphoid neoplasms such as small lymphocytic lymphoma. The karyotype is 45,X, − Y, − 13,del(9)(q13 or q13q34),del (11)(q14q23),t(12;?)(p13;?),t(11;14)(q13;q32), + mar 1. The rearranged and missing chromosomes are identified with arrows. Courtesy of Michelle M. LeBeau.

total function of the *BCL2* gene is not known, but its expression is undetectable in resting lymphocytes and rises rapidly after mitogenic stimulation. The BCL2 protein is localized to the inner mitochondrial membrane and appears to be important in cell survival. Also, 20–30% of diffuse large cell lymphomas exhibit t(14;18), indicating their relationship to follicular center cells. Utilization of the polymerase chain reaction can detect minimal numbers of malignant lymphoma cells in biopsies that demonstrate the t(14;18).

Splenic lymphoma with villous lymphocytes demonstrates immunophenotypic markers similar to those of follicular lymphomas, and histologically the spleen shows white pulp disease. Therefore, these rare lymphomas would be expected to exhibit a t(14;18)(q32.3;q21.3) karyotype as observed in follicular lymphomas.

Cytogenetic studies on WM and CLL-associated macroglobulinemia suggest that trisomy 12 may be the primary karyotypic change in malignant macroglobulinemia, whereas the appearance of minute or marker chromosomes as well as loss of G-group chromosomes or

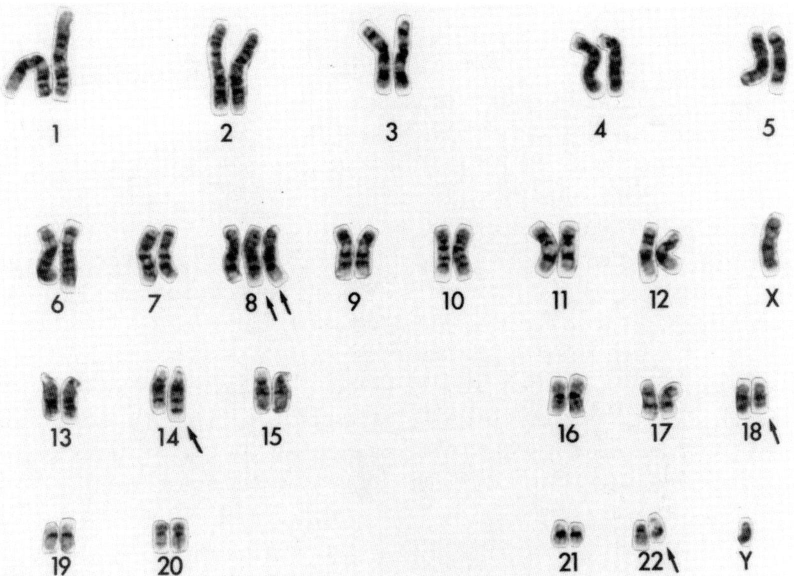

Figure 7-8 Trypsin-Giemsa banded karyotype from a bone marrow aspirate of a patient who has a follicular small cleaved cell lymphoma illustrating the recurring 14;18 translocation characteristcs of this disease. The karyotype of this cell is 47,XY,t(8;22)(q24;q11),t(14;18)(q32;q21),+der(8)t(8;22)(q24;q11). The rearranged chromosomes are identified with arrows. Courtesy of Michelle M. LeBeau.

chromosome 9 may be secondary karyotypic changes resulting from clonal evolution in these malignancies. Such clonal abnormalities further imply that chromosome changes may be more frequently associated with WM or CLL macroglobulinemia than with typical CLL without macroglobulinemia.

The most consistent structural abnormality in plasma cell leukemia and multiple myeloma is a 14q+ marker chromosome with a breakpoint at 14q32 within the IgH locus. The most common rearrangement is a reciprocal translocation involving chromosomes 11 and 14 in the t(11;14)(q13;q32); 11q13 → qter is relocated to chromosome 14, adjacent to the IgH V_H sequences.

Virtually all chromosomes have exhibited abnormalities in patients with multiple myeloma. Karyotypes are often very complex, with numerous structural anomalies involving mainly chromosomes 1, 11, 14, 17, and numerical anomalies involving mainly chromosome 3, 7, 9, and 11. Partial or complete trisomy for 1q is nearly as common as rearrangements affecting 14q. Some myeloma patients have the t(2;8), a variant of the t(8;14) observed in some Burkitt's lymphomas associated with increased κ chain production.

Although the majority of cases of myeloma demonstrate hyperdiploid clones prior to treatment, most are hypodiploid or pseudodiploid after treatment. Also, the addition of structural or numerical anomalies of chromosomes 5 and 7 may be indicative of subsequent therapy-induced myeloid leukemia.

Since T-CLL may not exist, and many cases in the literature undoubtedly represent TGLD, chronic ATLL, T-PLL, or leukemic phase of T-NHL, cytogenetic findings previously reported in the literature may not represent T-CLL. However, 14q aberrations have been touted as the hallmark of idiopathic T-CLL and other T-cell disorders. Unlike B-cell lymphomas and leukemias, in which terminal region translocations occur at the 14q32 breakpoint, chromosomal arrangements in previously reported T-CLL cases involve breaks in the proximal region of 14q (14q11.2). Such translocations involving the T-cell receptor α-and δ (14q11.2), β-(7q34), or γ-(7p15) chain loci are seen in T-cell leukemias and lymphomas and may activate the putative protooncogenes *TCL1* (at 14q32 centromeric to the IgH locus), *TCL2* (at 11p13), or *TCL4* (9q34), depending on the reciprocal translocation site.

In general, structural or numerical abnormalities of chromosomes 2 and 8 are most often observed in T-PLL, whereas aberrations of chromosome 14 seen in nearly 80% of B-PLL have not been observed in T-PLL. Also, T-PLL usually displays marked chromosome instability, with multiple deletions and hypodiploidy, characteristic of more aggressive disease. Clonal marker chromosomes are present in most metaphase cells, but the karyotypes are dissimilar in virtually every case.

Abnormal leukemic clones have been reported in the marrows of more than 90% of Japanese patients with HTLV-I-induced ATLL. Karyotypic aberrations, including trisomy 3, trisomy 7, trisomy 21, del(6)(q21), del(10)(p13), 14q11 translocations, and loss of the X chromosome, are frequently observed in HTLV-I-associated ATLL. They have also been observed in HTLV-I-negative ATLL. Some series have described trisomy 7 or 7q deletion as the dominant abnormality; others have observed abnormal rearrangement in the long arm of chromosome 6 to be the most common.

Immunohistochemical analysis of cells from patients with SS disclosed that approximately 90% exhibit helper T4(CD4) cells and 10% show T8 (CD8) cells. The karyotypic pattern by SS is typically complex with multiple chromosomal abnormalities. Moderately frequent abnormalities of chromosomes 6 and 1 have been reported, as have trisomy 7q and i(17q), which occur in the small cell variant of SS and

ATLL. However, one case that demonstrated interesting cytogenetic abnormalities had a t(7;14) involving bands 7p13–15 and 14q11. Molecular analysis revealed rearrangements of the α (14q11), β (7q34), and γ (7p15) receptor genes. Rearrangements of the α and β genes probably resulted from the translocation between chromosomes 7 and 14. Karyotypic and oncogenetic evaluations of a cell line derived from a patient with SS have shown trisomy 8 with an associated 3′ *MYC* anomaly that supposedly caused deregulation of the expression of the *MYC* gene. The postulated pathogenetic molecular mechanisms in SS seem to vary in different studies. Additional cytogenetic analyses seem indicated to determine a more exact frequency of various chromosomal aberrations in this disorder.

INTERPHASE CYTOGENETIC ANALYSIS

Cytogenetic information is usually obtained by direct analysis of chromosomes from cells arrested in metaphase. However, recent ad-

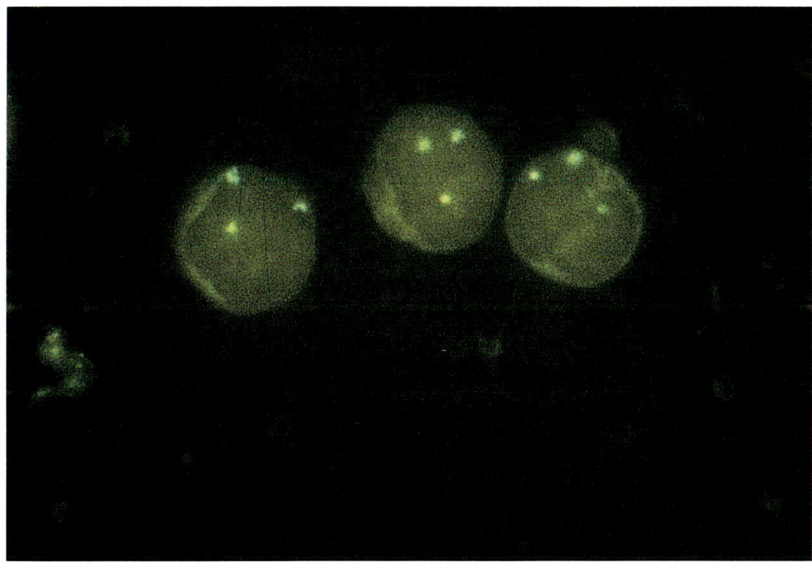

Figure 7-9 In situ hybridization with a biotinylated DNA probe to the alpha-satellite centomeric repeat sequences to chromosome 12(D12Z1). The hybridized probe was detected with fluoresceinated avidin. The three signals in each cell indicate three copies of chromosome 12, or trisomy 12. This is the most common cytogenetic abnormality in CLL and identifies such cells as leukemic lymphocytes. (×1000). Courtesy of John Anastasi.

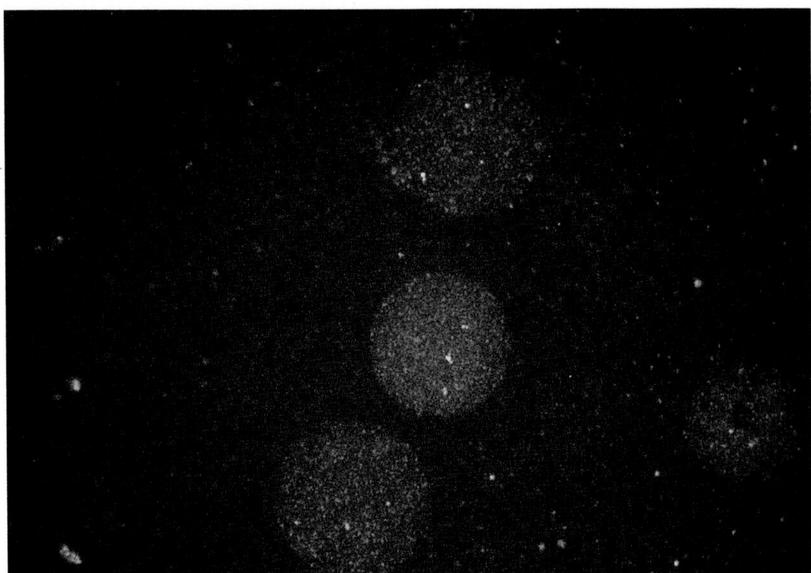

Figure 7-10 Detection of the *BCR-ABL* fusion gene in interphase CML cells by fluorescence in situ hybridization. Probes specific for the abl region of chromosome 9 distal to the breakpoint and the bcr region of chromosome 22 proximal to the breakpoint were labeled with biotin and digoxigenin-modified nucleotides, respectively. After hybridization, the ABL probe was detected with Texas red and the BCR probe with FITC (green). The locations of the normal copies of BCR and ABL in the nuclei are indicated by the isolated red and green signals. The *BCR-ABL* fusion gene produces closely spaced red and green signals, sometimes appearing yellow. The fusion is detectable even if it does not result from the process that produces a Ph^1. About 1% of normal nuclei have closely spaced red and green signals by chance. Some of the signals appear as double spots, presumably indicating that DNA synthesis has occurred in this region of the genome so that the genes on both chromatids are visible. The outlines of the nuclei are visible due to background hybridization signals. From Tkachuk DC et al: Detection of *BCR-ABL* fusion in chronic myelogenous leukemia by in-situ hybridization. *Science* 250:559–562, copyright 1990 by the AAAS.

vances in molecular genetics have made it possible to acquire cytogenetic information through the study of interphase and terminally differentiated cells. Use of chromosome-specific DNA probes or probes that are specific for certain chromosomal regions, and techniques of in situ hybridization along with nonradioactive detection methods, allow detection of numerical and structural chromosomal abnormalities from interphase cells. Such techniques eliminate the need for dividing cells for analysis, permit analysis of large and small numbers of cells not just in metaphase, do not require culturing, and can be performed within 24–36 hr. They would be ideally suited for detecting minimal residual disease. Peripheral blood lymphocytes from a patient with CLL are shown in Fig. 7.9 and CML cells in Fig. 7.10 using these techniques.

The burgeoning investigation in the realm of cytogenetics and molecular biology with the resultant accumulated knowledge has spawned a fusion of these two disciplines with an improved fundamental understanding of leukemogenesis. A convergence of these fields is quite evident in this and the next two chapters.

BIBLIOGRAPHY

Articles

Anastasi J, Le Beau MM, Vardiman JW, Rowley JD. Detection of trisomy 12 in chronic lymphocytic leukemia by in situ hybridization: A simple and sensitive method. *Lab Invest* 64:67A, 1991.

Bauchinger M, Mezger J: A case of malignant mastocytosis with near-haploid, near-diploid, and polyploid cells in the bone marrow. *Cancer Genet Cytogenet* 48:13–21, 1990.

Bearman RM, Kjeldsberg CR, Pangalis GA, et al: Chronic monocytic leukemia in adults. *Cancer* 48:2239–2255, 1981.

Benítez J, Santos M, Rivas C, et al: Sézary syndrome: morpho-immuno-phenotypic, cytogenetic and molecular characterization. *Med Clin (Barc)* 93:103–107, 1989.

Boveri T: Uber mehrpolige Mitosen als Mittel zur Analyse der Zellkerns. *Verh Phys Med Ges* 35:67–88, 1902.

Caspersson T, Farber S, Foley GE, et al: Chemical differentiation along metaphase chromosomes. *Exp Cell Res* 49:219–222, 1968.

Cuneo A, Tomasi P, Ferrari L, et al: Cytogenetic analysis of different cellular populations in chronic myelomonocytic leukemia. *Cancer Genet Cytogenet* 37:29–37, 1989.

De Braekeleer M: Breakpoint distribution in variant Philadelphia translocations in chronic myeloid leukemia. *Cancer Genet Cytogenet* 23:167–170, 1986.

Di Donato C, Croci G, Lazzari S, et al: Chronic neutrophilic leukemia: Description of a new case with karyotypic abnormalities. *Am J Clin Pathol* 85:369–371, 1986.

Fujita K, Yamasaki Y, Sawada H, et al: Cytogenetic studies on the adult T-cell leukemia in Japan. *Leuk Res* 13:535–543, 1989.

Gauwerky CE, Huebner K, Isobe M, et al: Activation of *MYC* in a masked t(8;17) translocation results in an aggressive B-cell leukemia. *Proc Natl Acad Sci USA* 86:8867–8871, 1989.

Goh KO, Anderson FW: Cytogenetic studies in basophilic chronic myelocytic leukemia. *Arch Pathol Lab Med* 103:288–290, 1979.

Groffen J, Stephenson JR, Heisterkamp N, et al: Philadelphia chromosomal breakpoints are clustered within a limited region, bcr, on chromosome 22. *Cell* 36:93–99, 1984.

Hagemeijer A, Bartram CR, Smit EM, et al: Is the chromosomal region 9q34 always involved in variants of the Ph[1] translocation? *Cancer Genet Cytogenet* 13:1–16, 1984.

Han T, Sadamori N, Takeuchi J, et al: Clonal chromosome abnormalities in patients with Waldenström's and CLL-associated macroglobulinemia: Significance of trisomy 12. *Blood* 62:525–531, 1983.

Han T, Henderson ES, Emrick LJ, et al: Prognostic significance of karyotypic abnormalities in B-cell chronic lymphocytic leukemia: An update. *Semin Hematol* 24:257–263, 1987.

Heisterkamp N, Stam K, Groffen J, et al: Structural organization of the *bcr* gene and its role in the Ph[1] translocation. *Nature* 315:758–761, 1985.

Huang CS, Gomez GA, Kohno SI, et al: Chromosomes and causation of human cancer and leukemia: 34. A case of "hypereosinophilic syndrome" with unusual cytogenetic findings in a chloroma, terminating in blastic transformation and CNS leukemia. *Cancer* 44: 1284–1289, 1979.

Juliusson G, Robért KH, Ost A, et al: Del(3)(p13) in B-prolymphocytic leukemia—A new nonrandom chromosomal aberration possibly related to the c-*ras* oncogene. *Cancer Genet Cytogenet* 14:191–195, 1985.

Klein G: Specific chromosomal translocations and the genesis of B-cell-derived tumors in mice and men. *Cell* 32:311, 1983.

Kubo A, Kawanami M, Matsuyama E, et al: Chronic neutrophilic leukemia associated with monoclonal gammopathy (IgA, kappa type). *Rinsho Ketsueki* 30:858–862, 1989.

Kunishima S, Mizuno R, Fujishiro N, et al: A case of chronic neutrophilic leukemia with abnormal karyotype. *Rinsho Byori* 37:943–947, 1989.

Lorente JA, Pëna JM, Ferro T, et al: A case of chronic neutrophilic leukemia with original chromosomal abnormalities. *Eur J Haematol* 41:285–288, 1988.

McKeithan TW, Ohno H, Diaz MO: Identification of a transcriptional unit adjacent to the breakpoint in the 14;19 translocation of chronic lymphocytic leukemia. *Genes Chromo Cancer* 1:247–255, 1990.

Mitelman F: Catalog of chromosome aberrations in cancer. In Sandburg AA: *Progress and Topics in Cytogenetics,* ed 2, vol 5. New York, Alan R Liss, 1985.

Nowell PC, Hungerford DA: A minute chromosome in human chronic granulocytic leukemia. *Science* 132:1497, 1960.

Ohno H, Takimoto G, McKeithan TW: The candidate proto-oncogene bcl-3 is related to genes implicated in cell lineage determination and cell cycle control. *Cell* 60:991–997, 1990.

Okada S, Miyoshi Y, Takizawa Y, et al: Neutrophil dysfunction in chronic neutrophilic leukemia without rearrangements of bcr and immunoglobulin heavy chain genes. *Rinsho Ketsueki* 30:1881–1885, 1989.

Ohyashiki K, Ohyashiki JH, Kinniburgh AJ, et al: Transposition of breakpoint cluster region (3′bcr) in CML cells with variant Philadelphia translocations. *Cancer Genet Cytogenet* 26:105–115, 1987.

Pugh WC, Pearson M, Vardiman JW, et al: Philadelphia chromosome–negative chronic myelogenous leukaemia: A morphological reassessment. *Br J Haematol* 60:457–467, 1985.

Reed JC, Tsujimoto Y, Alpers JD, et al: Regulation of bcl-2 proto-oncogene expression during normal human lymphocyte proliferation. *Science* 236:1295–1299, 1987.

Rowley JD: A new consistent chromosomal abnormality in chronic myelogenous leukaemia indentified by quinacrine fluorescence and Giemsa staining. *Nature* 243:290–293, 1973.

Rowley JD: Chromosome studies in the non-Hodgkin's lymphomas: The role of the 14;18 translocation. *J Clin Oncol* 6:919–925, 1988.

Saglio G, Emanuel BS, Guerrasio A, et al: 3′ c-*myc* rearrangement in a human leukemic T-cell line. *Cancer Res* 46:1413–1417, 1986.

Seabright M: A rapid banding technique for human chromosomes. *Lancet* 2:971–972, 1971.

Sherman SI, Abdulkadyrov KM, Shandlorenko SK, et al: Clinical morphological, cytogenetic and genealogical studies of patients with chronic monocytic leukemia. *Vopr Onkol* 25:38–43, 1979.

Shimoyama M, Abe T, Miyamoto K, et al: Chromosome aberrations and clinical features of adult T cell leukemia-lymphoma not associated with human T cell leukemia virus type I. *Blood* 69:984–989, 1987.

Shtivelman E, Lifshitz B, Gale RP, et al: Fused transcript of abl and bcr genes in chronic myelogenous leukaemia. *Nature* 315:550–554, 1985.

Theil E, Bauchinger M, Rodt H, et al: Evidence for monoclonal proliferation in prolymphocytic leukemia of T-cell origin. A cytogenetic and quantitative immunoautoradiographic analysis. *Blut* 35:427–436, 1977.

Tohyama K, Ohmori S, Ueda T, et al: Chronic neutrophilic leukemia with 7q− and the responses of CFU-GM. *Rinsho Ketsueki* 29:738–742, 1988.

Ueshima Y, Alimena G, Rowley JD, et al: Cytogenetic studies in patients with hairy cell leukemia. *Hematol Oncol* 1:215–226, 1983.

Yunis JJ: High resolution of human chromosomes. *Science* 191:1268–1270, 1976.

Van Den Berghe H: Chromosomes in plasma-cell malignancies. *Eur J Haematol* 51 (suppl):47–51, 1989.

Venti G, Mecucci C, Donti E, et al: Translocation t(11;14) and trisomy 11q13-qter in multiple myeloma. *Ann Genet* 27:53–55, 1984.

Yanagisawa K, Fukuoka T, Fujita S: Evidence for the neoplastic involvement of monocytic, eosinophilic and basophilic lineages in acute myelomonocytic leukemia with eosinophilia. *Acta Haematol* 83:145–148, 1990.

Yunis JJ, Bloomfield CD, Ensrud K: All patients with acute nonlymphocytic leukemia may have a chromosomal defect. *N Engl J Med* 305:135–139, 1981.

Review Articles

Anastasi J, LeBeau MM, Vardiman JW, et al: Detection of trisomy 12 in chronic lymphocytic leukemia by fluoresence in situ hybridization to interphase cells: A simple and sensitive method. *Blood* 79:1796–1801, 1992.

Bernstein R: Cytogenetics of chronic myelogenous leukemia. *Semin Hematol* 25:20–34, 1988.

Block AW: Cytogenetic analysis of B-cell chronic lymphoproliferative diagnosis: New technology, complexities, and promises. *Prog Clin Biol Res* 368:145–173, 1991.

Campbell ML, Arlinghans RB: Current status of the BCR gene and its involvement with human leukemia. *Adv Cancer Res* 57:227–256, 1991.

Dobrovic A, Peters GB, Ford JM: Molecular analysis of the Philadelphia chromosome. *Chromosoma* 100:479–486, 1991.

Dreazen O, Cananni E, Gale RP: Molecular biology of chronic myelogenous leukemia. *Semin Hematol* 25:35–48, 1988.

Juliusson G, Gahrton G: Chromosome aberrations in B-cell chronic lymphocytic leukemia. Pathogenetic and clinical implications. *Cancer Genet Cytogenet* 45:143–160, 1990.

Juliusson G, Oscier DG, Fitchett M, et al: Prognostic subgroups in B-cell chronic lymphocytic leukemia defined by specific chromosomal abnormalities. *N Engl J Med* 323:720–724, 1990.

Kantarjian HM, Keating MJ, Walters RS, et al: Clinical and prognostic features of Philadelphia chromosome–negative chronic myelogenous leukemia. *Cancer* 58:2023–2050, 1986.

Kantarjian HM, Kurzrock R, Talpaz M: Philadelphia chromosome negative chronic myelogenous leukemia and chronic myelomonocytic leukemia. *Hematol Oncol Clin North Am* 4:389–404, 1990.

Kaplan JC, Aurias A, Julier C, et al: Human chromosome 22. *J Med Genet* 24:65–78, 1987.

Kurzrock R, Gutterman JU, Talpaz M: The molecular genetics of Philadelphia chromosome–positive leukemias. *N Engl J Med* 319:990–990, 1988.

Levine EG, Bloomfield CD: Cytogenetics of non-Hodgkin's lymphoma. *Monogr Natl Cancer Inst* 10:7–12, 1990.

Mills KI, Benn P, Birnie GD: Does the breakpoint within the major breakpoint cluster region (M-bcr) influence the duration of the chronic phase in chronic myeloid leukemia? An analytical comparison of current literature. *Blood* 78:1155–1161, 1991.

Rabbitts TH: Translocations, master genes, and differentiation between the origins of acute and chronic leukemia. *Cell* 67:641–644, 1991.

Tanzer J: Molecular biology of chronic myelogenous leukemia. *Nouv Rev Fr Hematol* 33:197–220, 1991.

Van Den Berghe H: Chromosomes in plasma-cell malignancies. *Eur J Haematol* 51 (suppl):47–51, 1989.

Willman CL: Diagnosis of hematopoietic diseases of the myeloid lineage utilizing molecular probes in molecular diagnostics in pathology. In Fenoglio-Preiser CM, Willman CL: *Molecular Diagnostics in Pathology.* Baltimore, Williams & Wilkins, 1991, pp 111–122.

CHAPTER 8

Gene Rearrangement and Polymerase Chain Reaction

INTRODUCTION

The diagnosis of most CMLs and CLLs and related entities can usually be accomplished by use of the techniques already described in previous chapters. However, the more difficult cases may require molecular diagnostic studies that should be interpreted within the context of all available data.

The Ph[1] is found in 90–95% of patients with CML, 2% of adults with AML, and 20% of adults and 5% of children with ALL; however, a small percentage (<5%) of patients with classic clinical and morphologic features of CML are Ph[1]-negative. Despite negative cytogenetic studies, many of these patients have molecular fusion of the *BCR* and c-*ABL* genes that can be demonstrated by Southern blotting and restriction mapping. The c-*ABL* protooncogene was mapped to chromosome 9 band q34 and is involved in a reciprocal translocation in CML; it fuses with the *BCR* gene on chromosome 22 band q11. Currently, the function of the *BCR* gene in normal cells is still unknown. This *BCR-ABL* fusion is pathognomonic for CML and is an important observation in establishing the diagnosis of Ph[1]-negative CML.

In addition to *BCR-ABL* rearrangement analysis, Ig gene rearrangement and T-cell receptor analysis have been used to more clearly delineate lymphoid malignancies. Molecular genetic techniques employing Southern blot analysis are useful when clinical, morphologic, and immunophenotypic studies are inconclusive; however, the data must be interpreted in light of all other investigative facts. Indeed, in a recent analysis of 27 cases of acute leukemia and related entities by numerous parameters including gene rearrangement analysis, this technique, although supportive, was not needed to establish the final diagnosis. Although this was a small study and predominately myeloid cases, it emphasized caution in relying too heavily on molecular analysis.

Recently, the polymerase chain reaction (PCR) has been used in the diagnosis and in posttherapy monitoring of leukemias and lymphomas. Utilizing this technique, it is possible to detect minimal residual disease (MRD) in the order of 1 malignant cell in 100,000 total cells. Two chromosomal translocations, the t(9;22) in CML and the t(14;18) of follicular B-cell lymphomas, have been extensively analyzed for this purpose. Undoubtedly, this reaction will be applied to numerous hematologic malignancies in the near future to more accurately define MRD and "cure." Currently, PCR of CMLs with t(9;22) have not yielded clear cut results. Long term follow up of these cases seems indicated.

GENE REARRANGEMENT: GENERAL

Lymphocyte-specific antigen receptors, Ig, and TCRs are made up of several segments that are coded by different genes on different chromosomes. These segments include the IgH and IgL (kappa and lambda) and TCR α, β, γ, and δ chains. The gene controlling the IgH is on chromosome 14; kappa light chain, chromosome 2; lambda light chain, chromosome 22; TCR β and γ chains, chromosome 7; TCR α and δ chains, chromosome 14. A generalized schematic of the manner in which the Ig and TCR genes rearrange as the cell matures is depicted in Fig. 8.1.

These genes share a common evolutionary structure theme. They are organized into distinct regions: termed variable (V), diverse (D), junctional (J), and constant (C). Unlike other genes, the regions composing Ig and TCR genes must move into close proximity by intrachromosomal rearrangement before a functional protein can be produced. Since there are multiple V, D, J, and C regions that can be rearranged in numerous combinations, the end result is a diversified array of proteins and, therefore, antigen-binding specificities are produced from a relatively limited quantity of DNA.

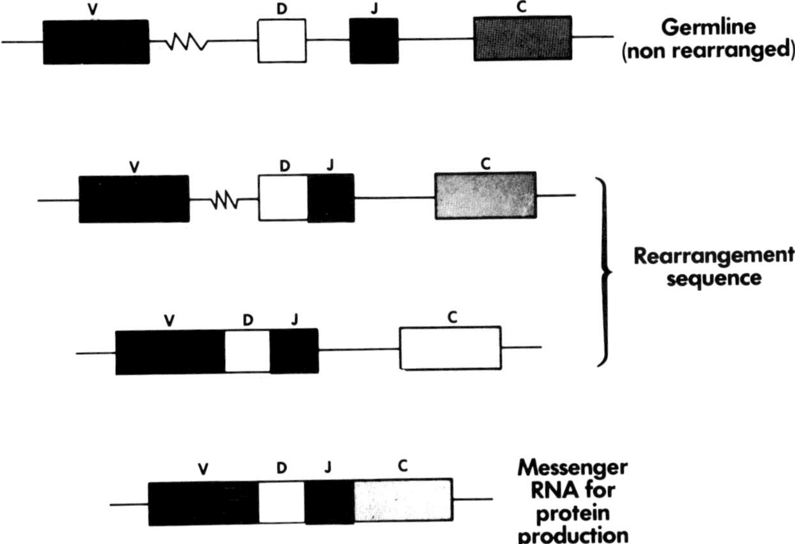

Figure 8-1 Generalized schematic of the manner in which the T-cell and B-cell genes rearrange as the cell matures. From Love JD et al: DNA probes to characterize leukemia and lymphoma cells. *Am Clin Prod Rev* 4:15, 1985. Copyright 1985 by International Scientific Communications, Inc.

TECHNICAL DETECTION OF GENE REARRANGEMENT

In Southern blot analysis, DNA from cells is purified and cut with various restriction enzymes (e.g., *Eco*RI, *Hin*dIII, *Bam*Hi, *BGl*II) that cleave DNA at very precise sequences. The fragments, whose lengths are measured in kb pairs, are separated by agarose gel electrophoresis. Following electrophoresis, the separated fragments are transferred to nitrocellulose paper, where they are identified by hybridization to a radiolabeled DNA probe (Fig. 8.2). The test is based on the principle that as a gene undergoes rearrangement, the relative positions of restriction sites at the site of the rearrangement are also affected. Consequently, a probe to the rearranging portion of the gene will detect a restriction fragment in a nongermline position if sufficient numbers of cells (1–5% of the total) share the same rearrangement. Such a high percentage of genetically identical cells implies clonality, and the pattern of gene rearrangements may indicate either a T-cell or a B-cell lineage. Usually, two sets of Southern blots are performed, one for Ig gene rearrangement and the other for

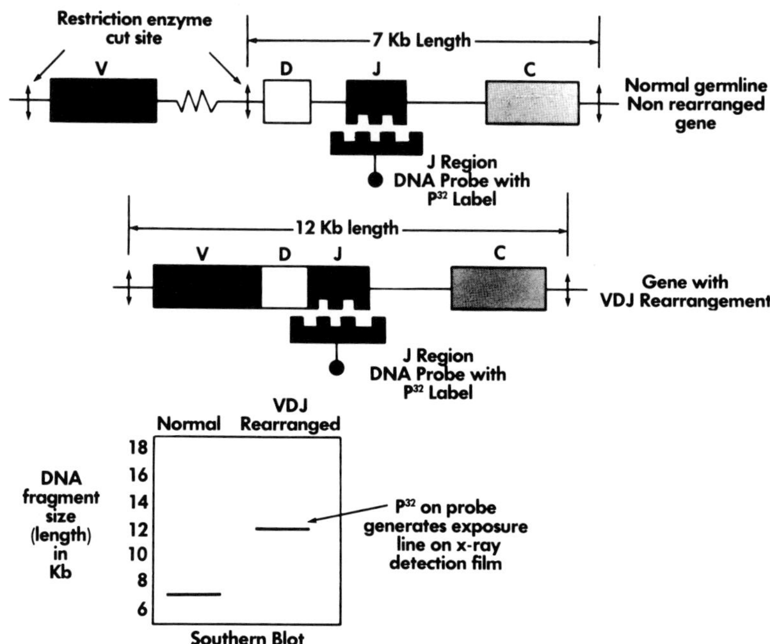

Figure 8-2 Southern blot analysis for gene rearrangement in T and B cells. Cellular DNA from blood specimens is cut with the appropriate restriction enzymes, and the size (length) of the fragments is analyzed by using a Southern blot format. Any deviation in fragment length, either larger or smaller from the germline, indicates that the genes are rearranged. The vertical arrows (↕) indicate restriction enzyme cut sites. From Love JD et al: DNA probes to characterize leukemia and lymphoma cells. *Am Clin Prod Rev* 4:16, 1985. Copyright 1985 by International Scientific Communications, Inc.

TCR gene rearrangement. The Ig genes rearrange in hierarchical order: IgH precedes IgL, and kappa precedes lambda. A similar hierarchical progression exists for the TCR genes: TCR γ and δ occur first in parallel followed by TCR β and TCR α. Some investigators have shown that the products of the genes are apparently expressed in mutually exclusive pairs (TCR γ, δ) or (TCR α, and β).

Most leukemias appear to be clonal expansions representing the progeny of a single cell. Therefore, every cell in the population will bear the same gene rearrangement and same-size DNA fragments. Since multiple copies of the same gene rearrangements are present in a clonal leukemia population, this enables detection by Southern blot analysis. In contrast, in a polyclonal population of normal cells with multiple gene rearrangements, none of the rearranged genes in this collective population will be ascertained by Southern blot analysis since they fall below the threshold of detection.

Although gene rearrangement analysis was thought initially to be the court of final appeal to identify clonal proliferation of lymphoid cells, unfortunately, this has not been the case. B cells have demonstrated TCR rearrangements; T cells have shown IgH and IgL gene rearrangement, and even some myeloid leukemias have manifested both IgH and IgL gene rearrangements, though rarely. Additional caution is needed in interpretation, since false-positive results may occur with partial digests or resistant digestion sites. If a restriction enzyme lacks suficient activity, the finished blot will reflect a mixture of fully and partially digested DNA fragments. Frequently, one or several aberrant-sized fragments predominate that produce new nongermline fragments on the autoradiogram, which may be mistaken for rearranged genes. Also, restriction fragment length polymorphisms (RFLPs), which are normal variations in the size of restriction fragments that arise due to single base changes in restriction enzyme recognition sites or variations in the amount of DNA between restriction enzyme recognition sites, may lead to normal germline bands that may migrate like clonally rearranged DNA. Finally, false-positive results may be interpreted if the gene has only a few variable regions available for recombination with joining and constant regions, as is the case with the TCR gamma gene. Consequently, a polyclonal population of cells with rearranged TCR gamma produces seven or eight discrete, new nongermline bands rather than a broad, often invisible smear of rearranged bands as is the usual situation for the other receptor genes. False-negative results may be seen because of (1) lack of sensitivity (<1 cell in 100), (2) comigration of the rearranged and germline fragments, (3) technical errors, (4) deletions of both alleles at an antigen receptor locus resulting in only germline bands of the nonneoplastic tissue being apparent, or (5) antigen receptor rearrangements occurring at many possible sites over a long distance that cannot be readily assayed by conventional Southern blot analysis, as is the case with the TCR α gene. Standard electrophoresis efficiently separates DNA fragments from 0.1 to 25 kb; however, special restriction enzymes and pulse-field gel electrophoresis are required to accommodate unusually large genes.

POLYMERASE CHAIN REACTION (PCR): GENERAL

The amount of genomic DNA required for the detection of single-copy genes by typical Southern blot analysis is approximately 0.1–0.5

μg; therefore, when 10 μg of DNA is analyzed by such a technique, its sensitivity is limited to detecting a clone of cells representing approximately 1–5% of the cells in a heterogeneous population. PCR circumvents the problem of detecting small numbers of malignant cells by enzymatically amplifying target sequences prior to analysis. PCR amplification has been utilized to (1) detect rare, malignant cells (1 in 100,000) with a particular molecular aberration, such as a mutation or chromosomal translocation, (2) identify infectious organisms, (3) amplify target DNA sequences from human hairs and blood for forensic identification, and (4) amplify target sequences for allele-specific oligonucleotide probes, thereby improving Southern blot analysis.

POLYMERASE CHAIN REACTION (PCR): TECHNICAL ASPECTS

PCR is an in vitro means of enzymatically amplifying specific regions of DNA prior to detection analysis. A denatured target DNA is incubated with two oligonucleotide primers that flank the DNA segment and are complementary to opposite strands. In order to prepare these primers, it is necessary to have sequence information at the limits of the region of DNA to be amplified (Fig. 8.3). At a suitable annealing temperature and in an appropriate buffer containing the four deoxyribonucleotides and DNA polymerase, the oligonucleotides will prime DNA synthesis across the region of interest. The newly synthesized duplex DNA is then heat-denatured to provide template for subsequent rounds of DNA synthesis. Initially, a DNA polymerase was added every round of synthesis since it was destroyed during heat denaturation. Recently, however, efficient and specific amplification of DNA by PCR has been accomplished by the use of a DNA polymerase from the heat-stable bacterium *Thermus aquaticus.* This DNA polymerase, referred to as *Taq* polymerase, has the remarkable ability to maintain its function after heating to 94°C, a temperature at which double-stranded DNA is rapidly melted. In the presence of a large molar excess of nucleotides and primers, a single addition of *Taq* polymerase will enable amplification through more than 25 repeated rounds of heat denaturation, primer annealing, and DNA synthesis. In this way a target sequence can easily be amplified 10^5–10^6-fold, allowing one to detect a single malignant cell in a heterogeneous background of 100,000 normal cells!

The effective utilization of PCR depends in large part on the careful selection of primers. In general, oligonucleotide primers are 15–30 bases in length and fully complementary to DNA of known sequence. Specifically, the amplification of only the desired DNA fragment re-

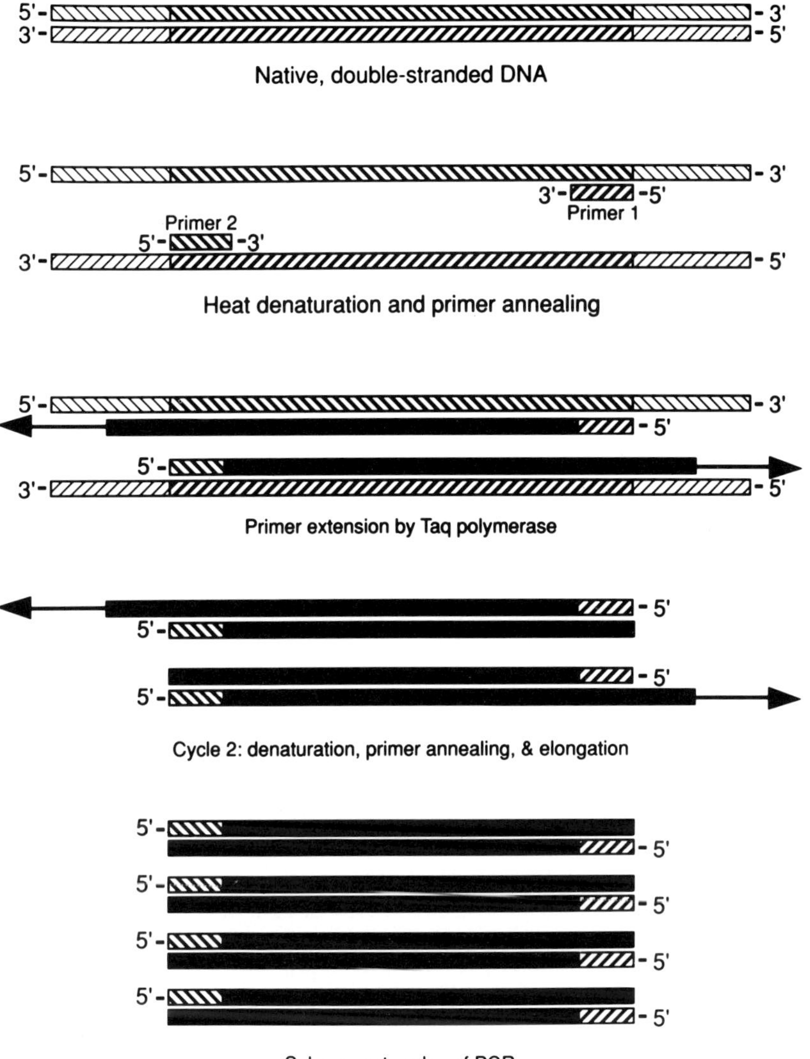

Figure 8-3 Subsequent cycles of PCR. From Bunn FH: Molecular genetics: Clinical and research use of the polymerase chain reaction. Hematology 1990. Education Program: *American Society of Hematology*. Boston, Mass., p 105.

sults from the use of primers of the correct sequence, with minimal homology to other sequences in the sample, and by maintaining optimum temperature and buffer conditions during the reaction. The specificity of the technique may be enhanced by a process called *nesting,* in which the initial primers are replaced after a few cycles of amplification with primers located within the desired amplification product. Amplification is then allowed to proceed from these internal sites. If the internal nucleotide sequences of unintended products of the first amplification are unrelated to the anticipated fragment (which is usually the case), then it is highly unlikely that any region of DNA other than the intended target will allow sequential amplification with both sets of primers.

In order to perform PCR, the sequence of the target must be partially known so that appropriate primers can be synthesized. Since the primer annealing sites on the target DNA are known, the size of the fragment amplified between primers is predictable. Often this amplified DNA fragment can be analyzed on a gel and visualized by ethidium bromide staining for the presence of a diagnostic product. Alternatively, greater specificity may be achieved by subsequent hybridization with a probe to the internal sequences of the amplified product.

Unlike a number of techniques used in molecular biology, PCR can be readily performed on impure DNA templates. Also, even denatured and/or ancient and degraded or fragmented DNA specimens can be successfully amplified. Furthermore, PCR may be performed with RNA as the starting material. The RNA is first copied into a single cDNA strand with reverse transcriptase, and the cDNA copy is then amplified.

CHRONIC MYELOID LEUKEMIA AND RELATED DISEASES

CML is associated with a specific chromosomal abnormality, t(9;22), that results in a shortened chromosome 22, termed the Ph^1. The Ph^1 abnormality is a result of the translocation of the c-*ABL* protooncogene from chromosome 9 onto chromosome 22, where the break usually occurs within a limited 5.8-kb region of the *BCR* gene, designated the bcr. The well-defined area of the bcr locus permits detection of this translocation by Southern blot analysis; and although heterogeneity of breakpoints exists within the bcr locus and within the *BCR* gene, the translocations can be detected in most cases by screening with the universal bcr probe on multiple digests. Initial screening employs *Xba*I and *Bgl*II digests, with an algorithm for bcr analysis

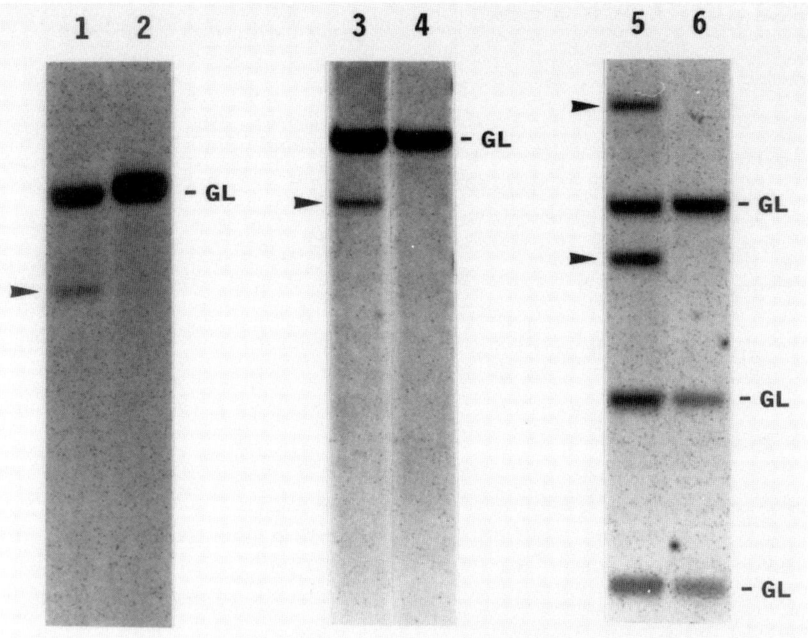

Figure 8-4 Southern blot analysis of clonal Ig gene rearrangements and *BCR-ABL* translocation in a case of CML in lymphoid blast crisis. Patient DNA is present in lanes 1, 3, and 5; control DNA is present in lanes 2, 4, and 6. Lanes 1 and 3 show clonal rearrangements of the IgH and kappa IgL genes, respectively. Lane 5 demonstrates a reciprocal translocation of the bcr of the *BCR* gene and the abl fragment of the *ABL* gene. Germline positions of the genes are designated "GL," and clonal rearrangements are indicated by arrows.

using additional digest combinations. Such a technique has clinical value because (1) Ph^1 cannot be detected in 5% of patients with CML; however, about half of these will demonstrate bcr rearrangements at the molecular level; (2) Ph^1-negative, bcr-negative CML patients may have a different prognosis and treatment response; and (3) although controversial, the presence or absence of the third exon of the bcr region in the fusion p210 protein may have prognostic impact, that is, its presence indicates earlier blast crisis. Such a screening strategy has established bcr analysis as a competitive technique with cytogenetic examination. Even though the turnaround time for bcr analysis may be slightly longer, the technique can detect bcr-positive, Ph^1-negative patients with CML and determine the breakpoint site that may have prognostic significance. A *BCR-ABL* rearrangement in a CML patient is shown in Fig. 8.4.

PCR UTILIZATION IN CML

Whereas *BCR* gene rearrangement analysis has been employed in diagnosis, cDNA-PCR of the *BCR-ABL* fusion mRNA with subsequent Southern blot analysis has been utilized to detect the presence of tumor cells after bone marrow transplant or in tissues considered devoid of tumor. Although many such studies have been reported that can detect 1 malignant cell in 100,000 cell population, extensive follow-up studies have yet to be carried out to determine the full clinical significance. Furthermore, PCR detects both viable and non-viable cells, and it is unclear whether generation of a PCR product should be equated with the potential for cell proliferation. Accurate assessment of cellular proliferative capability may be less of a concern when the target is RNA, given the reduced stability of those molecules compared with DNA. Nevertheless, extensive follow-up will be necessary to determine the exact significance of such a minuscule population of cells with malignant potential; yet some preliminary studies have indicated that those CML patients who have *BCR-ABL* rearrangements 6 months after bone marrow transplantation may have a reduced cure probability.

PHILADELPHIA CHROMOSOME IN ACUTE LEUKEMIAS

About 25% of adult ALL patients demonstrate the Ph^1 and have genomic breakpoints in the 5.8-kb bcr locus. Most of these patients are assumed to represent a lymphoid blast crisis of CML in patients with an undetected preexistent CML. However, the remaining adults with Ph^1-positive ALL and virtually all children with Ph^1-positive ALL are considered to be de novo ALL. In this situation, the c-*ABL* gene does not fuse with the *BCR* gene in the 5.8-kb bcr locus but is fused with the first intron of the *BCR* gene, nearly 100 kb upstream (Fig. 8.5). This translocation produces a 7.0-kb fusion mRNA product (Fig. 8.6), that codes for a 185–190 kda protein with elevated tyrosine kinase activity. Contrariwise, in classic CML fuction of c-*ABL* onto the 5.8-kb bcr locus produces an 8.5-kb fusion mRNA that endodes a 210-kd bcr-abl protein with elevated tyrosine kinase activity.

Ph^1 translocation also occurs rarely (<2%) in patients with de novo AML. Interestingly, these AML cases fuse c-*ABL* to intron I of the *BCR* gene, producing the 7.0-kb *BCR-ABL* fusion mRNA and the p190 fusion protein similar to what is seen in Ph^1-positive ALL.

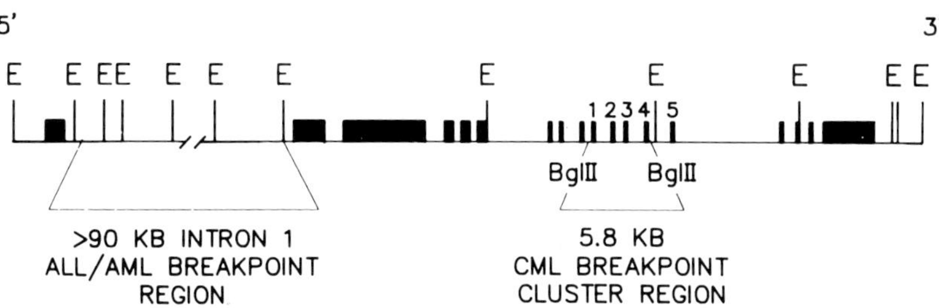

Figure 8-5 Map of the complete *BCR* gene. Exon map of the *BCR* gene reveals an upstream exon followed by a very large intron that is the site of fusion to c-*ABL* common exon II in Ph^1+ de novo ALL and AML. Over 100- kb downstream in the *BCR* gene is the site of the 5.8-kb CML bcr cluster, the site of fusion of c-*ABL* common exon II to the *BCR* gene in CML. From Willman CL: *Molecular Diagnostics In* Fenoglio-Preiser CM, Wilman CL (eds): *Pathology*. Baltimore, Williams & Wilkins, p 118, 1991.

It has been shown that the p190 bcr-abl fusion protein is more rapidly transforming in in vitro systems than is the p210 variant, which may relate to the more acute nature of the diseases in which it is found. However, the underlying mechanism controlling myeloid versus lymphoid morphology of the blasts in de novo Ph^1-positive acute leukemia is unknown at this time. Therefore, although the Ph^1 chromosomes in Ph^1-positive CML and the Ph^1-positive de novo

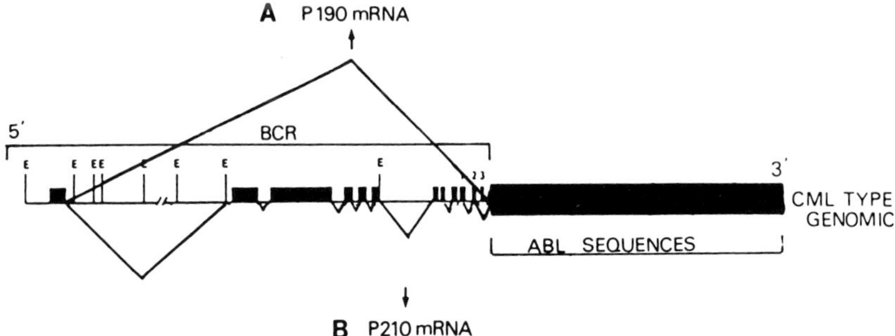

Figure 8-6 **(A)** Splicing of bcr exon I to common exon II of c-*ABL* produces a 7.0-kb BCR-ABL fusion mRNA and a p185–190 bcr-abl fusion protein. **(B)** Splicing of all *BCR* upstream exons including those of the 5.8-kb bcr cluster onto common exon II of c-*ABL* produces an 8.5-kb BCR-ABL fusion mRNA and p210 bcr-abl protein. From Willman CL: *Molecular Diagnostics In* Fenoglio-Preiser CM, Wilman CL (eds): *Pathology*. Baltimore, Williams & Wilkins, p 119, 1991.

acute leukemias appear identical, they have quite different molecular breakpoints that correlate with the different morphologic, cytochemical, and immunologic characteristics of these diseases and their differing clinical courses.

CHRONIC LYMPHOCYTIC LEUKEMIA AND RELATED DISORDERS

CLL and relatively well differentiated B-cell malignancies such as B-cell ALL, HCL, and well-differentiated B-cell lymphomas may show both IgH and IgL gene rearrangements, usually without TCR gene rearrangements. However, approximately 10% of B-cell leukemias and lymphomas may have nonfunctional rearrangements of TCR genes. This has been observed in some cases of CLL in which both Ig genes and TCR genes were rearranged; however, the latter rearrangements were nonfunctional.

Most follicular lymphomas (80–90%) exhibit a t(14;18) that juxtaposes the lgH gene to the 3′ region of *BCL*-2. In addition, approximately 10% of CLLs demonstrate a similar translocation cytogenetically. The chromosome 18 breakpoints in CLL, however, cluster at the 5′ flanking region of the *BCL*-2 gene, and no rearrangements have been found at the major or minor breakpoint regions in the 3′ portion of the *BCL*-2 gene, which is typical of the t(14;18) observed in follicular lymphomas. In addition, the *BCL*-2 gene in CLL has also been found juxtaposed to the Ig lambda chain gene on chromosome 22.

Richter's syndrome, manifested as immunoblastic lymphoma, arises in 10% of CLL patients., The question of whether the CLL lymphocytes and Richter lymphoma immunoblasts are clonally related has been addressed by immunophenotypic and gene rearrangement analyses. One study identified differences by two-color flow cytometric analysis and IgH gene analysis of blood and lymph specimens, which revealed nonidentical as well as identical nongermline bands in two populations. However, IgL gene analysis showed that both populations shared a common clonal origin! The authors emphasize the unreliability of using IgH genotype alone to identify clonal origin. Since postrearrangement deletion, point mutation, and IgH switching occur in lgH genes but are seldom seen in IgL genes, it is important to analyze both IgH and IgL genes to conclusively determine clonal origin. Such analysis is surely indicated in assigning clonal origin in Richter's syndrome and may help to clarify past literature.

A "prolymphocytic variant" of HCL showed both Ig and TCR β gene rearrangement without evidence of dual cellular populations.

In addition five cases of T-PLL have shown TCR β rearrangements supporting the existence of T-PLL.

HCL, being a relatively well differentiated B-cell malignancy, may show both IgH and IgL gene rearrangement, usually without TCR gene rearrangements. Such findings offer strong evidence for endogenous Ig synthesis in hairy cells and for the B-lymphocytic character of this leukemia in the overwhelming majority of cases. However, very rare cases of T-HCL have demonstrated TCR β rearrangement with IgH genes in germline configuration.

Less differentiated malignancies such as follicular or diffuse lymphomas and non-T, non-B ALL may show rearrangements of the IgH TCR loci, but usually not IgL loci. The most common lymphoma that frequently presents with a leukemia phase is follicular lymphoma. In the past these were described as "CLL-like syndromes"; however, in a significant number of cases, the morphologic features were different from those of CLL. The characteristic t(14;18) seen in follicular lymphomas usually occurs in clustered regions within the *BCL*-2 and IgH loci, facilitating molecular analysis by Southern blot or PCR.

Although WM may show IgH and IgL gene rearrangements, rarely a rearrangement of chromosome 14 may occur and involve chimeric DNA formation. Such a rearrangement may not only be between an Ig gene and a certain oncogene, but also between the IgH gene and IgL genes.

Multiple myeloma may show IgH and IgL gene rearrangements and also, more frequently, the aberrant chromosome 14 rearrangement mentioned above in WM. Rarely, TCR β gene may be rearranged in this disorder.

Relatively well differentiated T-cell malignancies usually have functional TCR gene rearrangements, without IgH and IgL gene rearrangements. However, T-cell neoplasms occasionally have nonfunctional IgH gene rearrangements.

TGLD is subdivided into two broad categories: those cases that are CD3 antigen–positive and exhibit clonal TCR β gene rearrangements, and those cases that are CD3 antigen–negative and exhibit the TCR β gene in germline configuration. Many cases of T-CLL reported in the past probably represent TGLD, ATLL, T-PLL, or a leukemic phase of a T-cell NHL.

The majority of cases of T-PLL demonstrate both TCR gamma and TCR β rearrangements, supporting the clonal T-cell nature of this malignancy. T-PLL is extremely rare, very aggressive, and characterized by massive splenomegaly, lymphadenopathy, and skin infiltration. It is refractory to most forms of therapy and is phenotypically distinct from ATLL.

ATLL is usually associated with HTLV-I and has been classified into acute, chronic, lymphomatous, and smoldering types by Japanese investigators. Studies of the TCR δ chain gene in patients with ATLL have revealed deletion of this locus in all cases of both ATLL-w (*with* monoclonally integrated HTLV-I proviral DNA) and ATLL-o (*without* integrated HTLV-I proviral DNA). Both forms of ATLL showed variable rearrangement of β and γ subunits of the TCR. Rearrangement was more frequent in ATLL-w than in ATLL-o and non-ATLL lymphoid malignancies. Therefore, TCR chain gene analysis and HTLV-I proviral DNA integration evaluation may help to differentiate ATLL from other T-cell malignancies. Needlesss to say, these results should be interpreted in the context of all the data.

SS and MF lymphocytes usually express pan-T-cell antigens CD2, CD5, and CD3, often lack pan-T-cell antigen CD7, and usually express the mature peripheral helper subset phenotype CD4+ and are CD8−. TCR rearrangements are usually found in the TCR β and TCR γ chain genes, but usually not in the plaque stage or suspected early cutaneous T-cell lymphoma. For this reason, some investigators have emphasized the importance of molecular analysis in lymphocytic skin infiltrates. However, caution is again emphasized since other investigators (Berger et al. 1988) have reported dual genotype in cutaneous T-cell lymphoma. In 4 of 13 cases, evaluation of peripheral blood lymphocytes from patients in the leukemic phase of their cutaneous T-cell lymphoma revealed TCR β chain gene and Ig gene J region rearrangements.

With few exceptions, Southern blot analysis in HCL reveals rearrangement of the IgH loci coupled to a reorganization of the IgL genes. In one study, none of the HCL cases demonstrated TCR β chain gene rearrangement. However, a rare case of the so-called prolymphocytic variant of HCL did show both IgH gene and TCR β chain gene rearrangement. Also, rare cases of an association between HCL and large granular lymphocytes with TCR rearrangements have been reported. Such findings at the genotypic level probably do not represent true cases of T-cell HCL.

From continuously accumulating data in the realm of gene rearrangement analysis, the watchword should be caution in the use of these studies in establishing a diagnosis. When the studies are used, they should be analyzed in relation to all the data!

PCR UTILIZATION IN LYMPHOID MALIGNANCIES

Although the use of the PCR has increased exponentially as a novel tool to detect point mutations, minor structural changes, rearrangements, and MRD, the t(14;18) translocation of follicular B-cell lymphoma has been extensively analyzed by this technique. The application of PCR must contend with the heterogeneity of breakpoint positions within the chromosomal DNA. In the t(14;18) in follicular B-cell lymphoma, the break in chromosome 14 occurs adjacent to or within any of the six homologous J-region gene segments of the IgH gene. Therefore, a single oligonucleotide complementary to conserved J-region sequences can be used for the chromosome 14 side of the translocation. On chromosome 18, the breaks occur scattered in or around the *BCL*-2 oncogene. Fortunately, breaks seem to be clustered predominantly within two small regions: the major breakpoint region (MBR) and the minor breakpoint region (mbr). Therefore, the majority of t(14;18) in these lymphomas can be detected by using several oligonucleotide primers complementary to sequences on the 5′ side of these bcrs.

Recently PCR has been used to evaluate MRD in childhood B-lineage lymphoblastic leukemia. In B lymphocytes, the process generates a hypervariable sequence known as the complementary determining region III (CDR III) of the IgH gene. Oligonucleotides complementary to these marker sequences have been used in combination with a flanking oligonucleotide to generate tumor-specific signals for detection of residual disease. Since ALL results from the clonal expansion of malignant B or T lymphocytes, these rearrangements can be exploited by the PCR as specific markers for the leukemic clone.

The PCR technique represents a threefold order of magnitude of detection capability over previously available methods and has revealed the presence of malignant cells in tissues from patients in "remission" and in post–bone marrow transplant individuals. Whether the presence of a single abnormal cell in 100,000 presages relapse, or absence of any malignant clone at this level of detection predicts cure, is not known at this time! Currently much effort is being extended in this area to resolve this question. PCR may also be used to detect viral DNA sequences such a HIV-1, HTLV-I, HTLV-II, and Epstein-Barr virus genomes. Furthermore, PCR can be used to detect mutations in oncogenes. Although the role of such mutations in the development or progression of hematologic malignancies has been controversial, utilization of PCR hopefully will lead to our improved understanding of oncogene aberrations in these conditions.

In summary, our original concepts of gene rearrangement analysis were imbued with some emotional fervor that we had found the magic bullet to differentiate benignity from malignancy. However, this has not been the case, since the complex biology of both normal and malignant tissue has thwarted our efforts to design the ultimate test. Therefore, molecular studies must be interpreted with caution and in the appropriate context to other data. As we embark on further investigations using the PCR, similar caution is indicated. Finally, good morphology, immunocytochemistry, flow cytometry, and cytogenetics, coupled with common sense, prevail as the cornerstone in the diagnosis of the chronic leukemias. Nevertheless, the new information provided by molecular biology will continue to impact on our diagnostic proficiency, and should be readily utilized in an appropriate manner.

BIBLIOGRAPHY

Articles

Adachi M, Tsujimoto Y: Juxtaposition of human *bcl*-2 and immunoglobulin lambda light chain gene in chronic lymphocytic leukemia is the result of a reciprocal chromosome translocation between chromosome 18 and 22. *Oncogene* 4:1073–1075, 1989.

Adachi M, Cossman J, Longo D, et al: Variant translocations of the *bcl*-2 gene to immunoglobulin lambda light chain gene in chronic lymphocytes leukemia. *Proc Natl Acad Sci USA* 86:2771–2774, 1989.

Adachi M, Tefferi A, Greippp PR, et al: Preferential linkage of *bcl*-2 to immunoglobulin light chain gene in chronic lymphocytic leukemia. *J Exp Med* 171:559–564, 1990.

Berenson J, Lichtenstein A: Clonal rearrangement of the beta-T cell receptor gene in multiple myeloma. *Leukemia* 3:133–136, 1989.

Berger CL, Eisenberg A, Soper L, et al: Dual genotype in cutaneous T cell lymphoma: Immunoglobulin gene rearrangement in clonal T cell malignancy. *J Invest Dermatol* 90:73–77, 1988.

Clearly ML, Wood GS, Warke R, et al: Immunoglobulin gene rearrangements in hairy cell leukemia. *Blood* 65:99–104, 1984.

Demeter J, Paloozi K, Foldi J, et al: Immunological and molecular biological identification of a true case of T-hairy cell leukemia. *Eur J Haematol* 43:339–345, 1989.

Dobrovic A, Trainor KF, Morley AA: Detection of the molecular abnormality in chronic myeloid leukemia by use of the polymerase chain reaction. *Blood* 72:2063–2065, 1988.

Foa, R, Pelicci PG, Migone N, et al: Analysis of T cell receptor beta chain (T beta) gene rearrangements demonstrates the monoclonal nature of T-cell chronic lymphoproliferative disorders. *Blood* 67: 247–250, 1986.

Giardina SL, Young HA, Faltynek CK, et al: Rearrangement of both immunoglobulin and T-cell receptor genes in a prolymphocytic variant of hairy cell leukemia patient resistant to interferon-alpha. *Blood* 72:1708–1716, 1988.

Haber LM, Childs CC, Hirsch-Ginsberg C, et al: Strategy for breakpoint cluster region analysis in chronic myelocytic leukemia in a routine clinical laboratory. *Am J Clin Pathol* 94:762–767, 1990.

Hooberman AL, Carrino JJ, Leibowitz D, et al: Unexpected heterogeneity of BCR-ABL fusion mRNA detected by polymerase-chain reaction in Philadelphia chromosome–positive acute lymphoblastic leukemia. *Proc Natl Acad Sci USA* 86:4259–4263, 1989.

Kawasaki ES, Clark SS, Coyne MY, et al: Diagnosis of chronic myeloid and acute lymphocytic leukemia by detection of leukemia-specific mRNA sequences amplified in vitro. *Proc Natl Acad Sci USA* 85:5698–5702, 1988.

Kimura N, Takihara Y, Akiyoshi T, et al: Rearrangement of T-cell receptor delta chain gene as a marker of lineage and clonality in T-cell lymphoproliferative disorders. *Cancer Res* 49:4488–4492, 1989.

Lai, JL, Aissaoui Z, Collyn-d'Hooghe C, et al: Chronic myeloid leukemia with unusual variant Ph translocation (22;22)(q11;q13). Two cases with chimeric BCR-ABL transcripts. *Cancer Genet Cytogenet* 48:209–216, 1990.

Lauria F, Foa R: Configuration of the immunoglobulin and T cell receptor gene regions in hairy cell leukemia and B-chronic lymphocytic leukemia. *Leukemia* 1:393–394, 1987.

Lee, MS, Chang KS, Cabanillas F, et al: Detection of minimal residual disease cells carrying the t(14;18) by DNA sequence amplification. *Science* 237:175–178, 1987.

Matnee K, Nakamura K, Mizutani S: Detection of minimal residual leukemia after bone marrow transplantation in patients with chronic myeloid leukemia using the polymerase chain reaction. *Rinsho Ketsueki* 31:603–608, 1990.

Migone N, Giubellino MC, Casorati G, et al: Configuration of the immunoglobulin and T-cell receptor gene regions in hairy cell leukemia and B-chronic lymphocytic leukemia. *Leukemia* 1:393–394, 1987.

Nishida K, Taniwaki M, Misawa S, et al: Nonrandom rearrangement of chromosome 14 at band q32.33 in human lymphoid malignancies with mature B-cell phenotype. *Cancer Res* 49:1275–1281, 1989.

Ohshima K, Yoshida T, Kikuchi M, et al: Rearrangement of human T cell receptor beta and gamma chain genes in adult T cell leukemia/lymphoma. *Hematol Oncol* 8:111–118, 1990.

Osada H, Seto M, Ueda R, et al: *bcl*-2 gene rearrangement analysis in Japanese B cell lymphoma; novel *bcl*-2 recombination with immunoglobulin kappa chain gene. *Jpn J Cancer Res* 80:711–715, 1989.

Perl A, Di Vincenzo JP, Ryan DH, et al: Rearrangement of the T-cell receptor alpha, beta, and gamma chain genes in chronic lymphocytic leukemia. *Leuk Res* 14:131–137, 1990.

Peters MS, Thibodeau SN, White JW Jr: Mycosis fungoides in children and adolescents. *J Am Acad Dermatol* 22:1011–1118, 1990.

Pignon JM, Henui, T, Armselam S, et al: Frequent detection of minimal residual disease by use of the polymerase chain reaction in long-term survivors after bone marrow transplantation for chronic myeloid leukemia. *Leukemia* 4:83–86, 1990.

Rolfkiser E, O'Connor NT, Crick J, et al: Genotypic analysis of cutaneous T-cell lymphoma. *J Invest Dermatol* 88:762–765, 1987.

Schnitzer B, Roth MS: Detection of Philadelphia chromosome–positive cells from glass slide smears using the polymerase chain reaction. *Am J Pathol* 137:1–6, 1990.

Schumacher HR, Shrit MA, Kowal-Vern A, et al: Acute leukemia and related entities: Impact of new technology. *Arch Pathol Lab Med* 115: 331–337, 1991.

Steis RG, Urba WJ, Mathieson BJ, et al: Rearrangement of both immunoglobulin and T-cell receptor genes in a prolymphocytic variant of hairy cell leukemia patient resistant to interferon alpha. *Blood* 72:1708–1716, 1988.

Stelet-Stevenson M, Raffeld M, Cohen P, et al: Detection of occult follicular lymphoma by specific DNA amplification. *Blood* 72:1822–1825, 1988.

Sun T, Susin M, Desner M, et al: The clonal origin of two cell populations in Richter's syndrome. *Hum Pathol* 21:722–728, 1990.

Tobinai K, Shimoyama M: Recent advances in clinical research on T-cell lymphoma. *Rinsho Ketsueki* 31:564–568, 1990.

Tohda S, Morio T, Suzuki T, et al: Richter syndrome with two B cell clones processing different suface immunoglobulins and immunoglobulin gene rearrangements. *Am J Hematol* 35:35–36, 1990.

Tycko B, Palmer JD, Link MP, et al: Polymerase chain reaction amplification of rearranged antigen receptor genes using junction-specific oligonucleoides: Possible application for detection of minimal residual disease in acute lymphoblastic leukemia. *Cancer Cell* 7:47–52, 1989.

Yamada M, Wasserman R, Lange B, et al: Minimal residual disease in childhood B-linkage lymphoblastic leukemia: Persistence of leukemic cells during the first 18 months of treatment. *N Engl J Med* 323:448–455, 1990.

REVIEW ARTICLES

Berliner N: T gamma lymphocytosis and T cell chronic leukemias. *Hematol Oncol Clin North Am* 4:473–487, 1990.

Chang KL, Stroup R, Weiss L: Hairy cell leukemia: Current status. *Am J Clin Path* 97:719–738, 1992.

Cossman J, Uppenkamp M, Sundeen J, et al: Molecular genetics and the diagnosis of lymphoma. *Arch Pathol Lab Med* 112:117–127, 1988.

Cossman J, Zehnbauer B, Garrett CT, et al: Gene rearrangements in the diagnosis of lymphoma/leukemia. *Am J Clin Pathol* 95:347–354, 1991.

Eisenstein BI: The polymerase chain reaction. A new method of using molecular genetics for medical diagnosis. *N Engl J Med* 322:178–183, 1990.

Fenoglio-Preiser CM, Willman CL: *Molecular Diagnostics in Pathology.* Baltimore, Williams & Wilkins, 1991.

Griesser H, Tkachuk D, Reis MD, et al: Gene rearrangements and translocations in lymphoproliferative diseases. *Blood* 76:1402–1415, 1989.

Hughes TP, Ambrosetti A, Barbu V, et al: Clinical value of PCR in diagnosis and follow up of leukemia and lymphoma: Report of the third workshop of the molecular biology/BHT study group. *Leukemia* 5:448–451, 1991.

Knowles DM: Immunophenotypic and antigen receptor gene rearrangement analysis in T cell neoplasia. *Am J Pathol* 134:761–785, 1989.

Mris MA, Gelfand DH, Sninsky JJ, White TJ: *PCR Protocols. A Guide to Methods and Applications.* San Diego, Academic Press, 1990.

Roth MS, Terry VH: Applications of the polymerase chain reaction for detection of minimal residual disease of hematologic malignancies. *Henry Ford Hospital Medical Journal* 39:112–116, 1991.

Willman CL, Griffith BB, Whitaker M: Molecular genetic approach for the diagnosis of clonality in lymphoid neoplasms. *Clin Lab Med* 10:119–149, 1990.

Yokota S, Abe T: Polymerase chain reaction (PCR)—A novel tool for the molecular diagnosis of neoplasms. *Gan To Kagaku Ryoko* 17:1395–1401, 1990.

CHAPTER 9

Oncogenes and Growth Factors: The Future

INTRODUCTION: ONCOGENES

Genes that are capable of inducing neoplastic transformation are termed *oncogenes*. Oncogenes, which currently number approximately 60–90, are involved in cellular proliferation, differentiation, and carcinogenesis in cells. Oncogene sequences in normal eucaryotic cells are referred to as *cellular oncogenes* (c-onc's) or *protooncogenes*, while the oncogene sequences transduced by viruses from normal cells are referred to as *viral oncogenes* or v-onc's. Cellular oncogenes may be activated by quantitative changes in their expression level or altered by qualitative structural changes in their genes and encoded proteins. The latter mechanisms of cellular oncogene activation include point mutation, gene deletion, chromosomal rearrangement, gene amplification, and insertional mutagenesis. Protooncogenes constitute a limited number of evolutionary conserved cellular genes that are apparently involved in normal cell growth and differentiation. Much of our knowledge about oncogenes has been acquired from the study of acute transforming retroviruses.

Retroviruses can be divided into two general categories based on their biological activities. In the first category, the acute transforming retroviruses efficiently transform cells and induce tumors in vivo within 2 to 3 weeks; in the other, slowly transforming retroviruses

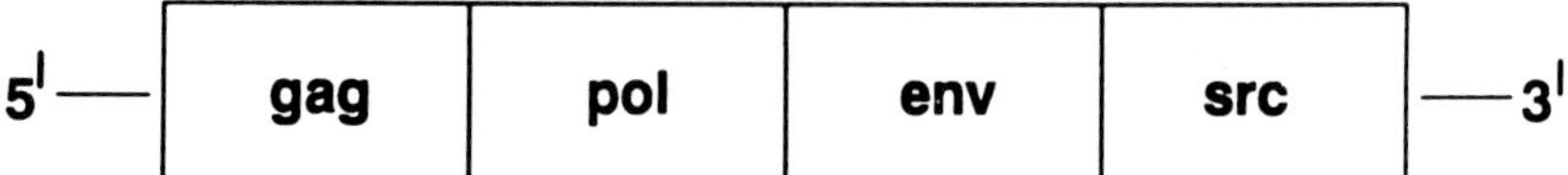

Figure 9-1 RNA genome of RSV, the quintessential replication-competent retrovirus: *gag* designates virion core proteins, *pol* encodes reverse-transcriptase, and *env* specifies viral envelope proteins; *src* is unique to RSV. Fenoglio-Preiser CM: *Molecular Diagnostics In Pathology*. Baltimore, Williams & Wilkins, p 81, 1991.

do not appear to transform cells in culture and only induce tumors in infected animals after long latency periods. Acutely transforming retroviruses such as the Rous sarcoma virus (RSV) provided the first clues implicating cellular genes in tumorigenesis. RSV, a prototype of acute transforming retroviruses, contains four genes within its RNA genome, and except for the oncogene sequence *src,* its genetic structure is typical of all replication-competent viruses (Fig. 9.1). The *gag* gene specifies viral core proteins; the *env* gene encodes viral envelope proteins; and the *pol* sequence encodes reverse transcriptase. The primary translocation products of the *gag* and *env* genes are protein precursors that are processed in the virion to yield multiple, functionally distinct polypeptides that lead to viral assembly.

The process of transformation involves the transcription of single-stranded RNA of the diploid viral genome into viral DNA by reverse transcriptase. This viral DNA is integrated into the cellular chromosomal DNA, the unique attribute of retroviruses! The retrovirus is then able to use the machinery of the host cell to express the viral genome. During this process of viral integration, replication, and assembly, retroviruses may incorporate certain genes from their hosts in a process known as *transduction.* This transfer of cellular DNA occurs during rare recombinational events between viral DNA and cellular DNA or RNA in retrovirus-infected cells. However, the viral oncogenes are never identical to the sequence of their normal cellular homologues since the process of transduction often results in mutation, translocation, truncation, and/or other alterations in the sequences of the normal cellular genes. Conceivably, transduction of cellular sequences into retroviruses removes the transferred genes from regulatory control, allowing the transduced gene to acquire transforming potential within the retrovirus (Fig. 9.2).

Besides the so-called *dominant* oncogenes that express nuclear or cytoplasmic-localizing oncogene products, *recessive* or *tumor-suppressive* oncogenes sometimes referred to as *antioncogenes* appear to play an important role in tumorigenesis. The idea that recessive mutations

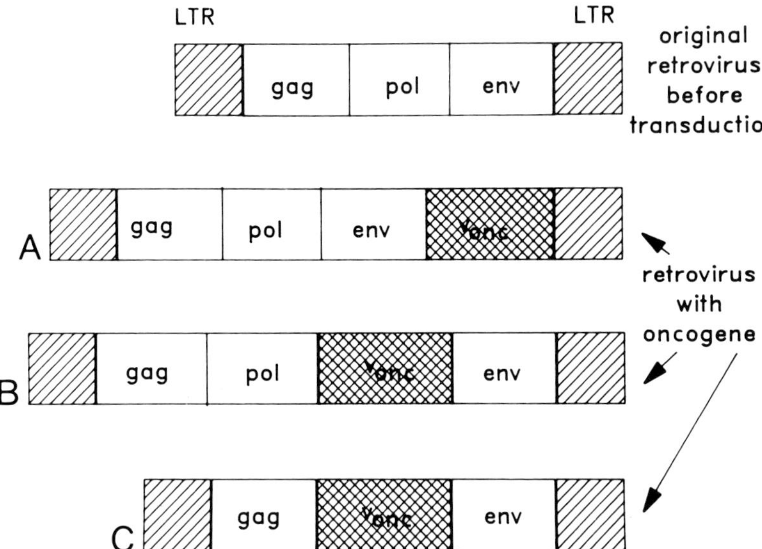

Figure 9-2 Recombination between the retroviral and host genomes can implant host genes anywhere in the viral genome. Native retroviral sequence at top. The addition of v-onc as depicted in (A) and (B) occurs without deletion of any native viral genome. In last figure (C), pol is deleted. Fenoglio-Preiser CM: *Molecular Diagnostics In Pathology.* Baltimore, Williams & Wilkins, p 83, 1991.

might underlie the tumorigenic phenotype in some cancers is supported by two observations. First, the neoplastic phenotype is often suppressed by fusion of cancer cells with normal cells, suggesting the presence of tumor suppressor genes in the normal genome. Second, karyotypic analysis of a variety of human tumors has shown consistent deletions of specific chromosomal regions suggesting loss of the normal allele of a tumor suppressor gene with a possible regulatory function. This potential expression of the recessive cancer phenotype by loss of normal alleles of certain genes has been observed not only in pediatric tumors but also in a wide variety of adult malignancies. Contrariwise, the dominant oncogenes acting by virtue of abnormal or elevated activity appear to be primarily operative in leukemias and lymphomas. There is no evidence yet that genetic predisposition to leukemia and lymphomas can be imported by oncogene mutations in the germline. However, there are conditions that predispose to these hematologic malignancies primarily through excessive chromosomal breakage and rearrangement (ataxia-telangiectasia, Bloom's syndrome, Fanconi's anemia, Kostmann's infantile agranulocytosis, glutathione reductase deficiency).

Utilization of studies on oncogenes has begun to impact on the diagnosis of the chronic leukemias and associated entities. *BCR-ABL* recombinant analysis has been most helpful in diagnosing Ph^1-negative CML and in detecting residual disease after treatment by PCR. In addition, as mentioned in the previous chapter, t(14;18) of follicular B-cell lymphoma with the associated disruption of the *BCL*-2 oncogene has been used to diagnose these cases and detect minimal residual disease by PCR. Undoubtedly, the use of aberrant oncogene function and rearrangement will be employed in multiple ways to diagnose chronic leukemias and related entities in the future.

Although it was initially thought that *activation* of homologous cellular oncogenes might lead directly to neoplasia, there is no evidence that activation of a single cellular oncogene acting alone is necessary or sufficient for production of carcinogenesis. Contrariwise to the rapid transformation to malignancy achieved by retroviruses, most human cancers develop from a succession of multiple steps occurring over many years, allegedly involving changes in expression of multiple genes. In support of this stepwise process are data that suggest that carcinogenesis results from the concerted action of several "activated" cellular oncogenes, and/or to the loss of other cellular genes that suppress the development of the tumor cell phenotype. Also, besides oncogenes, it would appear that immunosuppression of host T cells plays an important role in some hematopoietic malignancies as observed with the increased incidence of lymphoproliferative disorders in cardiac transplant recipients immunosuppressed with monoclonal antibody OKT3. Since leukemogenesis is a multistep process in which cellular oncogenes are activated by either point mutation, truncation, chromosomal translocations, overexpression, and/or underexpression, the study of oncogenes at various molecular levels will gain importance in diagnosis as our knowledge unfolds in this area.

ONCOGENE: FUNCTION, ACTIVATION, AND EXPRESSION

Oncogenes have nuclear functions and several encoding functions involving protein kinases, growth factors, growth factor receptors, G proteins, and signal transducers. Those oncogenes with nuclear function encode proteins located in the nucleus that are thought to regulate gene expression. Examples are *MYC, FOS,* and *JUN* genes. Of these the *MYC* gene is the most thoroughly studied and is intimately associated with control of proliferation and differentiation.

Those oncogenes that encode protein kinases can be divided into two functional groups: (1) those that code for intracellular protein kinases and (2) those that function as transmembrane growth factor receptors. Examples are *SRC, ABL, ERB,* and *HER* 2/neu (*ERB* B2) genes. Physiologic regulators of src-like kinase activity in any cell type are unknown; however, they are considered attractive candidates for components of signal transduction cascade. It is clear that mutated versions of these molecules, with increased kinase activity, can stimulate neoplastic growth in many cell types.

Oncogenes that encode growth factors when activated in an aberrant manner may lead to malignant transformation. Keating and Williams (1988) found that in contrast to receptor activation in normal cells, autocrine activation of platelet-derived growth factor (PDGF) receptors in v-sis transformed cells occurred in the intracellular compartments, disrupting receptor processing and diverting receptors and their precursors. Such findings demonstrate that intracellular activation of receptors by autocrine mechanisms may play a role in cell transformation. Examples of such oncogenes are *INT* and *SIS*. It has been shown that the v-sis gene is derived from genes encoding a PDGF that is 92% homologous to a potent mitogen for mesenchymal cells.

The *RAS* family of genes produce proteins that are involved in signal transduction. Ras proteins are found in a GTP-bound active state and a GDP-bound inactive state. Active ras proteins are converted to an inactive form by intrinsic guanosine triphosphatase (GTPase) activity that is stimulated by interaction with the GTPase-activating protein (GAP). Upon binding, GTP-ras proteins become activated and can stimulate cell proliferation through an unknown mechanism. Proteins encoded by oncogeneic alleles of cellular *RAS* are often mutated in a manner that decreases their intrinsic GTPase activity or their association with GAP, thus allowing the proteins to remain in an active form for a longer period of time. Examples of *RAS* genes include c-N-*RAS* on chromosome 1, c-Ha-*RAS*-1 on chromosome 11, and c-Ki-*RAS* on chromosome 12. *RAS* pseudogenes c-Ha-*RAS*-2 and c-Ki-*RAS*-1 exist on chromosomes X and 6, respectively.

Activation of c-onc's has been described at the molecular level by three basic mechanisms: (1) point mutation–insertion or deletion that changes primary structure, (2) gene amplification, and (3) gene rearrangement.

Point mutation in c-onc's may involve many oncogenes but frequently involves genes of the *RAS* family, which are the prototype. These mutations are commonly detected by DNA transfection technique (NIH/3T3) and subsequent restriction enzyme mapping or

DNA sequencing. Transfection involves transfer of donor high-molecular-weight DNA to recipient cells, usually NIH/3T3. The *RAS* genes include a family of genes that were mentioned above with further subdivisions occurring in each group. Compared with the normal cellular *RAS* protooncogene, the activated genes detected by the aforementioned assay have a single nucleotide mutation at position 12 or 13, or at position 59, 61, or 63. Apparently, this mutation renders the ras protein (p21) oncogenic.

About 15% of all human tumors including carcinomas, sarcomas, melanomas, and leukemias contain mutated c-*RAS* oncogenes that can be detected by various methods. *RAS* point mutations may be detected by PCR using mutation-specific oligonucleotide primers. Activated *RAS* genes are detected in 15–20% of patients with MDS and may be associated with transformation to acute leukemia. Also, *RAS* mutations are demonstrated in 20–30% of patients with AML, occurring more frequently in patients with acute myelomonocytic (M4) morphology. Mutations are most unusual in lymphoid malignancies, and when present usually correlate with the most undifferentiated ALL phenotype.

The incidence of *RAS* point mutations and their role in the CMLs is not entirely clear from the literature. Liu et al (1987) identified *RAS* mutations in four of six patients with Ph^1-positive CML, three occurring in the blast phase. However, larger series revealed a low incidence of *RAS* mutations (<5%), indicating that these molecular events played a minor role, if any, in Ph^1-positive CML transformation. Contrariwise, a significant incidence of *RAS* mutations has been reported in patients with CMML. Hirsh-Ginsberg et al. (1990) noted N- and K-*RAS* mutations in 14 of 24 (58%) patients with CMML, but in none among 9 patients with Ph^1-negative–*BCR*-gene-rearrangement-negative CML. In support, Padura et al. (1988) observed *RAS* mutations in 11 of 16 (69%) patients with CMML. Therefore, *RAS* mutations may play a role in the pathophysiology and diagnosis of CMML. The relationship between *RAS* mutations and the clinical course of CMML requires further investigation.

Although Ph^1-negative–*BCR*-gene-rearrangement-negative CML patients do not frequently demonstrate *RAS* gene mutations, some Ph^1-negative CMLs do show *ABL* insertion in the M-*BCR* on chromosome 22. The M-*BCR* sequences in the *BCR* gene are rearranged in these cases, and expression of one or other of the mRNA species characteristic of Ph^1-positive CML are observed. Analyzing such a case, Morris et al. (1990) were able to exclude transposon- or retroviral-mediated insertion of *ABL* into chromosome 22. Instead, they favored a two-translocation model in which a second translocation reconstituted a standard t(9;22)(q34;q11), but left the chromosome 9 insert, including 3′*ABL* in chromosome 22. In addition to the insertions noted above, rare cases of interstitial deletion and insertion in Ph[1]-positive CML have been reported. In such cases, the interstitial deleted material from chromosome 22 is inserted into another chromosome: 46,XX,der ins(11;22)(q13;q11q13). Such insertional deletions may have importance in evaluating the roles of oncogenes such as c-*ABL* and c-*SIS* in the Ph[1] rearrangement in the origin of leukemia.

Sometimes deletions of portions of oncogenes may be associated with malignancy. The t(9;22) resulting in the Ph[1] produces fusion DNA sequences consisting of the 5′ part of the major breakpoint cluster region–(M-*BCR*-1) and the *ABL* protooncogene that encodes for the p210 *BCR*/*ABL* phosphoprotein with tyrosine kinase activity implicated in the pathogenesis of CML. Rarely, detectable rearranged DNA homologous to the 5′ side bcr probe or abl-related fusion mRNA are not detected, suggesting that the bcr/abl fusion DNA has been deleted in these rare CML cases. It is suggested that replacement with other sequences occurred in a stepwise manner following the formation of the Ph[1] at any stage of the disease. Apparently, replacement of the N-terminal coding region of c-*ABL* gene is most important, since some evidence suggests that it results in a three- to fivefold increase of c-abl tyrosine kinase activity. Thus, it appears that N-terminal replacement is important in the activation of the c-*ABL* protooncogene.

Since rearrangement and amplification of c-*ABL* were described in the CML cell line K562, Daniel et al. (1987) evaluated leukemic cell DNA from 42 CML patients to determine if similar findings were present in these individuals. Surprisingly, none of the patients demonstrated amplification of c-*ABL*, and analysis of four patients during the course of their disease for c-*ABL* allele deletion was negative. Thus, amplification of c-*ABL* and loss of one c-*ABL* allele are both infrequent in CML and do not play a significant role in the course of this disease. Therefore, the K562 changes probably represent a cell line artifact. Similar findings with the c-*MYC* and c-*MYB* oncogene amplification probably also represent in vitro artifact.

While gene amplification rarely occurs in CLL, the *RAS* gene activation has been reported in infrequent cases of terminal prolymphocytic transformation of CLL.

Classic examples of oncogene rearrangement by chromosomal translocation are CML and Burkitt's lymphoma-leukemia. CML is characterized by translocation of c-*ABL* oncogene, which usually fuses into the bcr, a 5.8-kb region on the 22nd chromosome, and forms a novel chimeric *BCR-ABL* gene that produces a p210 protein.

In Burkitt's lymphoma-leukemia, one or both of the coding exons of c-*MYC* are translocated from chromosome 8 to the IgH locus on chromosome 14. This translocation is believed to cause inappropriate activation of c-*MYC* in cells that actively transcribe the IgH gene. Some cases of Burkitt's lymphoma-leukemia show translocation to chromosome 2, which contains the kappa IgL gene, or chromosome 22, which contains the lambda IgL genes. c-*ABL* and c-*MYC* are the most thoroughly studied and best understood translocated oncogenes.

Oncogene rearrangement in CLL must be rare, since Rechavi et al (1989) evaluated 38 cases of CLL for *BCL*-1, *BCL*-2, and c-*MYC* for rearrangement and none showed any abnormalities except one patient with aggressive, resistant disease with a c-*MYC* rearrangement. However, oncogene rearrangement is common in lymphomas derived from follicular center cells since 80–90% of cases evaluated reveal a t(14;18) (see Chapters 7 and 8). The IgH locus is the site of translocation that, in these cases, causes the *BCL*-2 protooncogene on chromosome 18 to be translocated and constitutively activated with resultant overproduction of the bcl-2 protein. This translocation arises, at least in part, as a result of mistakes in joining of the V, D, and J regions of the IgH locus on chromosome 14 during Ig gene rearrangemnent and a staggered double-stranded DNA break on chromosome 18.

BCL-2 encodes for an inner mitochondrial membrane protein that prolongs cell survival. It is strongly expressed in follicular lymphomas, both small cleaved cell and large cell type, and in the majority of diffuse large cell and immunoblastic lymphomas of B-cell immunophenotype. However, small lymphocytic lymphomas (well-differentiated and intermediate type) demonstrate significant, but less *BCL*-2 expression than follicular center cell lymphomas.

Those lymphocytic lymphomas formerly designated small lymphocytic lymphomas demonstrating t(11;14)(q13;q32.3) and its molecular counterpart bcl-1 rearrangements are rare outside the mantle cell lymphomas. However, there is probably a subset of PLL and multiple myeloma that contains these abnormalities. And bcl-1 sequences have been isolated from the t(11;14) breakpoint; however, these sequences do not encode a gene. Recently, a gene designated parathyroid adenomatosis 1 (*PRAD*-1) has been identified on chromosome 11q13 by virtue of its rearrangement with the parathyroid hormone locus on chromosome 11q15. The function of the *PRAD*-1 gene is deregulated by the rearrangement and has homology with cyclins, proteins implicated as regulators of the cell cycle. Interestingly, the *PRAD*-1 locus is about 200 kb from the bcl-1 locus, and the *PRAD*-1 gene apparently is overexpressed in lymphoproliferative disorders having the t(11;14). Thus, the bcl-1 locus formerly thought to represent a gene has been demoted to a mere sequence!

Translocations involving the TCR_{α} (14q11.2), TCR_{β} (7q34), or TCRγ (7p15) chain loci are seen in T-cell leukemias and lymphomas. Such translocations may activate putative protooncogenes *TCL*-1 (at 14q32 centromeric to the IgH locus), *TCL*-2 (at 11p13), or *TCL*-3 (at 10q24) depending on the reciprocal translocation site.

As discussed in Chapter 8, the PCR is ideally suited to detect small populations of malignant cells with such translocations. However, application of PCR must contend with the heterogeneity of breakpoint positions within chromosomal DNA. Since mRNA transcripts are less complex than the chimeric DNA genes, some investigators are performing PCR on mRNA. As mentioned earlier, the t(9;22) of CML and the t(14;18) of follicular B-cell lymphomas have been the most extensively analyzed by PCR techniques. The impact of such studies on prognosis in the leukemias and lymphomas awaits accumulation of more data. However, there is some evidence suggesting that oncogene implication may indicate a worse prognosis than would otherwise be expected by existing pathologic staging. Cellular oncogenes implicated in human leukemia with their chromosome location, c-onc-related protein, and cellular locale are depicted in Table 9.1.

Our future understanding of leukemogenesis will depend on our comprehension of the relationship of oncogenes to cell growth, division, and modulation. Some oncogene products are hematopoietic growth factors or growth factor receptors; others regulate cell proliferation or differentiation by diverse mechanisms. The balance between these processes currently seems to be the most likely mechanism of oncogene-related leukemogenesis. However, the answer to this conundrum is far from complete, and the numerous bits and pieces of information have fallen far short of any unifying hypothesis or central theme, if indeed one exists. Nevertheless, if the role of oncogenes in human leukemias can be more clearly defined, innovative diagnostic and therapeutic tactics may be forthcoming.

INTRODUCTION: GROWTH FACTORS

The mechanisms that control growth, differentiation, and division of hematopoietic cells remain poorly understood. In the 1960s, culture techniques utilizing semisolid microenvironments were developed that successfully supported the clonal growth of normal hematopoi-

Table 9-1 Cellular Oncogenes Implicated in Human Leukemias

Oncogenes	*Chromosome*	*Gene Product (kd)*	*Biochemical Activity*	*Function**	*Site*
MYC	8q24.1	67	Transcription factor	DNA binding	Nucleus
MYB	6q23	83	Transcription factor	DNA binding	Nucleus
ABL	9q34.1	145	Tyrosine kinase	Signal transduction	Cytoplasm
N*RAS*	1p11–13	21	GTPase	Signal transduction	Cytoplasm
H*RAS*	11p14–155	21	GTPase	Signal transduction	Cytoplasm
K*RAS*	12p12	21	GTPase	Signal transduction	Cytoplasm
FES	15q24–26	92	Tyrosine kinase	—	Cytoplasm
FOS	14q21–22	55	Transcription factor	DNA binding	Nucleus
FMS	5q34	140	Tyrosine kinase	M-CSF receptor	Membrane
SRC	1p36;20q13	60	Tyrosine kinase	—	Cytoplasm
SIS	22q11–21	28	Growth factor	PDGFB	Cytoplasm
MOS	8q11	37	Serine kinase	—	Cytoplasm
*ETS*1	11q23	51	Transcription factor	—	Nucleus
*ETS*2	21q22	56	Transcription factor	—	Nucleus
P53	17p13	53	—	—	Nucleus
PRAD-1	11q13	—	Cyclin	—	—
*BCL*2	18q21	26	—	—	Membrane/ cytoplasm
*TCL*1	14q32.1	—	—	—	—
*TCL*2	11p13	—	—	—	—
ERB B1	7p11–13		Tyrosine kinase	EGF receptor	Cytoplasm
ERB B2	17q21		Tyrosine kinase	EGF receptor	Cytoplasm
ERB A	17q21–22		—	Thyroid hormone receptor	Nucleus

Updated from Butturini A, Gale RP: Oncogenes and leukemia. *Leukemia* 4:138–160, 1990.
*M-CSF = macrophage colony-stimulating factor; PDGFB = platelet-derived growth factor beta; EGF = epidermal growth factor.

etic progenitor cells. Such systems added greatly to previous, more cumbersome in vivo assays of hematopoiesis, such as injecting hematopoietic cells into lethally irradiated mice and surveying their spleens for the appearance of hematopoietic colonies.

With the arrival of these in vitro systems, it was shown that specific glycoproteins are required for the survival, proliferation, and induction of lineage-specific differentiation in both normal and leukemic cells. Initially, growth factors defined on the myeloid differentiation pathways were termed colony-stimulating factors (CSFs) and those defined generally on lymphoid pathways were designated interleukins (ILs). However, as information accumulated, it became increasingly obvious that CSFs, ILs, and oncogenes are inextricably involved in cell growth, differentiation, and division. Indeed, even other cytokines not originally identified by their effects on hematopoietic cells such as tumor necrosis factor and transforming growth factor-beta may also have important regulatory effects on hematopoiesis.

GROWTH FACTORS: LOCATION AND FUNCTION

A number of hematopoietic factors have been identified, purified, and cloned by molecular recombinant techniques, thus enabling the production of these hematopoietic hormones in quantities sufficient for preclinical studies and for clinical application. They include erythropoietin (Ep), a physiologic regulator of erythropoiesis; granulocyte-macrophage colony-stimulating factor (GM-CSF); granulocyte colony-stimulating factor (G-CSF); interleukin-3 (IL-3); macrophage-monocyte colony-stimulating factor (M-CSF); interleukin-4 (IL-4); interleukin-5 (IL-5); and interleukin 6 (IL-6). The major growth factors are depicted in Table 9.2.

A high incidence of genes for growth factors and growth factor receptors occurs on the long arm of chromosome 5. The region 5q31 is now known to contain genes for IL-4, IL-5, c-*FMS* (the receptor for M-CSF), and PDGF receptor, in addition to the genes for IL-3, and GM-CSF. Deletions in the long arm of chromosome 5 are also frequently associated with the development of myeloid abnormalities and acute leukemias. One such disorder, the 5q− syndrome, is characterized by refractory macrocytic anemia and deletion of the region 5q31. Contrary to previous thinking, recent evidence suggests that the hematopoietic growth factors IL-3, IL-4, IL-5, IL-9, and GM-CSF loci are not deleted in the 5q− syndrome.

With the exception of Ep, the physiologic roles of these factors

Table 9-2 Growth Factors

Cytokines	*Cell sources*	*Functions*
IL-1	Monocytes-macrophages B cells Epithelial cells Fibroblasts, astrocytes Dendritic cells Keratinocytes	Endogenous pyrogen Growth factor for lymphocytes, fibroblasts, synovial cells, endothelial cells, haematopoietic cells Induction of acute-phase proteins
IL-2	Activated T cells	Growth and differentiation factor for lymphocytes and endothelial cells
IL-3, G-CSF, GM-CSF, M-CSF	Monocytes T cells	Growth factors for haematopoietic cells

Table 9-2 (continued)

Cytokines	*Cell sources*	*Functions*
IL-4	Activated T cells	Growth and differentiation factor for lymphocytes
IL-5	T cells	Eosinophil growth factor B-cell differentiation factor
IL-6	Monocytes-macrophages B cells Epithelial cells Fibroblasts, astrocytes Dendritic cells Keratinocytes	Endogenous pyrogen Growth factor for lymphocytes, fibroblasts, synovial cells, endothelial cells, haemopoietic cells Induction of acute-phase proteins Plasma cell growth factor
IL-7	Bone marrow stroma cells Spleen cells	Growth factor of pre-B and pre-T lymphocytes
IL-8	Monocytes T lymphocytes	Neutrophil chemotactic factor
IL-9	T lymphocytes	T-cell growth factor
IL-10	T lymphocytes	T-helper cell inhibitory factor Stem cell growth factor
IL-11	Stromal cells	Multifunctional regulator of hematopoiesis
Interferon (IFN)	T and NK cells	Differentiation factor for B cells Activator of NK cells and macrophages
Tumor necrosis factor (TNF) α/β	Monocytes T cells	Antivirus Cytotoxic factor Cachectin Septic shock Growth factor for haematopoietic and fibroblastic cells

Source: Fridman WH: Pathophysiology of cytokines, *Leukemia Research* 14(8):675–677, 1990, Pergamon Press.

have not yet been clearly established. However, in general (to name only a few important functions), GM-CSF stimulates granulocyte-macrophage, granulocyte, and macrophage colony factor formation in vitro and proliferation of normal human promyelocytes and myelocytes. G-CSF stimulates formation of granulocyte colonies in vitro and some granulocyte-macrophage progenitors, but the latter are not sustained beyond a few days. IL-3, also called multi-CSF, stimulates formation of the granulocyte, macrophage, eosinophil, mast cell, NK-like cell, and erythroid and multipotent colonies from murine fetal liver and bone marrow. M-CSF, CSF-1, stimulates predominantly macrophage colonies in vitro with some granulocyte component early in culture. IL-4, or B-cell stimulating factor, acts as a costimulant with anti-IgM antibodies for entry of resting B cells into DNA synthesis and increased expression of class II major histocompatibility (MHC) molecules on resting B cells. IL-5 promotes IgM secretion and proliferation by *BCL*-1 B-cell lines, induces hapten-specific IgG secretion in vitro by in vivo antigen-primed B cells, and promotes differentiation of normal B cells. It also stimulates eosinophil colony formation and differentiation in liquid culture and synergizes with GM-CSF and IL-3 in eosinophil induction in liquid culture. IL-6 has the ability to enhance Ig secretion by B lymphocytes and to induce B cells. It also supports growth of EBV infected B cells. To illustrate the complex interactions of growth factors, phagocytic modulation by CSFs is depicted in Fig. 9.3.

CHRONIC MYELOID LEUKEMIA AND RELATED DISEASES

Early in the 1980s a mechanism known as the autocrine hypothesis was formulated to explain malignant cellular proliferation. Simply stated, it postulates that malignant cells aberrantly produce self-active growth factors that exert a positive stimulatory effect on their own proliferation. Thus, the positive feedback loop formed could conceivably lead to the progressive uncontrolled cellular proliferation characteristic of the neoplastic state. With the advent of antioncogenes, this hypothesis has been expanded to include the possibility that abnormal cellular proliferation may result from the loss of normal mechanisms. Although the hypothesis is intellectually appealing, it is possible that the malignant cell growth phenomenon may occur by nonautocrine mechanisms that diminish the leukemic cells' need for CSF.

In CML, autocrine cellular growth has been postulated to be caused by the activation of c-*ABL*; however, other growth factors

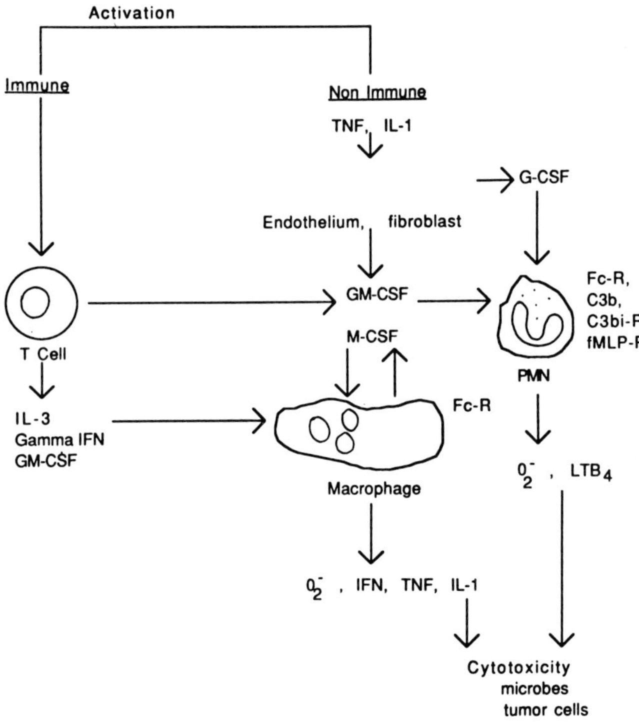

Figure 9-3 Phagocyte modulation by CSF. Weisbert RH: Hematopoietic growth factors, *Hemat Oncol Clinics* 3(3):405, 1989.

such as the PDGF encoded by c-*SIS* may also be responsible for the stimulation, progression, and variability seen during the course of this disease. Contrariwise, CML cells in culture apparently do not produce GM-CSF or IL-6 as autocrine growth factors in vitro. Also, CML cell growth in cell suspension culture in vitro appears to be independent of added GM-CSF and IL-1α. Studies using recombinant tumor necrosis factors on CML cell lines has revealed a heterogeneity of response.

In contrast, IL-6 and GM-CSF act in vitro as autocrine growth factors for CMML cells, and CMML cells in vivo may represent a GM-CSF-dependent autocrine growth system. Oncogenes *FMS* and *RAS* probably enter into the growth of CMML cells in that 20 to 58% of CMML patients show mutations of these oncogenes, respectively. Besides growth factors and oncogenes, CMML cell lines reveal a differential expression of MHC class II antigens. Such expression is linked to differential responsiveness of the cells to growth factors and inhibitors. These CMML cell lines may be a useful model to delineate the molecular basis of discordant MHC class II expression during myelomonocytic differentiation.

There is little information concerning the function of growth factors in chronic neutrophilic, monocytic, eosinophilic, basophilic, or mast cell leukemia. Nevertheless, various human lymphokines including IL-3, G-CSF, and IL-4 have been utilized to evaluate factors influencing proliferation and histamine content of cultured human bone marrow cells. Only IL-3 produced an increase in histamine in these cultured cells. The authors of this investigation concluded that basophil–mast cell differentiation in terms of augmentation of cellular histamine levels may be achieved by exposure to certain growth-inducing cytokines.

CHRONIC LYMPHOCYTIC LEUKEMIA AND RELATED DISORDERS: B-CELL DISORDERS

Recent studies on B-CLL from low-, intermediate-, and high-risk groups using methylcellulose as a semisolid media with feeder cells and/or growth factors revealed colony formation in 25 of 28 CLLs. Clonogenic cells from patients with low-risk CLL required either irradiated unstimulated T cells, with or without conditioned media, or irradiated activated T cells alone for colony formation. In contrast, clonogenic cells from patients with intermediate- and high-risk CLL required the combination of both irradiated activated T cells and conditioned media. Both the number and the size of the colonies in the intermediate- and high-risk groups were less than those of the low-risk group. This suggests that the mean cloning efficiency was reduced in these groups. None of the recombinant cytokines (IL-1–IL-7), tumor necrosis factor, alpha and gamma interferon, B-cell growth factor, and GM-CSF alone or in combination with each other could entirely replace the stimulatory effect of the activated T cells. Therefore, the clinical progression of B-CLL is associated with a loss of clonogenic potential in the circulating pool of neoplastic cells, which require as-yet-undefined factors provided by activated T cells and conditioned media. In addition to these clonogenic studies, investigations evaluating human high-molecular-weight (60 kd) B-cell growth factor by different methods have revealed that B-CLL cells are stimulated by this growth factor. Other studies have shown that CLL cells do not proliferate in response to B-cell growth factor or IL-2 when costimulated with Ig ligands. Although the mechanism is unclear, defective signaling via surface Ig cross-linking may be responsible. There is much evidence in the literature suggesting the clonal heterogeneity of CLL B-cell populations. Therefore, all data concerning growth factors on B-CLL must be interpreted with this in mind.

Studies concerning growth factors are sparse in PLL; however, B-PLL cells, like CLL B-cells, are activated when exposed to human high-molecular-weight (60 kD) B-cell growth factor. A study in one patient with B-PLL revealed that in the presence of phorbol myristate acetate, native and recombinant γ inteferon act as growth factors for B cells, and that IL-2 is not involved in this process.

HCL cells are activated when exposed to human high-molecular-weight (60 kd) B-cell growth factor. Studies involving a wide range of growth factors with HCL cells have shown that hairy cells mediate DNA synthesis of IL-4, IL-5, and IL-6 in vitro and suggest a possible autocrine in vivo role for these growth factors in the pathophysiology of HCL. Apparently, alpha interferon used as one of the treatment modalities in this disease impairs response to B-cell growth factors and induces further cellular differentiation of HCL cells.

Follicular B-cell lymphoma (large cell) cell lines have been studied from SJL mice to characterize their growth factor requirements. Numerous growth factors and cytokines with the exception of IL-7 and gamma interferon failed to have any detectable effect on the lymphoma cell line. IL-1 and gamma interferon appeared to affect B-cell growth factor–induced growth of the lymphoma cells by different mechanisms, and their combined effects were greater than that of IL-1 or gamma interferon alone.

Freshly isolated human myeloma cells have their growth augmented by IL-6, a B-cell differentiation factor, which has a wide variety of biological functions on various cells. It has been shown that myeloma cells constitutively produce IL-6 and express IL-6 receptors. Moreover, it has been revealed that anti-IL-6 antibody can inhibit the in vitro growth of the myeloma cells. These findings are direct evidence that an autocrine loop is operating in freshly isolated myeloma cells, and that a constitutive production of IL-6 and activation of the IL-6 gene could be involved in the oncogenesis of human myeloma. In addition, significant proliferation of myeloma cells after exposure to not only IL-6, but to IL-3 and IL-5, independently suggests that heterogeneity in the in vitro response of myeloma cells exists in concordance with other hematopoietic malignancies.

CHRONIC LYMPHOID LEUKEMIAS AND RELATED DISORDERS: T-CELL DISORDERS

Large granular lymphocyte (LGL) leukemia, or T-gamma lymphoproliferative disease (TGLD), represents a heterogeneous disease that is characterized by an increase of NK cells or T cells, most having the morphology of LGLs. Several cytokines have been shown to effect NK cell proliferation or cytolytic activity. Of these, IL-2 and the interferons have been the most extensively studied. The effects of IL-2 that ultimately produce augmented cytolytic activity are poorly understood. The initial reports that IL-2 exerts its effects on NK cells by stimulating autocrine secretion of interferons have been mistaken. IL-2 induces increased expression of some NK cell surface adhesion molecules, increases the number and size of NK cell cytolytic granules, and stimulates NK cell expression of mRNA for serine proteases. Elucidation of the mechanisms of NK cell activation by IL-2 is currently an area of active investigation.

T-PLLs express surface markers that are characteristic of resting mature T-helper lymphocytes. Woods et al. (1985) studied a case of T-PLL, and consistent with their helper phenotype, the leukemic cells did not produce suppressor factors but provided help for the normal B-enriched lymphocytes to respond to pokeweed mitogen as assessed by both blast transformation and IgG production. T-lymphocyte colonies developed when the leukemic cells were treated with phytohemagglutinin during a 20-hr liquid culture prior to being seeded into semisolid agar medium containing either phytohemagglutinin or an IL-2–containing lymphokine. There was no growth when untreated cells were directly seeded into IL-2–containing agar. Such findings demonstrate that in this particular case the helper T PLs share the functional capabilities of normal mature T lymphocytes as predicted from their helper phenotype. Additional investigation of growth factors in PLL are indicated to further understand the biology of this malignancy.

ATLL is endemic in Southern Japan, and some cases have been reported from the Southeastern United States, and the Caribbean Basin. The ATLL cells exhibit a number of unique growth factor interrelationships. They produce an ATLL-derived factor (ADF) that was purified from HTLV-I–infected leukemic T-cell line (ATL-2) and reported to be IL-2-receptor–inducing factor. Apparently, ADF exhibits marked synergism with other cytokines, such as IL-1 and IL-2, allowing virally infected lymphocytes to respond to suboptimal amounts of a variety of growth factors via autocrine stimulation. Additionally, a GM-CSF promoter appears to be activated by HTLV-I and HTLV-II *TAX* genes. The product of the *TAX* gene, the *TAX* protein, results in a constitutive GM-CSF production by HTLV-infected T cells. Such high levels of GM-CSF in HTLV cell lines may be due to transactivation of the GM-CSF promoter by the HTLV *TAX* protein. Expression of GM-CSF by HTLV-I–infected lymphocytes may have clinical implications since granulocytosis and eosinophilia are frequently seen in patients with HTLV-I–induced ATLL.

Rare studies on keratinocytes isolated from SS patients failed to demonstrate increased amounts of transforming growth factor alpha as observed in other patients with only psoriatic plaques. Other studies on growth factors in Ki-1 lymphoma, a cutaneous T-cell lymphoma, revealed that the malignant cells secrete transforming growth factor beta that suppresses the growth of activated human T lymphocytes. This paradox is explained by the fact that the Ki-1 lymphoma cells continue to proliferate because of defective suppression of IL-2 and related lymphokine-dependent DNA synthesis.

NEWER GROWTH FACTORS

Interleukin-7 (IL-7), a stromal cell–derived cytokine, stimulates DNA synthesis in ALL cells of B- and T-cell precursor origin. Apparently, IL-7 is involved in the complex regulation of ALL cell production. How it will relate to ALL blast crisis of CML remains to be investigated.

Interleukin-8 (IL-8), a keratinocyte-derived molecule, also known as neutrophil attractant-activation protein (NAP-1) attracts and activates human neutrophils but is not a chemoattractant for human monocytes. The role of IL-8, especially in CML, remains to be elucidated.

Interleukin-9 (IL-9) has a genomic sequence homology with a human IL-9 cDNA isolated from HTLV-I–transformed T cells by expression cloning. The IL-9 gene has been mapped to the long arm of human chromosome 5 at band 5q31–32, a region found to be deleted in a number of patients with acquired 5q− abnormalities and hematologic disorders. The 5′ regulatory region of human IL-9 gene also contains sequences identified in the 5′ flanking regions of other cytokine genes mapped to the long arm of human chromosome 5, including IL-3, IL-4, IL-5, and GM-CSF and other T-cell growth factor genes, including IL-2 and IL-6. The IL-9 gene is constitutively expressed in the HTLV-I–transformed human T cells, and the expression of IL-9 in these cells can be further induced by 12-*0*-tetradecanoylphorbol 13-acetate. Undoubtedly, understanding of IL-9 gene expression will allow us to study the regulatory mechanisms in normal and leukemic human T cells.

Interleukin-10 (IL-10) exhibits strong DNA and amino acid sequence homology to an open reading frame in the Epstein-Barr virus, BCRFI. Both human IL-10 and the BCRFI product inhibit cytokine synthesis by activated human peripheral blood mononuclear cells. Also, both human and mouse IL-10 sustain the viability of a mouse mast cell line in culture, and therefore this cytokine has implications in modulation of mastocytosis and mast cell leukemia

Interleukin-11 (IL-11), a stromal cell–derived cytokine, is capable of stimulating plasmacytoma proliferation and T-cell-dependent development of Ig-producing B cells and synergizes with IL-3 in supporting murine megakaryocyte colony formation. These properties implicate IL-11 as an additional multifunctional regulator in the hematopoietic microenvironment.

Interleukin-12 (IL-12) is a novel cytokine which, like IFN-γ and IFN-α, may be involved in protective immunity against infectious agents such as viruses. Previously known as natural killer cell stimulatory factor or cytotoxic lymphocyte maturation factor , IL-12 is a 75-kD heterodimeric glycoprotein displaying several in vitro activities including: (1) enhancement in synergy with IL-2 (2) increase in the cytotoxic activity of natural killer cells (3) promotion of the proliferation of activated T and natural killer cells (4) induction of IFN-γ production by resting or activated peripheral blood T and natural killer cells.

Indubitably, this burgeoning field of cellular biology will continue to expand at an exponential rate and most assuredly will increase our insights and understandings of this disease we call leukemia.

BIBLIOGRAPHY

Articles: Oncogenes

Ayscue LH, Ross DW, Ozer H, et al: *Bcr/abl* recombinant DNA analysis versus karyotype in diagnosis and therapeutic monitoring of chronic myeloid leukemia. *Am J Clin Pathol* 94:404–409, 1990.

Bartram CR, Ludwig WD, Hiddemann W, et al: Acute myeloid leukemia: Analysis of *ras* gene mutations and clonality defined by polymorphic X-linked loci. *Leukemia* 3:247–256, 1989.

Browett PJ, Norton JD: Analysis of *ras* gene mutations and methylation state in human leukemias. *Oncogene* 4:1029–1036, 1989.

Cooper GM: Cellular transforming genes. *Science* 217:801–806, 1982.

Daniel L, Ahmed CM, Bloodgood RS, et al: Polymorphism of the human c-*abl* gene: Relation to incidence and course of chronic myelogenous leukemia. *Oncogene* 1:193–200, 1987.

Gahrton G, Juliusson G, Robert KH, et al: Role of chromosomal abnormalities in chronic lymphocytic leukemia. *Blood Rev* 3:183–192, 1987.

Ganesan TS, Rassool F, Guo AP, et al: Rearrangement of the *bcr* gene in Philadelphia chromosome–negative chronic myeloid leukemia. *Blood* 68:957–960, 1986.

Hecht F, Morgan R, Schrier SL, et al: The Philadelphia (Ph) chromosome in leukemia: I. A new mechanism due to interstitial deletion and insertion in chronic myelocytic leukemia. *Cancer Genet Cytogenet* 14:3–10, 1985.

Heisterkamp J, Stephenson JR, Groffen J, et al: Localization of c-*abl* oncogene adjacent to a translocation break point in chronic myelocytic leukaemia. *Nature* 306:239–242, 1983.

Hirsch-Ginsberg C, LeMaistre AC, Kantarjian H, et al: *RAS* mutations are rare events in Philadelphia chromosome–negative/*bcr* gene rearrangement–negative chronic myelogenous leukemia, but are prevalent in chronic myelomonocytic leukemia. *Blood* 76:1214–1219, 1990.

Janssen JW, Steenvoorden AC, Lyons J, et al: *RAS* gene mutations in acute and chronic myelocytic leukemias, chronic myeloproliferative disorders, and myelodysplastic syndromes. *Proc Natl Acad Sci USA* 84:9228–9232, 1987.

Jin XM, Miao J, Xu Y, et al: Amplification and rearrangement of proto-oncogene c-*abl* in human leukemia cells. *Chung Hua Chung Liu Tsa Chih* 10:167–170, 1988.

Keating MT, Williams LT: Autocrine stimulation of intracellular PDGF receptors in v-*sis*-transformed cells. *Science* 239:914–916, 1988.

Knudson AG: The genetics of childhood cancer. *Bull Cancer (Paris)* 75:135–138, 1988.

Kobayashi T, Kita K, Ohno T, et al: Chronic lymphocytic leukemia in Japan. *Rinsho Ketsueki* 31:554–563, 1990.

LeMaistre A, Lee MS, Talpaz M, et al: *Ras* oncogene mutations are rare late stage events in chronic myelogenous leukemia. *Blood* 73:889–891, 1989.

Liu E, Hjelle B, Morgan R, et al: The role of mutant *ras* genes in preleukemic states (abstract). *Blood* 70:282a, 1987.

Masuda H, Battifora H, Yokota J, et al: Specificity of proto-oncogene amplification in human malignant disease. *Mol Biol Med* 4:213–217, 1987.

Morris CM, Heisterkamp N, Kennedy MA, et al: Ph-negative chronic myeloid leukemia: Molecular analysis of *ABL* insertion into M-*BCR* on chromosome 22. *Blood* 9:1812–1818, 1990.

Ohyashiki K, Ohyashiki JH, Iwabuchi H, et al: Philadelphia chromosome–positive chronic myelogenous leukemia with deleted fusion of *BCR* and *ABL* genes. *Jpn J Cancer Res* 81:35–42, 1990.

Padua RA, Carter G, Hughes D, et al: *RAS* mutations in myelodysplasia detected by amplification, oligonucleotide hybridization, and transformation. *Leukemia* 2:503–510, 1988.

Piwnica-Worms H, Saunders KB, Roberts TM, et al: Tyrosine phosphorylation regulates the biochemical and biological properties of pp60c-svc. *Cell* 49:75–82, 1987.

Rabbitts RH, Forster A, Matthews JG: The breakpoint of the Philadelphia chromosome 22 in chronic myeloid leukaemia is distal to the immunoglobulin lambda light chain constant region genes. *Mol Biol Med* 1:119–129, 1983.

Rassool F, Martiat P, Taj A, et al: Interstitial insertion of varying amounts of *ABL*-containing genetic material into chromosome 22 in Ph-negative CML. *Leukemia* 4:273–277, 1990.

Rechavi G, Katzir N, Brok-Simoni F, et al: A search for bcl1, bcl2, and c-*myc* oncogene rearrangements in chronic lymphocytic leukemia. *Leukemia* 3:57–60, 1989.

Swinnen LJ, Constanzo-Nordin MR, Fisher SG, et al: Increased incidence of lymphoproliferative disorder after immunosuppression with the monoclonal antibody OKT3 in cardiac-transplant recipients. *N Engl J Med* 323:1723–1728, 1990.

Tabin CJ, Bradley SM, Bargmann CI, et al: Mechanism of activation of a human oncogene. *Nature* 300:143–149, 1982.

Varmus HE: Form and function of retroviral proviruses. *Science* 216:812–820, 1982.

Wang JY: Negative regulation of c-*abl* tyrosine kinase by its variable N-terminal amino acids. *Oncogene Res* 3:293–298, 1988.

Willman CL, Whittaker MH: The molecular biology of acute myeloid leukemia. *Clin Lab Med* 10:769–796, 1990.

Review Articles: Oncogenes

Bishop JM: Viral oncogenes. *Cell* 42:23–38, 1985.

Bos JL: The *ras* gene family and human carcinogenesis. *Mutat Res* 195:255–271, 1988.

Butturini A, Gale RP: Oncogenes and human leukemias. *Int J Cell Cloning* 6:2–24, 1988.

Butturini A, Sthivelman E, Canaani E, et al: Oncogenes in human leukemias. *Acta Haematol (Basel)* 78 (suppl 1):2–10, 1987.

Butturini A, Sthivelman E, Canaani E, et al: Oncogenes in human leukemias. *Cancer Invest* 6:305–316, 1988.

Fenoglio-Preiser CM, Listrom MB: Oncogenes: Introduction. In Fenoglio-Preiser CM, Willman CL: *Molecular Diagnostics in Pathology.* Baltimore, Williams & Wilkins, 1991, pp 81–110.

Gahrton G, Juliusson G, Robert KH, et al: Role of chromosomal abnormalities in chronic lymphocytic leukemia. *Blood Rev* 1:183–192, 1987.

Nowell PC, Croce CM: Chromosomal approaches to oncogenes and oncogenesis. *FASEB J* 2:3054–3060, 1988.

Rattfield M, Jaffe ES: bcl-1, t(11;14) and mantle cell derived lymphomas: *Blood* 78:259–263, 1991.

Zbar B: Evidence for a recessive oncogene on human chromosome 3. In Cossman J: *Molecular Genetics in Cancer Diagnosis*. New York, Elsevier, 1990, pp 369–380.

Articles: Growth Factors

Barut BA, Cochran MK, O'Hara C, et al: Response patterns of hairy cell leukemia to B-cell mitogens and growth factors. *Blood* 76:2091–2097, 1990.

Brantschen S, de Weck AL, Stadler BM: Factors influencing proliferation and histamine content of cultured human bone marrow cells. *Immunobiology* 179:271–282, 1989.

Brodsky I, Hubbel HR, Strayer DR, et al: Implications of retroviral and oncogene activity in chronic myelogenous leukemia. *Cancer Genet Cytogenet* 26:15–23, 1987.

Dadmarz R, Rabinowe SN, Cannistra SA, et al: Association between clonogenic cell growth and clinical risk group in B-cell chronic lymphocytic leukemia. *Blood* 76:142–149, 1990.

Everson MP, Brown CB, Lilly MB: Interleukin-6 and granulocyte-macrophage colony-stimulating factor are candidate growth factors for chronic myelomonocytic leukemia cells. *Blood* 74:1472–1476, 1989.

Kiniwa M, Gately M, Gubler U, et al: Recombinant interleukin-12 suppresses the synthesis of immunoglobulin E by interleukin-4 stimulated human lymphocytes. *J Clin Invest* 90:262–270, 1992.

Lee F, Yokota T, Otsuka T, et al: Isolation and characterization of a mouse interleukin cDNA clone that expresses B-cell stimulatory factor 1 activities and T-cell- and mast-cell-stimulating activities. *Proc Natl Acad Sci USA* 83:2061–2065, 1986.

Lin FK, Suggs S, Lin CH, et al: Cloning and expression of the human erythropoietin gene. *Proc Natl Acad Sci USA* 82:7580–7584, 1985.

Nagata S, Tsuchiya M, Asano S, et al: Molecular cloning and expression of cDNA for human granulocyte colony-stimulating factor. *Nature* 319:415–418, 1986.

Newcom SR, Kadin ME, Ansari AA: Production of transforming growth factor-beta activity by Ki-1 positive lymphoma cells and analysis of its role in the regulation of Ki-1 positive lymphoma growth. *Am J Pathol* 131:569–577, 1988.

Nickoloff BJ, Mitra RS, Elder JT, et al: Decreased growth inhibition by recombinant gamma interferon is associated with increased transforming growth factor-alpha production in keratinocytes cultured from psoriatic lesions. *Br J Dermatol* 121:161–174, 1989.

Nimer SD, Gasson JC, Hu K, et al: Activation of the GM-CSF promoter by HTLV-I and -II tax proteins. *Oncogene* 4:671–676, 1989.

Ridge SA, Worwood M, Oscier D, et al: FMS mutations in myelodysplastic, leukemic, and normal subjects. *Proc Natl Acad Sci USA*

87:1377–1380, 1990.
Sanderson CJ, O'Garra A, Warren DJ, et al: Eosinophil differentiation factor also has B-cell growth factor activity: Proposed name interleukin 4. *Proc Natl Acad Sci USA*. 83:437–440, 1986.
Sporn MB, Roberts AB: Autocrine growth factors and cancer. *Nature* 313:745–747, 1985.
Uckun FM, Fauci AS, Chandan-Langlie M, et al: Detection and characterization of human high molecular weight B cell growth factor receptors on leukemic B cells in chronic lymphocytic leukemia. *J Clin Invest* 84:1595–1608, 1989.
Wakasugi N, Tagaya Y, Wakasugi H, et al: Adult T-cell leukemia derived factor/thioredoxin, produced by both human T-lymphotropic virus type I and Epstein-Barr virus transformed lymphocytes, acts as an autocrine growth factor and synergizes with interleukin 1 and interleukin 2. *Proc Natl Acad Sci USA* 87:8282–8286, 1990.
Wang Z, Gao XZ, Preisler HD: Studies of the proliferation and differentiation of immature myeloid cells in vitro: I. Chronic myelogenous leukemia. *Am J Hematol* 30:77–81, 1989.
Wong GG, Temple PA, Leary AC, et al: Human CSF-1: Molecular cloning and expression of 4-kb cDNA encoding the human urinary protein. *Science* 235:1504–1508, 1987.
Wong GG, Witek-Giannotti JS, Temple PA, et al: Stimulation of murine hemopoietic colony formation by human IL-6. *J Immunol* 140:3040–3044, 1988.
Woods GM, Sawyer PJ, Kirov SM, et al: Functional and phenotypic analysis of a T cell prolymphocytic leukemia. *Leuk Res* 9:587–596, 1985.
Yang YC, Ciarletta AB, Temple PA, et al: Human IL-3 (multi-CSF): Identification by expression cloning of a novel hematopoietic growth factor related to murine IL-3. *Cell* 47:3–10, 1986.

Review Articles: Growth Factors

Andreeff M, Welte K: Hematopoietic colony stimulating factors. *Semin Oncol* 16:211–229, 1989.
Chiu IM: Growth factor genes as oncogenes. *Mol Chem Neuropathol* 10:37–52, 1989.
Clark SC, Kamen R: The human hematopoietic colony-stimulating factors. *Science* 236:1229–1237, 1987.
Demetri GD, Griffin JD: Hemopoietins and leukemia. *Hematol Oncol Clin North Am* 3:535–553, 1989.
Fridman WH, Michon J: Pathophysiology of cytokines. *Leuk Res* 14:675–677, 1990.
Goldstone AH, Khwaja A: The role of haemopoietic growth factors in bone marrow transplantation. *Leuk Res* 14:721–729, 1990.

Kawano M, Kuramoto A, Hirano T, et al: Cytokines as autocrine growth factors in malignancies. *Cancer Surv* 8:905–919, 1989.

Kelleher K, Bean K, Clark SC, et al: Human interleukin-9: Genomic sequence, chromosomal location, and sequences essential for its expression in human T-cell leukemia virus (HTLV)-I-transformed human T cells. *Blood* 77:1436–1441, 1991.

Lang RA, Burgess AW: Autocrine growth factors and tumorigenic transformation. *Immunol Today* 11:244–249, 1990.

Lee F: Growth factors controlling the development of hemopoietic cells. *Prog Clin Biol Res* 352:385–390, 1990.

Leonard EJ, Yoshimura T: Human monocyte chemoattractant protein-1 (MCP-1). *Immunol Today* 11:97–101, 1990.

Metcalf D: Haemopoietic growth factors 2: Clinical applications. *Lancet* 1:885–887, 1989.

Metcalf D: The molecular control of cell division, differentiation commitment and maturation in haemopoietic cells. *Nature* 339:27–30, 1989.

Moore MA: Hematopoietic growth factors in cancer. *Cancer* 65:836–844, 1990.

Olsson I, Olofsson T: Tumor associated myelopoiesis inhibiting factors. *Leuk Res* 14:715–716, 1990.

Paul SR, Bennett F, Calvetti JA, et al: Molecular cloning of a cDNA encoding interleukin 11, a stromal cell–derived lymphopoietic and hematopoietic cytokine. *Proc Natl Acad Sci USA* 87:7512–7516, 1990.

Paul SR, Yang YC, Donahue RE, et al: Stromal cell–associated hematopoiesis: Immortalization and characterization of a primate bone marrow–derived stromal cell line. *Blood* 77:1723–1733, 1991.

Quesenberry P, Souza L, Krantz S: *Growth Factors.* Education Program. American Society of Hematology, 1989, pp 98–113.

Raso V: Growth factors and other ligands. *Cancer Treat Res* 37:297–320, 1988.

Robertson MJ, Ritz J: Biology and clinical relevance of human natural killer cells. *Blood* 76:2421–2438, 1990.

Testa NG, Dexter TM: Haemopoietic growth factors and haematological malignancies. *Baillieres Clin Endocrinol Metab* 4:177–189, 1990.

Thompson-Snipes L, Dhar V, Bond MW, et al: Interleukin 10: A novel stimulatory factor for mast cells and their progenitors. *J Exp Med* 173:507–510, 1991.

Touw I, Pouwels K, van Agthoven T, et al: Interleukin-7 is a growth factor of precursor B and T acute lymphoblastic leukemia. *Blood* 75:2097–2101, 1990.

Vieira P, de Waal-Malefyt R, Dang MN, et al: Isolation and expression of human cytokine synthesis inhibitory factor cDNA clones: Homology to Epstein-Barr virus open reading frame BCRFI. *Proc Natl Acad Sci USA* 88:1172–1176, 1991.

CASE 1

PATIENT: 39-year-old white male.

CHIEF COMPLAINT: Abdominal discomfort, night sweats, and weakness of 4 weeks' duration.

MEDICAL HISTORY: The patient was a librarian and maintained a full and energetic routine prior to onset of symptoms.

PHYSICAL EXAMINATION: Nontender splenomegaly was detected 6.0 cm below the left costal margin. No evidence of hepatomegaly, adenopathy, or bone tenderness.

LABORATORY RESULTS:

A. *Screening Procedure*
   WBC of 46.7 × 10^9/L with a differential count of segmented neutrophils 32%, band forms 5%, metamyelocytes 4%, myelocytes 15%, promyelocytes 2%, myeloblasts 3%, eosinophils 4%, basophils 5%, monocytes 9%, and lymphocytes 21%. HGB 10.6 g/dL. HCT 0.31 L/L. MCV 99 fL, MCH 31.0 pg, MCHC 33.7 g/dL, RDW 13.5. Platelets 510 × 10^9/L, MPV 7.1 fL.

HOSPITAL COURSE: Following examination of the peripheral blood film (Case 1.1A), a diagnosis of CML was considered, and a fresh blood sample obtained for cytochemical analysis. A unilateral iliac crest bone marrow biopsy was performed, and an aliquot was

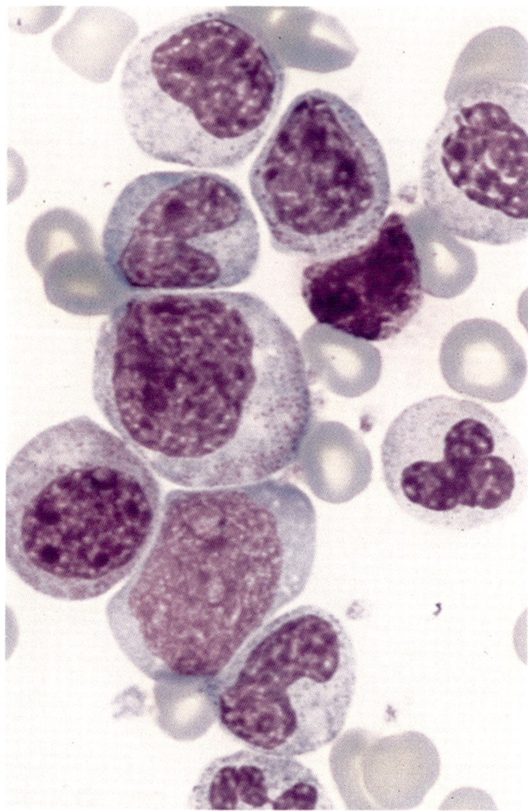

Case 1-1 (a) Peripheral blood film at diagnosis, with myeloblast, myelocytes, and metamyelocytes. (×1000).

submitted for cytogenetic evaluation. Following the retrieval of confirmatory laboratory data, the patient was started on a course of busulfan. This resulted in a drop in the white cell count and reduction of spleen size. Subsequently, the patient was followed in the oncology clinic and had not undergone metamorphosis 24 months from diagnosis.

QUESTIONS:

1. On examination of the peripheral blood film, what is the differential diagnosis?
2. What tests performed on the day of admission can be used to make a preliminary diagnosis?
3. What laboratory test firmly establishes the diagnosis?

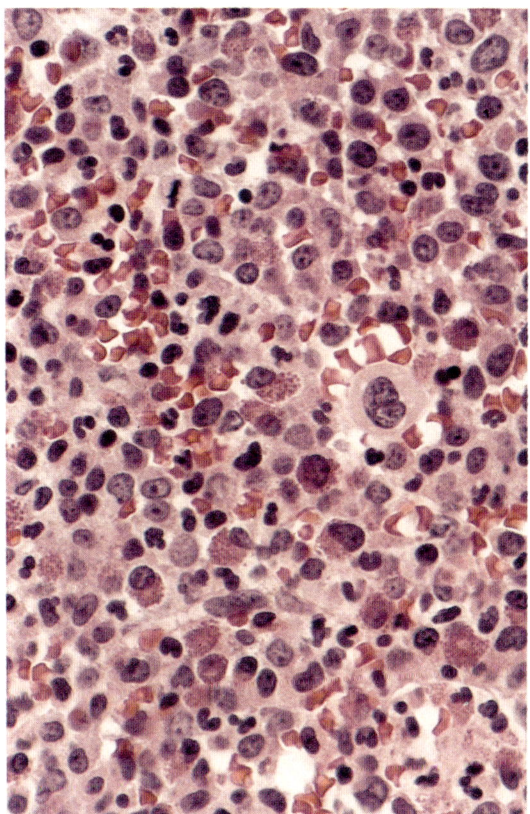

Case 1-1 (b) Hypercellular bone marrow biopsy with myeloid predominance. (×400).

LABORATORY RESULTS:

B. *Confirmatory Results*

Cytochemical evaluation: The leukocyte alkaline phosphatase score was 8.

Bone marrow examination: The marrow was hypercellular (Case 1.1B) with a fat/cell ratio of 20:80, and was myeloid predominant with a myeloid/erythroid ratio of 12:1. The myeloblast count was 3%, and myelocyte and neutrophil numbers were increased. No Auer rods, sea-blue histiocytes, or myelofibrosis was identified.

Cytogenetics: 46XY. Ph^1 chromosome identified.

DIAGNOSIS: Chronic myeloid leukemia.

DISCUSSION: CML is a clonal neoplasm of pleuripotential hematopoietic stem cell origin and accounts for about 15–20% of all human leukemia. The earliest descriptions of this myeloproliferative disease were by Bennett and Virchow in 1845. CML is slightly more prevalent in males, and each year about 3400 new cases are diagnosed in the United States. The median age at diagnosis is 53 years. Although CML is primarily a disease of adults, 10% of cases occur in childhood and adolescents and account for about 3% of childhood leukemias.

The characteristic features of CML are splenomegaly, leukocytosis with decreased LAP activity, myeloid predominance of the bone marrow, presence of the Ph^1 chromosome, and an increase in serum B_{12} binding proteins.

In most cases, the natural history of CML evolves through a chronic and accelerated phase and ultimately terminates in the clinicopathologic state of blast crisis. It is not unusual, however, for the diagnosis to be first established in accelerated phase or during blast crisis and, rarely, with Auer rods in circulating myeloblasts. Splenomegaly develops in about 90% of patients, and adenopathy is usually a manifestation of leukemic infiltration or chloroma. Other than the long-term results of bone marrow transplantation, which are too early to ascertain at this time, the overall prognosis of CML for all age groups is about 36 months.

Leukocytosis is invariably present at diagnosis, and the total leukocyte count is usually $>25.0 \times 10^9/L$. In >50% of cases the total leukocyte count is above $100.0 \times 10^9/L$. Concurrent eosinophilia, basophilia, or monocytosis may be present, and such changes, especially in patients with a normal or minimally elevated white count, may be a clue to the diagnosis. "Pelgeroid" granulocytic changes with round or bilobed nuclei may be evident, and the cytoplasmic content of basophils decreased. Occasionally, granulocytes with abnormal eosinophilic and basophilic granules are present. During the chronic phase of CML, the peripheral blood smear reveals myeloid immaturity, usually with less than 3% myeloblasts, and varying number of promyelocytes, myelocytes, metamyelocytes, band forms, and neutrophils. Invariably, myelocytes and neutrophils predominate. In >50% of cases, the platelet count is increased, and counts as high as $1{,}000{,}000 \times 10^9/L$ may be encountered. Occasionally, platelet clumping and giant platelets are observed. The presence of poikilocytosis, tear drop erythrocytes, and circulating NRBC are often a sign of evolving myelofibrosis. LAP activity is characteristically decreased in CML, and the presence of a low LAP score can serve as an adjunct to rapid diagnosis. Other cytochemical reactions including the myeloperoxidase, specific esterase (Leder), and SBB remain unaffected in CML, and immunophenotyping of leukemic cells is generally not necessary to establish the diagnosis in the chronic and accelerated phases of disease.

The bone marrow in CML is myeloid-predominant, and the M/E ratio is usually >10:1. The profile of myeloid maturation may be strikingly similar to that in the peripheral blood, with myelocytes and neutrophils predominating, and <5% myeloblasts. Megakaryocyte numbers are usually increased, and they are mostly small, mature, and lacking in the prominent nuclear lobation (endoreduplication) observed in some of the other myeloproliferative disorders. Erythropoiesis is often decreased and normoblastic, but may occasionally be megaloblastoid or megaloblastic. Mast cell numbers are generally increased, and less frequently, large blue histiocytes (pseudo-Gaucher cells) may be interspersed between other cellular elements. As with the other chronic leukemias, a unilateral iliac crest bone marrow biopsy is adequate to evaluate quantitative abnormalities in CML. Hypercellularity is common and may approach 100%. In about 50% of patients, varying degrees of reticulin fibrosis may be first observed during the chronic and accelerated phases of disease (Case 1.2A).

Several staging systems have been proposed for CML and are discussed further in Chapter 3. It is particularly important, however, to identify CML that has undergone metamorphosis to an accelerated, acute, or blastic growth phase and thereby avert misdiagnosis. Metamorphosis has been well described by Spiers (1979) and is of both therapeutic and prognostic significance. During the accelerated phase, the myeloblast content in the bone marrow increases to between 5 and 30% and on transition to blast crisis is >30%. Progressive splenomegaly, anemia, and thromobocytosis invariably accompany metamorphosis, and additionally fever and resistance to therapy are often manifest. Blast crisis is myeloblastic in about 70% of cases (Case 1.2B) and lymphoblastic in 20–30%. In fewer instances, blast crisis is either erythroblastic, megakaryoblastic, monoblastic, or of mixed lineage. In most examples of lymphoblastic crisis (Case 1.3A), blast forms display FAB L1 or L2 morphology, and are usually pre-B phenotye, CALLA+, and Tdt+ (Case 1.3B) and reveal Ig gene rearrangement. Less frequently, the process is of T phenotype and, on Southern blot analysis, reveals β-TCR gene rearrangement. Additional cytochemical analysis, immunophenotyping, and electron microscopy may be necessary to accurately classify blast crisis in any given case. The phenotypic diversity observed in blast crisis is ex-

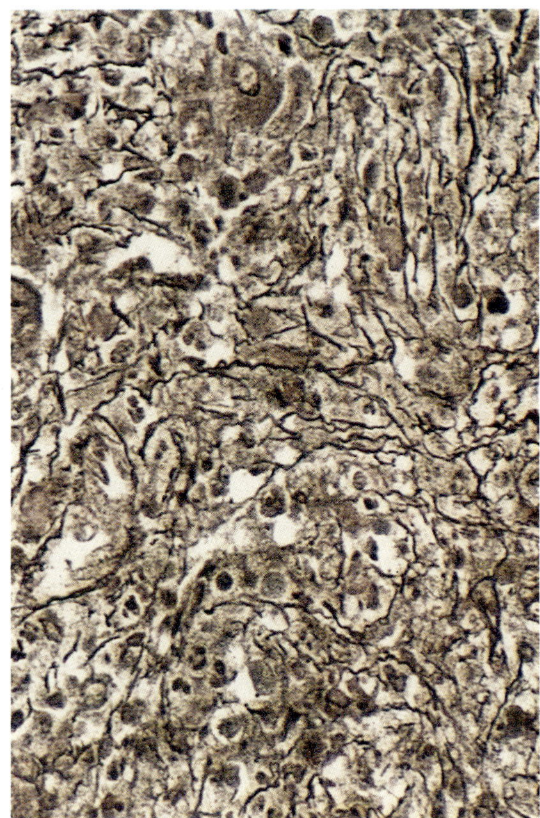

Case 1-2 (a) Increased reticulin in bone marrow biopsy during chronic phase of CML. (×400).

plained by the monoclonal origin of CML from a pleuripotential stem cell, and by the ability of tumor cells to differentiate along one or more cell lines.

In 1960, Nowell and Hungerford described an abnormal G-group chromosome in two patients with CML. This was named the Philadelphia chromosome and abbreviated Ph^1 in anticipation of other likely companion abnormalities. Thirteen years later, using banding techniques, Rowley (1973) ascertained that the Ph^1 chromosome results from a translocation abnormality involving chromosome 22. More recently, molecular genetic studies have confirmed that the basic abnormality is reciprocal translocation of genetic material between the proto oncogene c-*abl* on the long arm of chromosome 9,

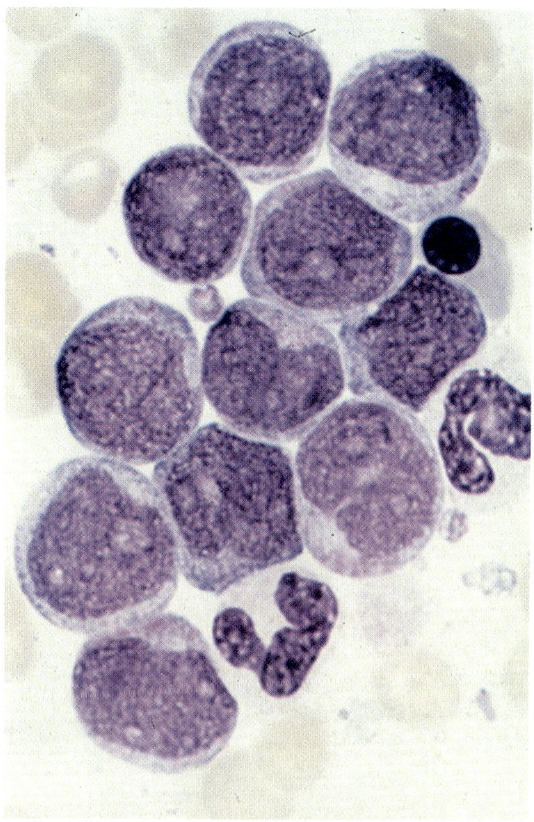

Case 1-2 (b) Myeloblastic crisis of CML. Bone marrow aspirate. (×1000).

and a portion of the *BCR* gene on the long arm of chromosome 22, resulting in the formation of a chimeric *BCR-ABL* gene on chromosome 22 in all hemtaopoietic marrow elements. In studies predating the era of *BCR* technology, the Ph^1 chromosome remained undetectable by conventional karyotyping in about 8% of patients with CML. In the majority of such cases, *BCR-ABL* fusion can be identified. Hence the number of true Ph^1-negative CML cases is either very small or nonexistent according to some observers. It is important, therefore, that all suspected cases that are Ph^1-negative by conventional karyotyping be further tested for *BCR-ABL* fusion. During metamorphosis and blast crisis, additional chromosomal abnormalities develop and include increase in the modal chromosome numbers to between 47 and 50, acquisition of a second Ph^1 chromosome, an isochromosome for the long arm of chromosome 17 [i(17q)], +8 (tri-

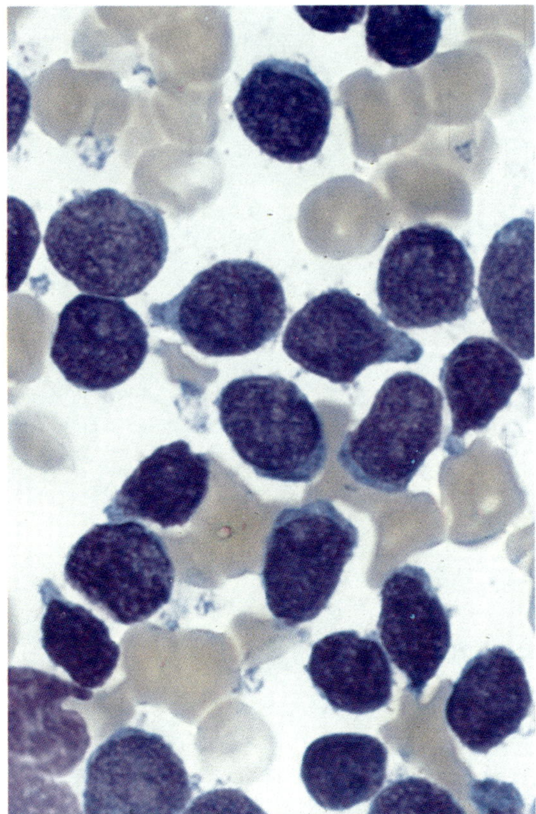

Case 1-3 (a) Lymphoblastic crisis of CML with ALL-L1 morphology. (×1000).

somy 8), +19, and t(15;17). Rarely, chromosome loss, such as, −7 and Y chromosomal deletion, may be observed.

The pathogenesis of CML is poorly understood at the present time. However, following G6PD isoenzyme studies in female heterozygotes, karyotypic analysis in constitutional mosaics, and chromosome 22 satellite studies in parents and propositi, the monoclonal nature of CML has been established. Since *BCR-ABL* fusion is known to precede leuocytosis in the evolution of CML, it is apparent that the events that precede the development of this chimeric gene remain uncertain. No viral or chemical leukemogen has been identified. However, in persons exposed to radiation from atomic detonation and therapeutic radiation, the incidence of CML is greater than in comparable populations. Transcription of a hybrid 8.5-kb mRNA which is controlled by the chimeric *BCR-ABL* gene results in the pro-

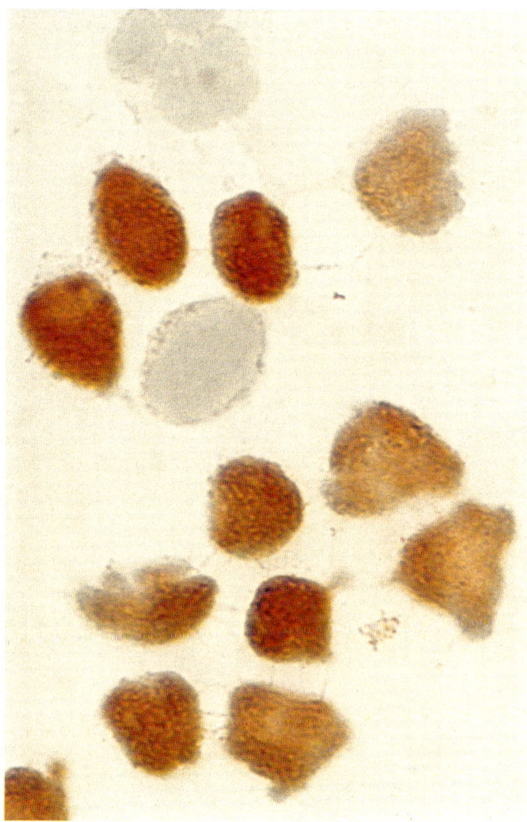

Case 1-3 (b) Lymphoblastic crisis of CML. Note Tdt+ cells. PAP (×1000).

duction of a p^{210} bcr-abl protein with enhanced tyrosine kinase activity. This has been associated with CSF, PDGF, and possibly other growth-regulating properties and appears to be responsible for increasing the granulocyte pool up to 150 times normal in CML. The role, if any, of the HLA antigens CW3 and CW4, which are more prevalent in patients with CML, remains uncertain, and the recent identification of a chimeric *BCR-ABL* gene in transgenic mice with a disease similar to human CML is of additional interest.

Since a variety of heterogeneous disorders may simulate CML, careful clinicopathologic correlation is recommended in every case. Included in the differential diagnosis are other cases of granulocytosis such as infections, granulocytic leukemoid reactions, CNL; other causes of eosinophilia, basophilia, and monocytosis; and alterations in bone marrow cellularity and composition resulting in myeloid hyperplasia, maturation arrest, and panmyelosis.

In granulocytic leukemoids, toxic granulation and Döhle bodies may be present, and in leukoerythroblastic reactions, associated causes such as myelofibrosis, metastatic carcinoma, or granulomata involving the bone marrow are usually apparent. Due to their tinctorial properties and relative sparsity of distribution in the bone marrow, pseudo-Gaucher cells may be distinguished from Gaucher cells. However, cytochemical stains may occasionally be necessary to make this distinction and are discussed further by Ulirsch (1985). Mast cells in the bone marrow may also be increased in certain low-grade lymphomas and Waldenströms macroglobulinemia. Distinguishing these entities from CML is, however, seldom a problem. Appearances of the bone marrow biopsy may be occasionally indistinguishable from those of polycythemia vera, agnogenic myeloid metaplasia, and essential thrombocythemia. In these disorders, and particularly in essential thrombocythemia, megakaryocytic endoreduplication may be quite prominent. In this latter disorder, megakaryocytic abutment is often striking and perimegakaryocytic reticulin frequently present. Myelophthisic red cell changes in the peripheral blood are frequently present in agnogenic myeloid metaplasia, and in polycythemia vera stainable iron usually absent. It is noteworthy that the Ph^1 chromosome is absent in these other examples of myeloproliferative disease.

As monocytosis is also a feature of CMML and may clinically simulate CML, differentiating these disorders is important. Trilineage myelodysplasia is frequently apparent in CMML and is seldom if ever observed in CML. Furthermore, the Ph^1 chromosome is absent in CMML. Cases hitherto designated as Ph^1-negative CML may in some instances be more appropriately classified as CMML. Such cases have hitherto accounted for about 8% of patients originally classified as CML and when lacking basophilia and pronounced monocytosis have been considered atypical forms of CML. Unexplained basophilia and eosinophilia should always arouse suspicion of associated CML. Some such cases have been designated as chronic basophilic leukemia and chronic eosinophilic leukemia. In the evaluation of such cases, testing for the Ph^1 chromosomes and *BCR-ABL* rearrangement is invaluable.

Occasionally, extramedullary forms of blast crisis (chloroma) may be the first manifestation of CML. In some such cases, although the microscopic appearances of the peripheral blood and bone marrow may not be diagnostic of CML, the Ph^1 chromosome is invariably demonstrable. Chloromas may develop in lymph nodes, skin, breast, bone, nervous system, serous membranes, and gastrointestinal tract and are composed of a myeloblastic proliferation with interspersed eosinophilic myelocytes. Since the Ph[1] chromosome has been identified in such chloroma-associated eosinophils, their identity as neoplastic components has now been established. The specific esterase (Leder) stain which is positive in chloroma remains the most effective means of differentiating this entity from lymphoma. In some cases, however, immunophenotyping may be of additional value.

SUMMARY

Peripheral Blood Film	**Leukocytosis with myeloid immaturity and <5% myeloblast**
Bone Marrow Biopsy	**Hypercellular marrow with myeloid predominance and variable reticulin fibrosis at diagnosis**
Cytochemistry	**Decreased LAP score on peripheral blood neutrophils**
Cytogenetics	**Ph[1] chromosome or *BCR-ABL* rearrangement in virtually all cases**
Serum B_{12} Binding Proteins	**Increased**
Diagnosis	**Chronic myeloid leukemia**

ANSWERS:

1. Reactive granulocytosis, leukemoid reaction, CMML, and CML.
2. The bone marrow aspirate and LAP score. Correlative data from these studies are valuable in making a preliminary diagnosis.
3. Detection of the Ph[1] chromosome or *BCR-ABL* rearrangement firmly establishes a diagnosis of CML and excludes other considerations from the differential diagnosis.

BIBLIOGRAPHY

Articles:

Battelheim P, Lutz D, Majdic O, et al: Cell lineage heterogeneity in blast crisis of chronic myeloid leukemia. *Br J Haematol* 59:395–409, 1985.

Bennet JH: Case of hypertrophy of the spleen and liver in which death took place from suppuration of the blood. *Edin Med Surg J* 64: 413, 1845.

Bloomfield CD, Lindquist LL, Brunning RD, et al: The Philadelphia chromosome in acute leukemia. *Virchows Arch Cell Pathol* 29:81–91, 1978.

Canaani E, Gale RG, Steiner-Saltz D, et al: Altered transcription of an oncogene in chronic myeloid leukemia. *Lancet* 1:593–595, 1984.

Chikkappa G, Wang GJ, Santella D, et al: Granulocyte colony-stimulating factor (G-CSF) induces synthesis of alkaline phosphatase in neutrophilic granulocytes of chronic myelogenous leukemia patients. *Leuk Res* 12:491–498, 1988.

Cutler, SJ, Young JL: *Third National Cancer Survey: Incidence Data.* National Cancer Institute Monograph 41. Washington, DC, US Government Printing Office, 1975.

Dakmezian R, Katarjian HM, Keating MJ: The relevance of reticulin stain measured fibrosis at diagnosis in chronic myelogenous leukemia. *Cancer* 59:1739–1743, 1987.

Fialkow PJ, Gartler SM, Yoshida A: Clonal origin of chronic myeloid leukemia in man. *Proc Natl Acad Sci, USA* 58:1468–1471, 1967.

Fialkow PJ, Jacobson RJ, Papayannopoulou T: Chronic myeloid leukemia: Clonal origin in a stem cell common to the granulocyte, erythrocyte, platelet and monocyte/macrophage. *Am J Med* 63:125–130, 1977.

Fitzgerald PH, Beard ME, Morris CM, et al: Ph-negative chronic myeloid leukemia. *Br J Haematol* 66:311–314, 1987.

Freedman MH, Estrov Z, Chan HSL: Juvenile chronic myelogenous leukemia. *Am J Pediatr Hematol Oncol* 10:261–267, 1988.

Galbraith PR, Abu-Zahra HT: Granulopoiesis in chronic granulocytic leukaemia. *Br J Haematol* 22:135–143, 1972.

Ganesan TS, Rassool F, Guo A-P, et al: Rearrangement of the *bcr* gene in Philadelphia chromosome–negative chronic myeloid leukemia. *Blood* 68:957–960, 1986.

Groffen J, Voncken JW, van-Schaick, et al: Animal models for chronic myeloid leukemia and acute lymphoblastic leukemia. *Leukemia* 6:44–46, 1992.

Heisterkamp N, Stephenson JR, Groffen J, et al: Localization of the c-*abl* oncogene adjacent to a translocation breakpoint in chronic myelocytic leukaemia. *Nature* 306:239–242, 1983.

Inokuchi K, Inoue T, Tojo A, et al: A possible correlation between the type of *bcr-abl* hybrid messenger RNA and platelet count in Philadelphia-positive chronic myelogenous leukemia. *Blood* 78: 3125–3127, 1991.

Jacknow G, Frizzera G, Gajl-Peczalska K, et al: Extramedullary presentation of the blast crisis of chronic myelogenous leukemia. *Br J Haematol* 561:225–236, 1985.

Kapadia SB, Krause JR, Pan SF, et al: Chronic granulocytic leukemia occurring in blast crisis. *Arch Pathol Lab Med* 103:291–292, 1979.

Kantarjian HM, Keating MJ, Smith TL, et al: Proposal for a simple synthesis prognostic staging system in chronic myelogenous leukemia. *Am J Med* 88:1–8, 1990.

Kantarjian HM, Kurzrock R, Talpaz M: Philadelphia chromosome-negative chronic myelogenous leukemia and chronic myelomonocytic leukemia. *Hematol Oncol Clin North Am* 4:389–404, 1990.

Kowal-Vern A, Birdsong BA, Dizikes G, et al: Lymphoblastic crisis of chronic myelogenous leukemia. *Arch Pathol Lab Med* 114:676–678, 1990.

Kurzrock R, Kantarjian HM, Shtalrid M, et al: Philadelphia chromosome–negative chronic myelogenous leukemia without breakpoint cluster region rearangement: A chronic myeloid leukemia with a distinct clinical course. *Blood* 75:445–452, 1990.

Lazzarino M, Morra E, Castello A, et al: Myelofibrosis in chronic granulocytic leukaemia: Clinicopathological correlation and prognostic significance. *Br J Haematol* 64:227–240, 1986.

Lee RE, Ellis LD: The storage cells of chronic myelogenous leukemia. *Lab Invest* 24:261–264, 1971.

Mills KI, Benn P, Birnie GD: Does the breakpoint within the major breakpoint cluster region (M-*bcr*) influence the duration of chronic phase myeloid leukemia? An analytical comparison of current literature. *Blood* 78:1155–1161, 1991.

Moloney WC: Natural history of chronic granulocytic leukaemia. *Clin Haematol* 6:41–53, 1977.

Montefusco E, Mauro FR, LoCocco F, et al: Long term remission of T-lymphoid extramedullary blast crisis of chronic myelogenous leukemia following allogeneic bone marrow transplantation. *Haematologica* 75:391–393, 1990.

Nowell PC, Hungerford DA: A minute chromosome in human chronic granulocytic leukemia. *Science* 132:1497, 1960.

Rosner F, Schreiber ZR, Parise F: Leukocyte alkaline phosphatase: Fluctuations with disease status in chronic granulocytic leukemia. *Arch Intern Med* 130:892–894, 1972.

Rowley JD: A new consistent chromosomal abnormality in chronic myelogenous leukemia identified by quinacrine fluorescence and Giemsa staining. *Nature* 243:290–293, 1973.

Saglio G, Guerrasia A, Rosso G, et al: A new type of *bcr/abl* junction in Philadelphia chromosome–positive chronic myelogenous leukemia. *Blood* 76:1819–1824, 1990.

Shepherd PC, Ganesan TS, Galton DA: Haematological classification of the chronic myeloid leukaemias. *Bailliere's Clin Haematol* 1:887–906, 1987.

Spiers ASD: Metamorphosis of chronic granulocytic leukemia: Diagnosis, classification and management. *Br J Haematol* 41:1–7, 1979.

Travis LB, Pierre RV, DeWald GW: Ph[1]-negative chronic granulocytic leukemia: A nonentity. *Am J Clin Pathol* 85:186–193, 1986.

Ulirsch RC: *Sea-Blue Histiocytosis in Chronic Myelogenous Leukemia.* ASCP Tech Sample H-4, American Society of Clinical Pathologists, Chicago, Ill, 1985.

Vélez-Garcia E, Fradera J, Telmont MDL, et al: Megakaryoblastic transformation of Ph positive chronic granulocytic leukemia. *Am J Clin Pathol* 84:228–233, 1985.

Virchow R: Weisses Blut. *Frorieps Notizen* 36:151, 1845.

Review Articles:

Cannistra SA: Chronic myelogenous leukemia as a model for the genetic basis of cancer. *Hematol Oncol Clin North Am* 4:337–357, 1990.

Georgi A, Vykoupil KF, Buhr T, et al: Chronic myeloproliferative disorders in bone marrow biopsies. *Pathol Res Pract* 186:3–27, 1990.

Kreipe H, Felgner J, Jaquet K, et al: DNA analysis to aid in the diagnosis of chronic myeloproliferative disorders. *Am J Clin Pathol* 98:46–54, 1992.

Polliack A, Leizerowitz R, Kornberg A, et al: Blastic transformation of chronic granulocytic leukemia and other myeloproliferative disorders. A study of 26 cases emphasizing the importance of cytochemistry and ultrastructure in defining the cell phenotype. In *Human Leukemia.* Boston, Martinus-Nijhoff, 1984, pp 105–121.

Silver RT: Chronic myeloid leukemia. A perspective of the clinical and biologic issues of the chronic phase. *Hematol Oncol Clin North Am* 4:319–335, 1990.

CASE 2

PATIENT: 52-year-old white male.

CHIEF COMPLAINT: Increasing fatigue, decreased exercise tolerance, and a dragging sensation in the left upper abdomen.

MEDICAL HISTORY: The patient was in excellent health until 4 weeks prior to examination.

PHYSICAL EXAMINATION: Mild right cervical and left axillary lymphadenopathy present. The spleen tip was palpable 2.0 cm below the left costal margin. No hepatomegaly detected.

LABORATORY RESULTS:

A. *Screening Procedure*
   WBC of 54.5 × 10^9/L with a differential of segmented neutrophils 13%, eosinophils 2%, basophils 1%, monocytes 5%, lymphocytes 71%, prolymphocytes 5%, and atypical lymphocytes 2%. HGB 10.9 g/dL. HCT 33.2 L/L, MCV 95.7 fL, MCH 32.4 pg, MCHC 33.9 g/dl, RDW 15.2. Platelets 173 × 10^9/L.

HOSPITAL COURSE: Examination of the peripheral blood smear revealed a marked increase in small mature lymphocytes, with coarse clumped chromatin and scant cytoplasm. Similar cells were observed in the bone marrow aspirate (Case 2.1). The bone marrow biopsy (Case 2.2) demonstrated an interstitial lymphocytic infiltrate, which

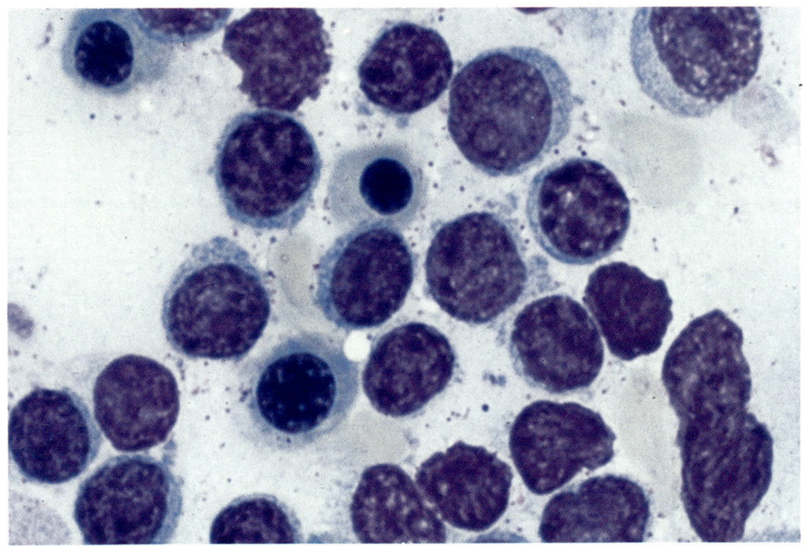

Case 2-1 Bone marrow aspirate. Increased numbers of mature small lymphocytes are present. (×1000).

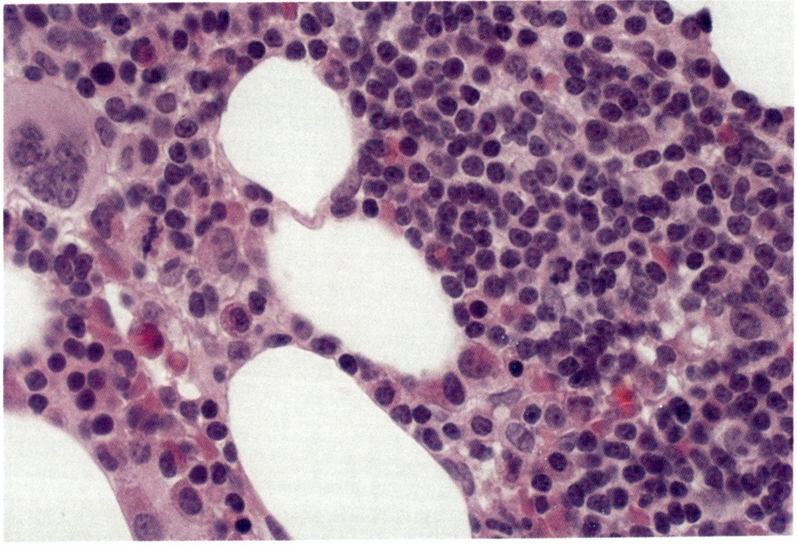

Case 2-2 Bone marrow biopsy. Focal interstitial infiltration by CLL is evident (×400).

constituted about 40% of cellular elements. The fat cell ratio was 40:60, and other hematopoietic elements were adequate and maturing. The patient was started on chlorambucil.

QUESTIONS:

1. What primary diagnosis should be considered from the peripheral blood and marrow findings?
2. Is a lymph node biopsy necessary to support the diagnosis?
3. Does the presence of 5% prolymphocytes in the peripheral blood change the diagnosis?

LABORATORY RESULTS:

B. *Confirmatory Results*

Flow cytometry on peripheral blood: CD5+, CD19+, CD20+, SIgM/kappa+, HLA-DR+. sIgM was of low intensity.

Cytogenetics: 46XY.

Gene rearrangement studies: High-molecular-weight DNA from homogenized peripheral blood lymphocytes was prepared for Southern blot analysis. Restriction digests probed for the beta and gamma subunit genes of TCR were germline. Clonal rearrangements were detected in digests probed for the IgH and IgL genes. Patterns and relative intensities of autoradiographic signals were compatible with a clonal B-cell proliferation.

DIAGNOSIS: Chronic lymphocytic leukemia (B phenotype).

DISCUSSION: CLL is the most common leukemia of adults and results from clonal expansion and failure of maturation of small lymphocytes, leading to their accumulation in the blood, marrow, and parenchymal tissues. In the western hemisphere, CLL accounts for up to 30% of all leukemias. It is rarer in Asia, where the incidence is below 5%. A male predominance is evident, and the M/F ratio is about 2.5:1. The median age at diagnosis is 55 years. Hereditary and immunologic factors appear to play a role in the pathogenesis, as first-degree relatives of patients are at three times greater risk to develop this disorder than the general population. CLL seldom develops before the age of 30.

Early in the natural history of CLL, lymphocytosis may be the only sign of evolving disease, and hence the diagnosis may be unexpected. According to two working groups, the International Workshop on CLL, and the National Cancer Institute–sponsored working group, a diagnosis of CLL early in the course of disease can be made when there is sustained lymphocytosis (absolute lymphocyte count $>5\ \times$

10^9/L) of at least 4 weeks' duration, with less than 55% atypical or immature forms, CD5 activity, evidence of light chain restriction, presence of low-density SIg, and greater than 30% lymphocytes in the bone marrow. However, in patients with a sustained absolute lymphocyte count of 10×10^9/L or greater, demonstration of a monoclonal B phenotype or evidence of bone marrow involvement as noted above are acceptable criteria.

In established CLL, WBC counts of 600×10^9/L or greater are not unusual. Lymphocytes may account for 99% of circulating white cells, and consequently neutropenia may be present. The lymphocytes of CLL are small and mature with scant cytoplasm. Nuclei are mostly round but may occasionally demonstrate minimal irregularity of the membrane and plasmacytoid distribution of chromatin. In less than 15% of B-CLL patients, shallow nuclear indentations may be present (Rieder cells); but in most instances, cytologic appearances are indistinguishable from those of normal and small lymphocytes. Due to the mechanical fragility of CLL lymphocytes, numerous stripped nuclei (basket cells) may be observed in wedge smears of the peripheral blood. This artifact is, however, virtually eliminated in smears prepared by a mechanical spinner. Up to 10% of circulating lymphocytes in CLL may be large, nucleolated, and classifiable as PLs. When present in greater numbers, a diagnosis of prolymphocytic transformation of CLL (mixed CLL-PLL of the FAB cooperative group) should be considered and implies an accelerated phase of growth. When PLs are ≥55% at presentation, a diagnosis of PLL is more likely.

Since the evaluation of tumor burden and patterns of infiltration in the bone marrow have an important role in diagnosis and prognosis, a unilateral iliac crest bone marrow biopsy is recommended in all new cases. Diagnosis from the bone marrow aspirate alone should be evaluated with caution, since benign lymphoid aggregates may manifest a monomorphic pattern indistinguishable from CLL. Additionally, in estimating the tumor burden, both aspirate and biopsy should be evaluated since the distribution of lesion may be focal. A minimum of 30% tumor cellularity is necessary to establish a diagnosis of CLL. Four well-recognized patterns of infiltration are observed and include nodular, interstitial, mixed nodular and interstitial, and diffuse types. Nodular lesions are present in about 10% of patients and may be either intertrabecular or paratrabecular. More frequently, the distribution is intertrabecular. Nodular lesions are monomorphic and lack germinal centers, which are usually present in nodular (follicular) hyperplasia. Interstitial lesions are observed in about 35% of cases, and do not result in architectural damage to the marrow. An interstitial pattern usually connotes early disease. A mixed nodular and interstitial pattern is seen in about 30% of cases and is associated with a favorable prognosis. Diffuse infiltration with extensive replacement of the marrow is present in about 25% of cases. This growth pattern connotes an aggressive clinical course. Occasionally, nucleolated prolymphocytes with larger nuclei and abundant cytoplasm may be interspersed within the infiltrate or proliferate as pseudofollicular aggregates, also know as *growth centers*. Appearances of these prolymphocytic components are similar to those observed in the lymph nodes of CLL, as characterized by Dick and Maca in 1978.

In CLL, thrombocytopenia and anemia eventually develop. In up to 30% of cases, such cytopenias may be present at diagnosis and signify a worse prognosis and more advanced clinical stage. Cytopenias may be secondary to marrow infiltration or, in a minority of cases, may be due to autoimmune mechanisms. In such cases, a Coombs-positive warm antibody hemolytic anemia may be present.

Each of the numerous systems that have been used to stage CLL have merit. In recent years, however, those of Rai and Binet have been most widely used and are tabulated in Tables C2.1 and C2.2.

Combining these systems into low-, intermediate-, and high-risk groups has now been found to be of clinical utility. Accordingly, the low-risk group includes patients in Rai stage 0 and Binet stage A. Median survival is greater than 10 years. The intermediate risk group includes Rai stages I and II, and Binet stage B. The worst prognostic high-risk group includes Rai stages III and IV, and Binet stage C, with a median survival of less than 2 years. However, as in this patient with Rai stage III and Binet stage A disease, placement into a specific risk group may not always be easy.

Investigation into the immunobiology of CLL arose when Dameshek in 1967 questioned the immunologic competence of the CLL lymphocyte. By 1972, it was clear that 95% of cases were B pheno-

Table C2-1 Rai Staging System for CLL

Stage	*Clinical Features*	*Survival** *(months)*
0	Lymphocytosis in blood and bone marrow only	>120
I	Lymphocytosis and enlarged lymph nodes	95
II	Lymphocytosis plus hepatomegaly, or splenomegaly, or both	72
III	Lymphocytosis and anemia (hemoglobin $<$ 110 g/L)	30
IV	Lymphocytosis and thrombocytopenia (platelets $<$ 100 $\times$ 10^9/L)	30

*Weighted mean survival derived from 8 different series that involved 952 patients.

Table C2-2 Binet Staging System for CLL

Stage	*Clinical Features*	*Survival** *(months)*
A	Hemoglobin $\geq$ 100 g/L; platelets $\geq 100 \times 10^9$/L; <3 areas involved†	>120
B	Hemoglobin $\geq$ 100 g/L; platelets $\geq 100 \times 10^9$/L; and $\geq$3 areas involved	61
C	Hemoglobin < 100 g/L, or platelets $< 100 \times 10^9$/L, or both (independently of the areas involved)	32

*Weighted median survival derived from 8 different series that involved 1117 patients.
†The three areas include cervical, axillary, and inguinal lymph nodes (unilateral or bilateral), spleen, and liver.

type. This incidence of B-CLL is actually higher since careful studies of cases previously reported as T-CLL have revealed that most could be better reclassified as TGLD, adult T-cell lymphoma-leukemia, T-PLL, or T–lymphosarcoma cell leukemia. Hence, true T-CLL is a rare disease. In contrast to normal circulating B lymphocytes, which are strong sIg+, C3d-R+, C3b-R+ and do not express murine erythrocyte receptors, those of B-CLL are weakly SIg+, C3d-R+, C3b-R−, and express murine erythrocyte receptors. In most instances, IgM can be demonstrated on the cell surface, and in fewer cases, IgD is additionally manifest. Median survival in both groups appear identical. When fluorescent microscopy and flow cytometry are used, SIg may be minimal, undetectable, or absent in less than 20% of patients with B-CLL. Such cases have been referred to as *null CLL* and are characterized as representing a stage of maturation between pre-B and early-B lymphocytes. Scant cytoplasmic Ig has also been demonstrated in some cases but appears to have little diagnostic significance. Clonality may be established in cases of B-CLL by demonstrating a restricted light chain pattern on the cell surface, and as with other lymphoproliferative disorders, those with lambda light chain expression appear to have a worse prognosis. B-CLL lymphocytes express the pan-B antigens CD19, CD20, CD24, and CD40 and are CD45+ (weak) and variably CD25+. Since the lymphocytes of B-CLL represent an intermediate stage of maturity, they are Tdt−, CD10−, CD38−, and PCA-1−. Paradoxically, the pan-T lymphocyte antigen CD5, a 67-kd glycoprotein, is also expressed in greater than 80% of B-CLL cases. Since it has also been found in other lymphoproliferative disorders, such as mantle zone lymphoma, in patients with rheumatoid arthritis, and following bone marrow transplantation, CD5 activity should be interpreted in tandem with other clinical and laboratory data. In B-CLL, sIg, CD 5 activity, and the ability to manifest mouse erythrocyte rosettes are expressed independently of each other and are present in greater than 70% of all cases. In virtually every case of B-CLL, at least two of these three immunologic markers are in evidence. It is of interest that in B-PLL, sIg activity is stronger and CD5 activity weaker that in B-CLL.

Most data on T-cell function in B-CLL are difficult to interpret. Although a minority of patients have a monoclonal Ig spike, almost all eventually develop hypogammaglobulinemia. The pathogenesis of hypogammaglobulinemia remains controversial. However, it appears to be multifocal and linked in part to regulatory abnormalities of T-cell function associated with altered T4/T8 ratios and diminished NK cell activity. T-cell gamma receptor gene rearrangement has been present in some cases of B-CLL, and, as in this patient, heavy and light chain gene rearrangement is invariably present.

Electron microscopy of the B-CLL lymphocytes reveals a round nucleus, clumped heterochromatin, and small nucleoli. Occasionally, a single linear nuclear invagination, folds, and nuclear pockets may be manifest. A few mitochondria, lysosomes, and polyribosomes are usually present. Rarely, ribosome-lamella bodies are observed, and the cell membrane may reveal a few short and blunt microvilli.

Approximately 50% of patients with CLL demonstrate chromosomal abnormalities. These frequently involve chromosomes that have either Ig-encoding genes such as in chromosome 14 (heavy chain), or oncogenes such as in chromosome 11 (C-*ras*-Kristen) and chromosome 12 (C-*ras*-Harvey). Trisomy 12 is the most frequent numeric karyotypic abnormality in CLL and is also known to accompany other complex abnormalities. In contrast to CML, the pattern of chromosomal abnormalities in CLL mostly tends to remain unchanged throughout the course of the disease. The next most frequently observed changes include translocation, deletion, or inversion abnormalities of chromosome 14. Karyotypic analysis at diagnosis is recommended, since 14q+ is the most common structural chromosomal abnormality in CLL with a breakpoint at band q32 and is associated with poorer response to therapy and an increased risk for prolymphocytic transformation. Also, patients with low- and intermediate-risk disease and trisomy 12 abnormality appear to have a poorer survival than those with a normal karyotype. Additionally, patients with a complex karyotype with or without trisomy 12 appear to be more susceptible to develop Richter's syndrome than those with either a simple trisomy 12 or a normal karyotype. *BCL*-2 gene rearrangement in CLL should be interpreted with caution, since these may represent examples of lymphosarcoma cell leukemia.

The differential diagnosis of CLL includes reactive lymphocytosis, monoclonal B lymphocytosis of unknown significance, lymphosarcoma cell leukemia, HTLV-I-associated lymphoma-leukemia, HCL, and TGLD.

Reactive lymphocytosis is invariably secondary to a viral illness, and the lymphocytes are mostly of T phenotype. Numerous immunoblasts are usually present in the peripheral blood, and the accompanying B lymphocytes are polyclonal.

It has been known for many years that some patients with monoclonal B lymphocytosis pursue an indolent course and tend to remain in Rai stage 0 for well over a decade. Such cases are believed to represent a benign or smoldering variant of CLL and can only be diagnosed with certainty on long-term follow-up. In most instances, such clonal lymphocytosis remains of unknown significance.

In recent years, greater attention has been focused on second malignancies in CLL. Included herein are melanomas, soft tissue sarcomas, and carcinomas of the large bowel and lung. Hybrid neoplasms, including CLL and HCL, CLL and PLL, and CLL and Hodgkin's disease, continue to be reported. More frequently manifest, however, is blastic transformation of CLL (Richter's syndrome), wherein the lymph node biopsy resembles large cell lymphoma. Immunophenotyping studies in such cases are most essential in establishing clonal identity of this process and the initial CLL.

Little information is available concerning the normal counterpart of the B-CLL lymphocyte. However, cells with many similar immunologic features have been detected at the periphery of germinal centers in lymph nodes, tonsil, and fetal spleen. The etiology of CLL remains unknown, and recent data indicate normal expression of most protooncogenes studied.

SUMMARY

Morphology	**Small mature lymphocytes**
Cytochemistry	**Not considered necessary to make the diagnosis**
Immunophenotyping	**CD5+, CD19+, CD20+, low-intensity sIgM/kappa+, HLA-DR+**
Cytogenetics	**46XY**
Molecular Genetics	**Clonal rearrangements of light and heavy chain genes**
Diagnosis	**Chronic lymphocytic leukemia (B phenotype)**

ANSWERS:

1. Based on the peripheral blood, marrow, and clinical findings, CLL is the most likely diagnosis.
2. A lymph node biopsy is unnecessary to establish a diagnosis of CLL. Biopsy is indicated in the event of progressive adenopathy to rule out transformation and the possibility of a second neoplasm.
3. No. Up to 10% prolymphocytes in the peripheral blood are acceptable in CLL. When prolymphocytes number between 11 and 55%, a diagnosis of prolymphocytic transformation of CLL (mixed CLL-PLL) should be considered.

BIBLIOGRAPHY

Articles:

Apostolopoulos A, Symeonidis A, Zoumbos N: Prognostic significance of immune function parameters in patients with chronic lymphocytic leukaemia. *Eur J Haematol* 44:39–44, 1990.

Batata A, Shen B: The importance of surface immunoglobulin, mouse rosettes, and CD5 in the immunophenotyping of chronic lymphocytic leukemia and reactive lymphocytosis. *Cancer* 68:355–361, 1991.

Bernard DJ, Bignon YJ, Pauchard J, et al: Genotypic analysis of Richter's syndrome. *Cancer* 67:997–1002, 1991.

Bezwoda WR, Bernstein R, Pinto M, et al: B-cell chronic lymphatic leukemia in Hodgkin's disease. *Cancer* 59:761–766, 1987.

Binet, JL, Auguier A, Dighiero G, et al: A new prognostic classification of chronic lymphocytic leukemia derived from a multivariate survival analysis. *Cancer* 48:198–216, 1981.

Brecher M, Banks PM: Hodgkin's disease variant of Richter's syndrome. Report of eight cases. *Am J Clin Pathol* 93:333–339. 1990.

Briggs PG, Kraft N, Atkins RC: T cells and CD45R expression in B-chronic lymphocytic leukemia. *Leuk Res* 14:155–159, 1990.

Burger T, Molnar L, Schmelczer M, et al: Changes in T-lymphocytic subsets and their consequences in B-CLL. *Folia Haematol (Leipz)* 117:115–125, 1990.

Butturini A, Gale RP: Oncogenes in chronic lymphocytic leukemia. *Leuk Res* 12:89–92, 1988.

Cutter J: Increased incidence of hematologic malignancies in first degree relatives of patients with chronic lymphocytic leukemia. *Cancer Invest* 10:103–109, 1992.

Dick FR, Maca RD: The lymph node in chronic lymphocytic leukemia. *Cancer* 41:285–292, 1978.

Freedman AS, Boyd AW, Bieber FR, et al: Normal cellular counterparts of B cell chronic lymphocytic leukemia. *Blood* 70:418–427, 1987.

Foucar K, Rydell RE: Richter's syndrome in chronic lymphocytic leukemia. *Cancer* 46:118–134, 1980.

Geisler C, Ralfkiaer E, Hansen MM, et al: The bone histological pattern has independent prognostic value in early stage chronic lymphocytic leukemia. *Br J Haematol* 62:47–54, 1986.

Gray JL, Jacobs A, Block M: Bone marrow and peripheral blood lymphocytosis of chronic lymphocytic leukemia. *Cancer* 33:1169–1178, 1974.

Hamblin T, Hough D: Chronic lymphocytic leukemia: Correlation of immunofluorescent characteristics and clinical features. *Br J Haematol* 36:359–365, 1977.

Han T, Barcos M, Emrich L, et al: Bone marrow infiltration patterns and their prognostic significance in chronic lymphocytic leukemia. Correlation with clinical, immunological, phenotypic and cytogenetic data. *J Clin Oncol* 2:562–570, 1984.

Han T, Ozer H, Gavigan M, et al: Benign monoclonal B-cell lymphocytosis—A benign variant of CLL, clinical, immunologic, phenotypic and cytogenetic studies in 20 patients. *Blood* 64:244–252, 1984.

Han T, Ozer H, Sandamori N, et al: Prognostic importance of cytogenetic abnormalities in patients with CLL. *N Engl J Med* 310:288–292, 1984.

Hanson CA, Gribbin TE, Schnitzer B, et al: CD11c (Leu M5) expression characterises a B-cell chronic lymphoproliferative disorder with features of both chronic lymphocytic leukemia and hair cell leukemia. *Blood* 76:2360–2367, 1990.

Hernandez-Nieto L, Montserrat-Costa E, Muncunill J, et al: Bone marrow patterns and clinical staging in chronic lymphocytic leukaemia. *Lancet* 1:1269, 1977.

International workshop on chronic lymphocytic leukemia. Recommendations for diagnosis, staging and response criteria. *Ann Intern Med* 110:236–238, 1989.

Kay NE, Zarling J: Restoration of impaired natural killer cell activity of B-chronic lymphocytic leukemia patients by recombinant interleukin-2. *Am J Hematol* 24:161–167, 1987.

Kimby E, Mellstedt H, Nilsson B, et al: Differences in blood T and NK cell populations between chronic lymphocytic leukemia of B cell type (B-CLL) and monoclonal B-lymphocytosis of undetermined significance (B-MLUS). *Leukemia* 3:501–504, 1989.

Larramendy ML, Peltomaki P, Salonen E, et al: Chromosomal abnormality limited to T4 lymphocytes in a patient with T-cell chronic lymphocytic leukemia. *Eur J Haematol* 45:52–59, 1990.

Leber BF, Murphy JJ, Norton JD: Abnormalities in T-cell associated rearrangement of T-cell receptor gamma chain genes in B-cell chronic lymphocytic. *Leuk Res* 13:259–266, 1989.

Lishner M, Hawker G, Amato D: Chronic lymphocytic leukemia in a patient with systemic lupus erythematosus. *Acta Haematol* 84:38–39, 1990.

Melo JV, Catovsky D, Galton DAG: The relationship between chronic lymphocytic leukemia: I. Clinical and laboratory features of 300 patients and characterization of an intermediate group. *Br J Haematol* 63:377–387, 1986.

Montserrat E, Rozman C, Binet JL, et al: Meeting report: Fifth international workshop on chronic lymphocytic leukemia. *Adv Leuk Lymphoma* 2:3–6, 1991.

Pangalis GA, Roussou PA, Kittas C, et al: Patterns of bone marrow involvement in chronic lymphocytic leukemia and small lymphocytic (well differentiated) non-Hodgkin's lymphoma. *Cancer* 54:702–708, 1984.

Pittman S, Catovsky D: Prognostic significance of chromosome abnormalities in chronic lymphocytic leukaemia. *Br J Haematol* 58: 649–660, 1984.

Rai KR: A critical analysis of staging in CLL. In Gale RP and Rai KR (eds): *Chronic Lymphocytic Leukemia: Recent Progress and Future Directions*. New York, Alan R Liss, 1987, pp 253–264.

Rai KR, Han T: Prognostic factors and clinical staging in chronic lymphocytic leukemia. *Hematol/Oncol Clin North Am* 4:447–456, 1990.

Rai KR, Montserrat E: Prognostic factors in chronic lymphocytic leukemia. *Semin Hematol* 24:252–256, 1987.

Rai KR, Sawitsky A, Cronkite EP, et al: Clinical staging of chronic lymphocytic leukemia. *Blood* 46:219–234, 1975.

Richter MN: Generalized reticular cell sarcoma of lymph nodes associated with lymphatic leukemia. *Am J Pathol* 4:285–292, 1928.

Rozman C, Montserrat JM, Rodriguez-Fernandez R, et al: Bone marrow histologic pattern—The best single prognostic parameter in chronic lymphocytic leukemia: A multivariate survival analysis of 329 cases. *Blood* 64:642–648, 1984.

Rywlin AM: Histopathology of Bone Marrow. Boston, Little, Brown, 1976, p. 110.

Scully RE, Mark EJ, McNeely WF (eds): Richter's syndrome. Case Records of the Massachusetts General Hospital (Case 18–1991). *N Engl J Med* 324:1267–1277, 1991.

Terstappen LW, de Grooth BG, Segers-Nolten I, et al: Cytotoxic lymphocytes in B-cell chronic lymphocytic leukemia. A flow cytometric study of peripheral blood, lymph nodes and bone narrow. *Blut* 60:81–87, 1990.

Totterman TH, Carlsson M, Simonsson B, et al: T-cell activation and subset patterns are altered in B-CLL and correlate with the stage of disease. *Blood* 74:786–792, 1989.

Touw I, Lowenberg B: Interleukin-2 stimulates chronic lymphocytic leukemia colony formation in vitro. *Blood* 66:237–240, 1985.

Zaknoen SL, Kay NE: Immunoregulatory cell dysfunction in chronic B-cell leukemias. *Blood Rev* 4:165–174, 1990.

Zucker-Franklin D: Virus like particles in the lymphocytes of a patient with chronic lymphocytic leukemia. *Blood* 21:509–512, 1963.

Review Articles:

Bennett JM, Catovsky D, Daniel M-T, et al: Proposals for the classification of chronic (mature) B and T lymphoid leukaemias. *J Clin Pathol* 42:567–584, 1989.

Cheson BD, Bennett JM, Rai KR, et al: Guidelines for classical protocols for chronic lymphocytic leukemia: Recommendations of the National Cancer Institute sponsored working group. *Am J Hematol* 29:152–163, 1988.

Freedman AS: Immunobiology of chronic lymphocytic leukemia. *Hematol/Oncol Clin North Am* 4:405–429, 1990.

Foon KA, Rai KR, Gale PG: Chronic lymphocytic leukemia: New insights into biology and therapy. *Ann Intern Med* 113:525–539, 1990.

Gale RP, Foon KA: Chronic lymphocytic leukemia. Recent advances in biology and treatment. *Ann Intern Med* 103:101–120, 1985.

Juliusson G, Oscier DG, Fitchett M, et al: Prognostic subgroups in B-cell chronic lymphocytic leukemia defined by specific chromosomal abnormalities. *N Engl J Med* 323:720–724, 1990.

Kay NE, Perri RT: Immunobiology of malignant B cells and immunoregulatory cells in B-chronic lymphocytic leukemia. *Clin Lab Med* 8:163–177, 1988.

Williams J, Schned A, Cotelingam JD, et al: Chronic lymphocytic leukemia with coexistent Hodgkin's disease. *Am J Surg Pathol* 15: 33–42, 1991.

CASE 3

PATIENT: 43-year-old white male.

CHIEF COMPLAINT: Intermittent fever and abdominal pain over a 3-week period.

MEDICAL HISTORY: 16 years earlier a diagnosis of seropositive rheumatoid arthritis was made. Four months prior to admission a right hemicolectomy was performed for diverticulitis. Postoperative complications included typhlitis, an abdominal abscess, and an enterocutaneous fistula. Treatment was with antibiotics, segmental resection of the ileum with jejunocolic anastomosis, and splenectomy.

PHYSICAL EXAMINATION: Temperature 99.7°F. Abdominal tenderness present. No organomegaly.

LABORATORY RESULTS:

A. *Screening Procedure*
   WBC of 14.9 × 10^9/L with a differential of segmented neutrophils 1%, eosinophils 1%, basophils 2%, monocytes 7%, and lymphocytes 89%. HGB 13.6 g/dL. HCT 0.41 L/L. MCV 87.2 fL, MCH 29.0 pg, MCHC 33.2 g/dL, RDW 17.6. Platelets 547 × 10^9/L.

HOSPITAL COURSE: Large lymphocytes with abundant pale cytoplasm and prominent azurophilic granules (Case 3.1) were observed in the peripheral blood film. Bone marrow aspirate revealed markedly

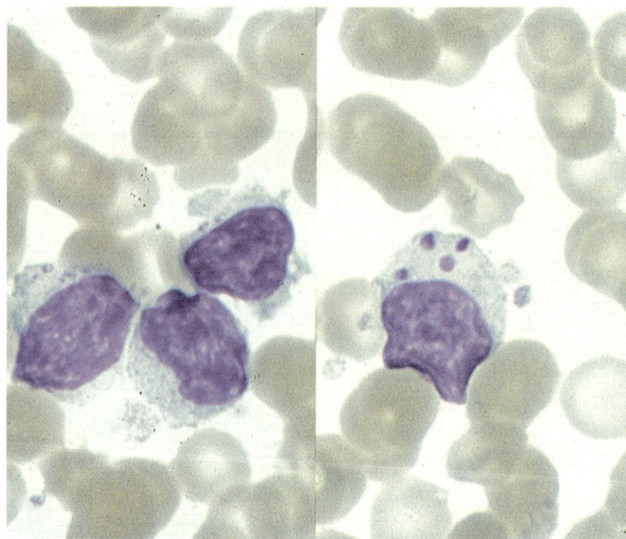

Case 3-1 LGLs in peripheral blood film. Note variation in granule size and content. (×1000).

decreased granulopoiesis with maturation arrest. LGLs were increased and constituted 78% of all cellular elements. An interstitial infiltrate (Case 3.2) and two nonparatrabecular lymphoid aggregates were observed in the biopsy. Erythropoiesis was normoblastic, and adequate megakaryocytes were present. A left lower abdominal abscess was located and drained. *Citrobacter diversus* was cultured. Under antibiotic treatment the fever defervesced.

QUESTIONS:

1. Can the diagnosis be suspected from the history and CBC?
2. Are the cytoplasmic granules in lymphocytes ribosome lamella bodies?
3. What is the differential diagnosis?

LABORATORY RESULTS:

B. *Confirmatory Results*

Cytochemistry: LGLs from a buffy coat preparation were acid phosphatase+ (tartrate-sensitive), and Tdt−.

Immunophenotyping studies: Performed on lymphocytes from pe-

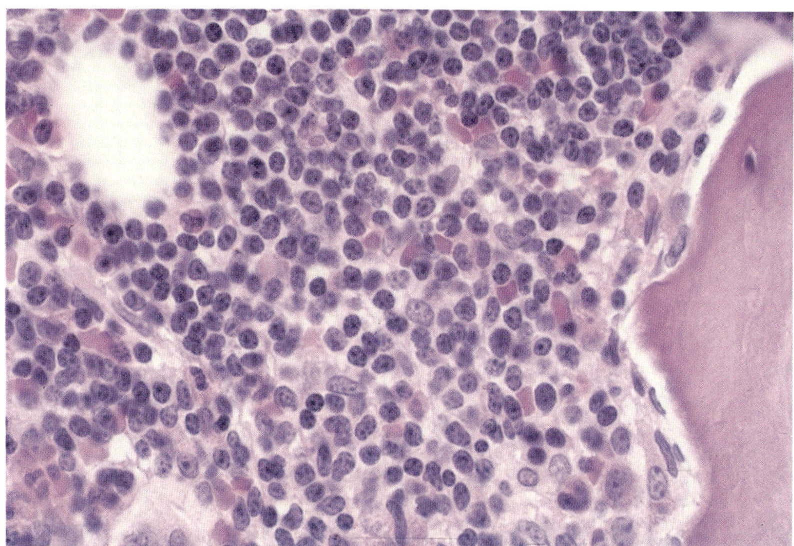

Case 3-2 Lymphocytic infiltrate in bone marrow biopsy. (×400).

ripheral blood sample: CD7+, CD8+, CD16+, and CD57+ in 80% of lymphocytes. CD4+ in 16%, and CD3−.

Cytogenetics: Normal karyotype 46XY.

Gene rearrangement studies: The genes for IgH, kappa light chain, and the beta and gamma subunits of the TCR were probed and were found without detectable rearrangement or deletion.

DIAGNOSIS: T-gamma lymphoproliferative disease.

DISCUSSION: Following the initial descriptions of Brody et al., Brouet et al., and McKenna et al. between 1975 and 1977, and numerous subsequent reports, it is now well established that TGLD is a distinct clinicopathologic entity within the spectrum of postthymic T-cell neoplasms. Included herein is a diverse group of chronic leukemias and lymphomas that differ in their clinical manifestations, predilection for tissue localization, and natural history. Entities other than TGLD in this group that manifest a leukemic component include HTLV-I-associated lymphoma-leukemia, T-PLL, mycosis fungoides with circulating Sézary cells, T-HCL, and true T-CLL.

TGLD is a heterogenous disorder classified by the FAB cooperative group as a form of T-CLL. However, manifestations range from those of an indolent and possibly reactive disease of immune regulation to that of an aggressive malignancy, thereby accounting for the bewildering plethora of designations in the literature. These include T-gamma lymphocytosis with neutropenia, T-cell lymphocytosis, T-CLL, CLL of T-cell origin, LGL leukemia, leukemia of LGLs, lymphoproliferative disease of LGLs, large granular T-cell lymphoproliferative disease, T-gamma lymphocytosis syndrome, and TGLD.

Although TGLD usually develops in individuals over the age of 50, pediatric cases have been reported. A slight male predilection is evident (M/F ratio 1.3:1). About 25% of cases are asymptomatic and diagnosed incidentally after a routine blood count. The association of lymphocytosis and neutropenia in a patient with chronic recurrent infections, however, often serves as a clue to diagnosis. In a multicenter international study of 151 cases, Pandolfi et al. found that 72% of patients were symptomatic. Included were weakness, joint pains, fever, symptoms of hepatic dysfunction, and skin infiltrates. Splenomegaly was present in 50% of cases, and hepatomegaly in 34%. Lymphadenopathy is uncommon, and seropositive rheumatoid arthritis has been reported in about one-third of patients. In most instances, TGLD purses an indolent course. However, <5% of cases develop progressive lymphocytosis within infiltration of parenchymal tissues and fatal infections secondary to neutropenia. Rarely, spontaneous regression of TGLD has been reported.

A characteristic finding in the peripheral blood is the presence of increased numbers of LGLs and neutropenia. In a well-stained peripheral blood film, the majority of lymphocytes are large, with abundant pale cytoplasm and varying numbers of prominent azurophilic granules. Although absolute LGL counts greater than 2,000/mm^3 (2×10^9/L) are usually characteristic of TGLD, counts greater than 7000/mm^3 have been reported in 19% of cases. Following splenectomy, counts may be further elevated. Neutropenia is present in over 60% of patients. This may be cyclic and secondary to antineutrophil antibodies. Mild anemia and thrombocytopenia are usually present. Rarely, an associated red cell aplasia has been observed.

The bone marrow is involved in the majority of patients with TGLD. In aspirate preparations, the appearances of LGLs are similar to those in the peripheral blood. In the biopsy, lesions may vary in appearance from small poorly defined lymphoid aggregates to larger nonparatrabecular, nodular, interstitial, and diffuse infiltrates, which may replace greater than 75% of hematopoietic elements. Lesions are composed of small lymphocytes with minimum irregularity of nuclear contours, inconspicuous or absent nucleoli, condensed chromatin, and scant cytoplasm. Interspersed larger transformed lymphocytes and plasma cells are occasionally present. Appearances may be indistinguishable from those of other reactive or low-grade lymphoproliferative disorders, emphasizing the need to correlate bone marrow appearances with findings in the peripheral blood and the clinical picture.

The LGLs observed in this condition were originally designated T-gamma (suppressor) cells, since they uniformly expressed Fc receptors for IgG (CD16) by rosetting techniques. LGLs are Tdt−, myeloperoxidase-positive, β-glucuronidase-positive, and A-EST+. In about 50% of cases, low-affinity receptors for sheep erythrocytes (CD2) are demonstrable. Under physiologic conditions, the T/B lymphocyte ratio in the peripheral blood is about 4:1, and the helper/suppressor cell ratio 2:1. Normally, between 14 and 40% of circulating lymphocytes are T suppressor cells, and most are CD8+/CD4− with NK activity and are large and granular. However, some are smaller and lack azurophilic granules. Only rarely have normal LGLs been found to express a helper CD4+ phenotype. In some cases of TGLD, NK activity may be absent in CD8+/CD4− LGLs, and in others, LGLs may be CD8−/CD4−, and CD3+. Rarely, a third subtype of LGL with "contrasuppressor" activity (Tcs) has been identified in patients with TGLD. Under physiologic circumstances, Tcs block the effect of T suppressor cells on T helper cells. Such activity has been retained in some cases with TGLD.

In the majority of cases, the LGLs of TGLD are CD7+, CD8+, CD11b+, CD16+, NHK-1(CD56)+ and HNK-1(CD57)+. However, LGLs with variable NK activity have also been found to be frequently CD2+, CD3+, CD11c+, CD38+, and CD45+, prompting the need to examine a battery of markers in suspected cases. In 1992 McDaniel et al proposed a classification of T-cell and NK cell TGLD into types 1 and 2, based largely on CD16 and CD57 expression. The clinical value of this system awaits further study.

Azurophilic granules in the cytoplasm of LGLs have often been located in the centrosomal region of the cell on electron microscopy, and vary between 1000 and 6000 Å in diameter. These inclusions are membrane-bound and contain parallel bundles of microtubule-like structures in a dense amorphous lattice of crystalloid material with a periodicity of 70–80 Å. These structures have been named *parallel tubular arrays* (PTAs) and are of unknown function and significance.

Although trisomy 8 and trisomy 14 have been reported in TGLD, no consistent cytogenetic abnormality appears to be present in the majority of patients. However, in most cases, clonal rearrangement of β or γ TCR genes has been present, suggesting that TGLD is likely to be neoplastic in most instances. It is of interest although of unknown significance that cases lacking TCR gene rearrangement and NK cell activity are also CD3−. The natural history of these cases, however, appears to be no different from those that are CD3+. Although fraught with considerable controversy at the present time, variations in the immunophenotypic profile (with the exception of HNK-1) appear to have little impact on prognosis.

Applying statistical analysis, Pandolfi et al. determined that bad prognostic indicators in TLS included (1) lymphadenopathy, hepatomegaly, and fever at diagnosis, (2) skin infiltration, (3) absolute LGL counts $<3000/\text{mm}^3$ or $>7000/\text{mm}^3$, (4) total WBCs $<5000/\text{mm}^3$ or $>20{,}000/\text{mm}^3$, (5) low percentage of HNK-1+ mononuclear cells. In their study, 7.9% of patients died of TGLD within 48 months of diagnosis.

Concomitant neoplasms reported in patients with TGLD include examples of malignant lymphoma (diffuse undifferentiated), AML, myelodysplasia evolving to AML, Ph^1+ CML, HCL, and plasma cell dyscrasia with primary amyloidosis. Hence, careful clinical and hematologic follow-up of all cases is recommended.

The differential diagnosis of TGLD includes reactive lymphocytosis, CLL, HCL, T-PLL, and LSCL. Although these conditions may be associated with infections and neutropenia, a definitive diagnosis should be based on a clinical, cytologic, morphologic, and immunophenotypic assessment. Reactive T-cell lymphocytosis is usually present in patients with several infections including those with the Epstein-Barr virus, cytomegalovirus, and also with toxoplasmosis and *Bordetella pertussis*. In this latter condition, most circulating lymphocytes are small, agranular, and mainly CD4+. In the viral group, distinctive immunoblastic features (cytologically similar to those observed in infectious mononucleosis) are often present, and LGLs may be lacking. Additionally, the application of two-color flow cytometric analysis with appropriate antibodies may be a valuable adjunct in distinguishing the aforementioned from TGLD. In this connection, we find a CD8−/CD16+/CD56+ profile of LGL in patients without neutropenia to be more supportive of a nonspecific NK cell hyperplasia than of TGLD.

A modest increase in circulating LGLs may be rarely observed in the peripheral blood of patients with Felty's syndrome. Since rheumatoid arthritis with neutropenia and splenomegaly are also features of TGLD, distinguishing these entities from each other may occasionally prove difficult. In TGLD, all clinical parameters are usually apparent at diagnosis. In contrast, the features of Felty's syndrome may become obvious many years after the onset of rheumatoid arthritis. Additionally, unlike the arthritis of TGLD, the arthritis of Felty's syndrome is quite severe. Following splenectomy, the neutropenia of Felty's syndrome usually improves, while there is seldom any consistent improvement in TGLD. Furthermore, the splenic lesion of TGLD is a red pulp infiltrate, while that of Felty's is primarily follicular hyperplasia.

The etiology of TGLD remains obscure. However, Starkebaum et al. have detected antibodies against HTLV-I core proteins p19 and p24 in the serum of 6 of 12 patients with TGLD, thus implicating this retrovirus in a possible etiologic role.

SUMMARY

Morphology	**Large granular lymphocytes**
Cytochemistry	**AP+, Tdt−**
Immunophenotyping	**CD7+, CD8+, CD16+, CD57+, CD3−**
Cytogenetics	**46XY**
Molecular Genetics	**No detectable rearrangement or deletion**
Diagnosis	**T-gamma lymphoproliferative disease (TGLD)**

ANSWERS:

1. Yes. Although neutropenia secondary to such conditions as drug toxicity and malignancy may be associated with infections and relative lymphocytosis, the presence of increased numbers of LGLs in the peripheral blood should prompt a consideration of TGLD in the differential diagnosis.
2. No. The cytoplasmic granules observed in a routine Wright-Giemsa stain are nonribosomal inclusions characterized by their distinctive electron microscopic appearance and named *parallel tubular arrays*. These inclusions are structurally different from *ribosome-lamella bodies* often present in HCL.
3. Reactive lymphocytosis, CLL, LSCL, HCL, and T-PLL are conditions that should enter the differential diagnosis during evaluation of the peripheral blood smear.

BIBLIOGRAPHY

Articles:

Abkowitz JL, Kadin ME, Powell JS, et al: Pure red cell aplasia: Lymphocyte inhibition of erythropoiesis. *Br J Haematol* 63:59–67, 1986.

Amparo E, Kaplan L, Rosenbloom B, et al: T-γ lymphoproliferative disorder arising in a background of autoimmune disease and terminating in plasma cell dyscrasia with primary amyloidosis. *Arch Pathol Lab Med* 115:74–77, 1991.

Bakri K, Ezdinli EZ, Wasser LP, et al: T-suppressor cell chronic lymphocytic leukemia. Phenotypic characterization by monoclonal antibodies. *Cancer* 54:284–292, 1984.

Bennett JM, Catovsky D, Daniel M-T, et al: Proposals for the classification of chronic (mature) B and T lymphoid leukemias. *J Clin Pathol* 42:567–584, 1989.

Berliner N: T-gamma lymphocytosis and T-cell chronic leukemias. *Hematol/Oncol Clin North Am* 4:473–487, 1990.

Berliner N, Dubey AD, Linch DC, et al: T-cell receptor gene rearrangements define a monoclonal T-cell proliferation in patients with T-cell lymphocytosis and cytopenia. *Blood* 67:914–918, 1986.

Bom-van Noorloos AA, Pegels HG, van Oers RHJ, et al: Proliferation of T-gamma cells with killer cell activity in two patients with neutropenia and recurrent infections. *N Engl J Med* 302:933–937, 1980.

Brody JI, Burningham RA, Nowell PC, et al: Persistent lymphocytosis with chromosomal evidence of malignancy. *Am J Med* 58:547–552, 1975.

Brouet J-C, Flandrin G, Saportes M, et al: Chronic lymphocytic leukemia of T-cell origin. *Lancet* 2:890–893, 1975.

Campion G, Maddison PJ, Goulding N, et al: The Felty syndrome: A case matched study of clinical manifestations and outcome, serological features and immunogenetic associations. *Medicine* 69: 69–80, 1990.

Chan WC: Large granular lymphocyte proliferation. *Am J Clin Pathol* 95:900, 1991.

Chan WC, Link S, Mawle A, et al: Heterogeneity of large granular lymphocyte proliferations. Delineation of two major subtypes. *Blood* 68:1142–1153, 1986.

Costello C, Catovsky D, O'Brien, et al: Chronic T-cell leukemias: I. Morphology, cytochemistry and ultrastructure. *Leuk Res* 4:463–476, 1980.

Downey H, McKinlay CA: Acute lymphadenosis compared with acute lymphatic leukemia. *Arch Intern Med* 32:82–112, 1923.

Kadin ME, Kamoum M, Lamberg J: Erythrophagocytic T gamma lymphoma. A clinicopathologic entity resembling malignant histiocytosis. *N Engl J Med* 304:648–653, 1981.

Kotlyo PK, Sample RB, Redmond NL, et al: Reference ranges for lymphocyte subsets. *Arch Pathol Lab Med* 115:181–184, 1991.

Kubic VL, Kubic PT, Brunning RD: The morphologic and immunophenotypic assessment of the lymphocytosis accompanying *Bordatella pertussis* infection. *Am J Clin Pathol* 95:809–815, 1991.

Lin CK, Liu HW, Tse PWT, et al: A patient with large granular lymphocytosis of unusual phenotype and polymorphic T-cell receptor beta-chain gene rearrangement. *Am J Clin Pathol* 94:211–216, 1990.

Loughran TP, Starkebaum G: Large granular lymphocyte leukemia. Report of 38 cases and review of the literature. *Medicine* 66:397–405, 1987.

Loughran TP Jr, Starkebaum G, Aprile JA: Rearrangement and expression of T-cell receptor genes in large granular lymphocyte leukemia. *Blood* 71:822–824, 1988.

Marolleau JP, Henni T, Gaulard P, et al: Hairy cell leukemia associated with large granular lymphocyte leukemia: Immunologic and genomic study, effect of interferon treatment. *Blood* 72:655–660, 1988.

McDaniel HL, MacPherson BR, Tindle BH, et al: Lymphoproliferative disorder of granular lymphocytes. *Arch Pathol Lab Med* 116:242–248, 1992.

McKenna RW, Arthur DC, Gajl-Peczalska KJ, et al: Granulated T-cell lymphocytosis with neutropenia: Malignant or benign chronic lymphoproliferative disorder? *Blood* 66:259–266, 1985.

Miller ML, Fishleder AJ, Tubbs RR: The expression of CD22(Leu 14) and CD11c(Leu M5) in chronic lymphoproliferative disorders using two-color flow cytometric analysis. *Am J Clin Pathol* 96:100–108, 1991.

Nagasawa T, Abe T, Nakagawa T: Pure red cell aplasia and hypogammaglobulinemia associated with T-cell chronic lymphocytic leukemia. *Blood* 57:1025–1030, 1981.

Newland AC, Catovsky D, Linch D, et al: Chronic T-cell lymphocytosis: A review of 21 cases. *Br J Haematol* 58:433–446, 1984.

Oshimi K: Granular lymphocyte proliferative disorders: Report of 12 cases and review of the literature. *Leukemia* 2:617–627, 1988.

Rambaldi A, Pelicci P-G, Allavena P, et al: T-cell receptor beta chain gene rearrangements in lymphoproliferative disorders of large granular lymphocytes/natural killer cells. *J Exp Med* 162:2156–2162, 1985.

Reynolds CW, Foon KA: T-gamma lymphoproliferative disease and related disorders in humans and experimental animals: A review of the clinical, cellular, and functional characteristics. *Blood* 64: 146–1158, 1984.

Saito H, Oshimi K, Akahoshi M, et al: Contrasuppressor T cell leukemia: Clonal proliferation of contrasuppressor T cells in a patient with granular lymphocyte-proliferative disorder. *Br J Haematol* 78: 5–13, 1991.

Semenzato G, Pandolfi F, Chisesi T, et al: The lymphoproliferative disease of granular lymphocytes. A heterogenous disorder ranging from indolent to aggressive conditions. *Cancer* 60:2971–2978, 1987.

Starkebaum G, Loughran TP Jr, Kalyanaraman VS, et al: Serum reactivity to human T-cell leukemia/lymphoma virus type 1 proteins in patients with large granular lymphocytic leukemia. *Lancet* 1:596–598, 1987.

Starkebaum G, Martin PF, Singer JW, et al: Chronic lymphocytosis with neutropenia: Evidence for a novel abnormal T-cell population associated with antibody-mediated neutrophil destruction. *Clin Immunol Immunopathol* 27:110–123, 1983.

Sun T, Cohen NS, Marino J, et al: CD3+, CD4−, CD8− large granular T-cell lymphoproliferative disorder. *Am J Hematol* 37:173–178, 1991.

Velasco CR, Kjeldsberg CR: Large granular lymphocyte leukemia. *ASCP Check Sample* 32:90-11(H-226) 1990.

Wallis WJ, Loughran TP Jr, Kadin ME, et al: Polyarthritis and neutropenia associated with circulating large granular lymphocytes. *Ann Intern Med* 103:357–362, 1985.

Zutter M: Gamma-delta T-cells in the immune response. *Am J Clin Pathol* 95:761–762, 1991.

Review Articles:

Agnarsson BA, Loughran TP Jr, Starkebaum G, et al: The pathology of large granular lymphocytic leukemia. *Human Pathol* 20:643–651, 1989.

Loughran TP Jr, Kadin ME, Starkebaum G, et al: Leukemia of large granular lymphocytes: Association of clonal chromosomal abnormalities and autoimmune neutropenia, thrombocytopenia and hemolytic anemia. *Ann Intern Med* 102:169–175, 1985.

McKenna RW, Perkin J, Kersey JH, et al: Chronic lymphoproliferative disorder with unusual clinical, morphologic, ultrastructural and membrane surface marker characteristics. *Am J Med* 62:588–596, 1977.

Otraldo JR, Longo DL: Human natural lymphocyte effector cells: Definition, analysis of activity, and clinical effectiveness. *J Natl Cancer Inst* 80:999–1010, 1988.

Pandolfi F, Loughran TP, Starkebaum G, et al: Clinical course and prognosis of the lymphoproliferative disease of granular lymphocytes: A multicenter study. *Cancer* 65:341–348, 1990.

Whiteside TL, Herberman RB: The role of natural killer cells in human disease. *Clin Immunol Immunopathol* 53:1–23, 1989.

CASE 4

PATIENT: 67-year-old white female.

CHIEF COMPLAINT: Weight loss, decreased appetite, and vague abdominal discomfort of 8 weeks' duration.

MEDICAL HISTORY: The patient had an appendectomy at age 15. She used nitroglycerine periodically for angina, but otherwise enjoyed good health. During the 8 weeks prior to examination she lost 5 pounds.

PHYSICAL EXAMINATION: Nonfebrile patient of moderate build. Splenomegaly present and palpable at 2.0 cm below left costal margin. No evidence of hepatomegaly, adenopathy, or arthritis.

LABORATORY RESULTS:

A. *Screening Procedure*
   WBC of 19.5 × 10^9/L with a differential count of segmented neutrophils 90%, band forms 3%, eosinophils 1%, basophils 1%, monocytes 2%, and lymphocytes 3%. Occasional Döhle bodies present. No myeloid immaturity identified. HGB 9.3 g/dL. HCT 28.4 L/L. MCV 83.4 fL, MCH 27.2 pg, MCHC 32.8 g/dL, RDW 15.8. Platelets 410 × 10^9/L. MPV 6.0 fL.

HOSPITAL COURSE: No parenchymal malignancy or inflammatory process was detected during careful clinical and radiologic ex-

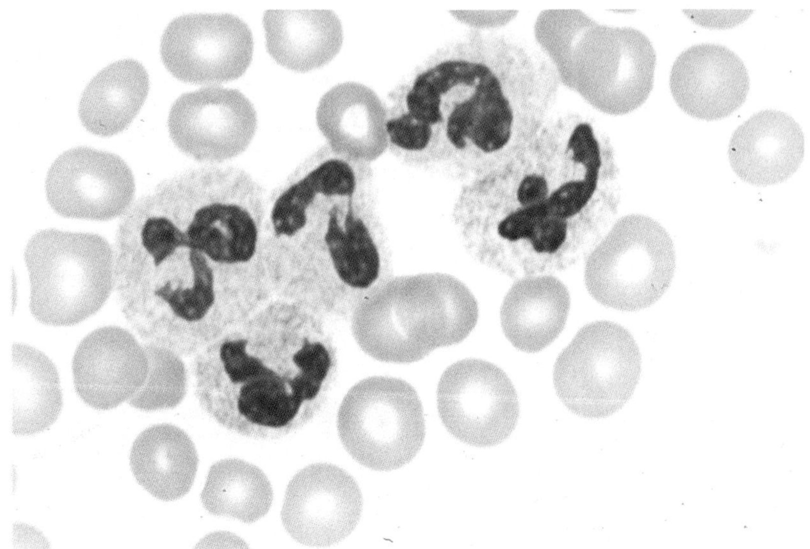

Case 4-1 Peripheral blood film at diagnosis. ($\times 1000$).

amination. The peripheral blood film revealed neutrophilia without immaturity (Case 4.1). Cytoplasmic neutrophil granules were unremarkable. No NRBC or tear drop cells were present. On bone marrow examination, the fat/cell ratio was 5:95, and the M/E ratio 8:1. Myeloid maturation was orderly, with a marked increase in neutrophilic granulocytes (Case 4.2). Blast forms and promyelocytes were not increased. Erythropoiesis was normoblastic, and no dysplastic features were present. Megakaryocytes were slightly increased, without abutment or prominent endoreduplication. Lymphocytes and plasma cells were unremarkable. No metastatic tumor or granuloma was present, and the reticulin framework was mildly accentuated. No collagen fibrosis was evident.

Additional confirmatory tests were performed. No specific therapy was administered at diagnosis, and the total white count continued to fluctuate between 18 and 23 $\times$ 10^9/L during subsequent clinic visits, over a 3-month period.

QUESTIONS:

1. What is the differential diagnosis?
2. How can the differential diagnosis be evaluated?
3. Is immunophenotyping indicated?

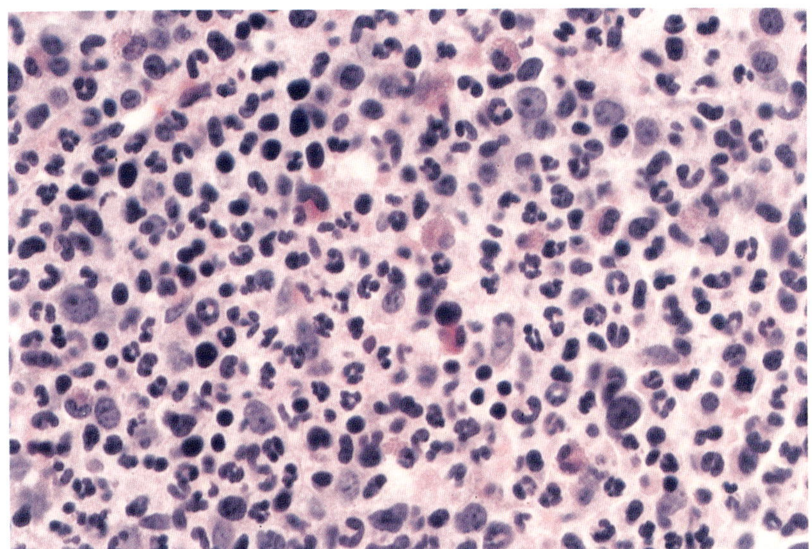

Case 4-2 Bone marrow biopsy. Note increased numbers of neutrophils. (×400).

LABORATORY RESULTS:

B. *Confirmatory Results*

Cytochemistry: The LAP score evaluated on a peripheral blood sample was increased at 210.

Erythrocyte sedimentation rate: Normal.

Serum B_{12} assay: 1700 ng/L (normal range 200–900 ng/L).

Serum protein analysis: Total and differential proteins were normal.

Serum uric acid: Normal.

Cytogenetics: 46XX

DIAGNOSIS: Chronic neutrophilic leukemia.

DISCUSSION: CNL is a rare disease. In 1920, Tuohy reported a case of hyperleukocytosis with splenomegaly, which is believed to be the earliest description of this entity in the English literature. In their report of two cases in 1932, however, Emile-Weil and See additionally cite two earlier cases from the turn of the century in the French and German literature. CNL is primarily a disease of adults. Incidence among men and women appears to be equal, and most reported patients have been over 50 years of age. In infancy and childhood, CNL does not appear to be a well-defined entity, and review of the literature leads us to believe that no more than 60 acceptable cases are documented at this time.

Recent reports reveal that in isolated instances, CNL has been preceded by polycythemia vera, thorotrast injection, and plasmacytoma. CNL has also been diagnosed with coexistent myelodysplastic features and with multiple myeloma; and a few patients have gone on to develop multiple myeloma several years following the diagnosis of CNL. In some instances, CNL has been reported to terminate in blast crisis, AML-M1, AMML, and AMoL.

At clinical presentation, abdominal discomfort, weight loss, fatigue, and anorexia are often present. Splenomegaly is a consistent manifestation, and in the case reported by Tuohy, extended 3 in. beyond the umbilicus. Hepatomegaly is also frequently associated. Easy bruisibility, ecchymosis, and gouty arthritis have been reported in some cases. Sustained neutrophilic hyperleukocytosis, a hypercellular myeloid predominant bone marrow, increased LAP score, increased levels of serum B_{12} and serum B_{12} binding protein, elevated levels of serum uric acid, and absence of the Ph^1 chromosome are other well-documented features.

The total leukocyte count is increased at diagnosis, and, in Tuohy's case, rose from 65,000 to 240,000 following splenectomy. However, since splenectomy has not been a consistent therapeutic modality in other reported cases, the relevance of the phenomenon remains uncertain. Neutrophils may constitute 99% of circulating white cells, and only rarely are accompanying band forms, metamyelocytes, and myelocytes present. Döhle bodies and hypogranular and hyposegmented "Pelgeroid" myelodysplastic features have been described in some instances. Zoumbos et al. (1989) believe that these cases should be designated "CNL with dysplastic features" and consider this subtype of CNL to overlap into the spectrum of the myelodysplastic disorders. Rarely, ring-shaped nuclei in neutrophils have also been observed. Since CNL is known to terminate in ANLL, sequential evaluation of the CBC, peripheral blood smear, and bone marrow with appropriate cytochemical, immunophenotypic, and cytogenetic studies should be performed commensurate with the detection of any increase in the blast count. Anemia in CNL is variable, and it is not unusual to observe some macrocytosis, polychromasia, stippling, tear drop forms, and circulating NRBC. Thrombocytopenia at diagnosis may correlate with a history of ecchymosis and easy bruisibility. However, no specific coagulation factor abnormally appears to be present.

In CNL, the bone marrow is hypercellular and myeloid predominant. Reports of M/E ratios have varied between 5:1 and 25:1. Myeloblasts are generally <5%, and neutrophils are the predominant cell type. Megakaryocyte numbers have been increased in some cases, but they lack the endoreduplication and abutment observed in some of the other myeloproliferative disorders. Erythropoiesis is generally normoblastic. However, megaloblastoid and dyskinetic maturation has been reported in cases of CNL with dysplastic features. Increased reticulin has been observed in some cases, and rarely focal fibrosis and osteosclerosis have been reported.

Since identification of neutrophils is made easily in the peripheral blood smears and the bone marrow aspirate, immunophenotyping and cytochemical analysis is unnecessary to make a diagnosis. However, the LAP score should be evaluated. Although this is consistently increased in CNL and leukemoid reactions and does not serve to distinguish these entities, it does exclude a diagnosis of CML during the preliminary workup.

No specific ultrastructural feature distinguishes normal neutrophils from those of CNL. It is of considerable significance that the Ph^1 chromosome by conventional karyotypic analysis has not been identified in a single case of CNL, and BCR rearrangement has not been reported. Although no specific chromosomal abnormality has yet been recognized in CNL, reported abnormalities include a missing chromosome 2, with replacement by an abnormal large single chromosome; trisomy 9 with partial deletion of the long arm of chromosome 20; and trisomy 8, which has also been frequently observed in myelodysplasia, particularly CMML. In the majority of cases, no chromosomal abnormality is present.

Splenic infiltrations in CNL involve the red pulp and have variably revealed an infiltration of mature neutrophils or complete myeloid metaplasia.

The differential diagnosis of CNL includes CML and neutrophilic leukemoid reactions. Hence, in the presence of a spontaneously normalizing neutrophilia, low LAP score, sepsis, or any condition considered capable of inducing a leukemoid reaction and the presence of a Ph^1 chromosome, the diagnosis of CNL should be reconsidered.

Alterations in the erythrocyte sedimentation rate, serum vitamin B_{12} and B_{12} binding protein levels, serum uric acid levels, and degree of marrow reticulin may be of additional correlative value. Furthermore, since polycythemia vera and multiple myeloma may coexist with CNL, evaluation and correlation of other relevent laboratory, radiologic, and clinical parameters should be considered within the context of the differential diagnosis.

The clinical course of CNL has extended over 5–80 months in different patients, and the risk factors heralding a worse prognosis remain uncertain. Preliminary functional studies have revealed that leukemic neutrophils have active bactericidal activity, reduced lysozyme and β-glucuronidase content, and a variable growth pattern in cell culture. As yet, no definite etiologic factors have been ascertained, but the association of polycythemia vera and multiple myeloma in some cases suggests failure of a yet-undetermined regulation of granulopoiesis. Since the protooncogene *abl* and the protooncogene *src* are located on chromosome 9 and chromosome 20, respectively, and have revealed abnormalities in CNL, their role, if any, prompts further consideration.

SUMMARY

Peripheral Blood	**Sustained and unexplained neutrophilia without accompanying immaturity**
Bone Marrow	**Hypercellular, with granulocytic predominance**
Cytochemistry	**Increased LAP score**
Serum B_{12}	**Increased**
Serum Proteins	**Gamma globulins variably increased**
Serum Uric Acid	**Variably increased**
Cytogenetics	**Absence of Ph^1 chromosome**
Diagnosis	**Chronic neutrophilic leukemia**

ANSWERS:

1. The differential diagnosis includes reactive neutrophilia, leukemoid reaction, and CML.
2. A careful history and clincial examination will exclude causes of neutrophilia and leukemoid reaction. Additionally, an elevated LAP score and absent Ph^1 chromosome exclude the possibility of CML
3. No. This is because the leukemic cell type is composed of mature neutrophils and can be readily identified by microscopy. However, in a case studied by Iurlo et al., reactivity with CD11a, CD11b, CD11c, CD13, CD14, CD15, CD18, CD33, and CD34 was observed.

BIBLIOGRAPHY

Articles:

Aoki I, Toyama K, Tsuchida T, et al: A case of chronic neutrophilic leukemia. *Rinsho Ketsueki* 20:777–785, 1979.

Bareford D, Jacobs P: Chronic neutrophilic leukemia. *Am J Clin Pathol* 73:837–838, 1980.

Boggs DR, Kaplan SS: Cytobiologic and clinical aspects in a patient with chronic neutrophilic leukemia after thorotrast exposure. *Am J Med* 81:905–910, 1986.

Cervantes F, Marti JM, Rozman C, et al: Chronic neutrophilic leukemia with marked myelodysplasia terminating in blast crisis. *Blut* 56:75–78, 1988.

Cervantes F, Rozman M, Vives-Corrons J-L, et al: Chronic neutrophilic leukemia with dysplastic features. *Acta Haematol* 84:109, 1990.

Dash S, Sarode R, Dey P, et al: Chronic neutrophilic leukemia with myelodysplastic features. *Indian J Pathol Microbiol* 33:182–184, 1990.

DiDonato C, Croci G, Lazzari S, et al: Chronic neutrophilic leukemia: Description of a new case with karyotypic abnormalities. *Am J Clin Pathol* 85:369–371, 1986.

Dotten DA, Pruzanski W, Wong D: Functional characterization of the cells in chronic neutrophilic leukemia. *Am J Hematol* 12:157–165, 1982.

Eichenhorn MS, Van Slyck EJ: Marked mature neutrophilic leukocytosis: A leukemoid variant associated with malignancy. *Am J Med Sci* 284:32–36, 1982.

Emile-Weil AN, See G: La Leucémie myélogène à polynucléaires neutrophiles. *Presse Med* 40:1071, 1074, 1932.

Foa P, Iurlo A, Saglio G, et al: Chronic neutrophilic leukemia associated with polycythemia vera: Pathogenetic implications and therapeutic approach. *Br J Haematol* 78:286–288, 1991.

Franchi F, Seminara P, Giunchi G: Chronic neutrophilic leukemia and myeloma: Report on long survival. *Tumori* 70:105–107, 1984.

Fremans W, Marcelis L, Ardichvili D: Chronic neutrophilic leukemia with enlarged lymph nodes and lysozyme deficiency. *J Clin Pathol* 36:324–328, 1983.

Hayashi K, Nakamura H, Onishi Y, et al: A case of chronic neutrophilic leukemia accompanied by the infiltration of mature neutrophils in liver sinusoids. *Rinsho Ketsueki* 24:600–606, 1983.

Iurlo A, Foa P, Maiolo AT, et al: Polycythemia vera terminating in chronic neutrophilic leukemia: Report of a case. *Am J Hematol* 35:139, 1990.

Jackson IMD, Clark RM: A case of neutrophilic leukemia. *Am J Clin Sci* 249:72–74, 1965.

Kanoh T, Saigo K, Yamagishi M: Neutrophils with ring shaped nuclei in chronic neutrophilic leukaemia. *Am J Clin Pathol* 86:748–751, 1986.

Kaplan SS, Chervenick PA: Leukocyte function in chronic neutrophilic leukemia (abstract). *Blood* 62:605, 1983.

Kreipe H, Felgner J, Jaquet K, et al: DNA analysis to aid in the diagnosis of chronic myeloproliferative disorders. *Am J Clin Pathol* 98:46–54, 1992.

Lewis MJ, Oelbaum MH, Coleman M, et al: An association between chronic neutrophilic leukaemia and multiple myeloma with a study of cobalamin-binding proteins. *Br J Haematol* 63:173–180, 1986.

Lorente JA, Pena JM, Ferro T, et al: A case of chronic neutrophilic leukaemia with original chromosomal abnormalities. *Eur J Haematol* 41:285–288, 1988.

Lugassy G, Farhi R: Chronic neutrophilic leukemia associated with polycythemia vera. *Am J Hematol* 31:300–301, 1989.

Orazi A, Cattoretti G, Sozzi G: A case of chronic neutrophilic leukemia with trisomy 8. *Acta Haematol (Basel)* 81:148–151, 1989.

Rovira M, Cervantes F, Nomdedeu B, et al: Chronic neutrophilic leukemia preceding for seven years the development of multiple myeloma. *Acta Haematol* 83:94–95, 1990.

Shindo T, Sakai C, Shibata A: Neutrophilic leukemia and blast crisis. *Ann Intern Med* 87:66–67, 1977.

Silberstein CB, Zellner DC, Shivakumar BN, et al: Neutrophilic leukemia. *Ann Intern Med* 80:110–111, 1974.

Standen Gr, Jasani B, Wagstaff M, et al: Chronic neutrophilic leukaemia and multiple myeloma. An association with lambda light chain expression. *Cancer* 66:162–166, 1990.

Tang DJ, Yu ZF, Song JZ, et al: Gaucher like cells in chronic neutrophilic leukemia. A case report. *Chin Med J* 100:988–989, 1987.

Tanzer J, Harel P, Boison M, et al: Cytochemical and cytogenetic findings in a case of chronic neutrophilic leukemia of mature cell type. *Lancet* 1:387–388, 1964.

Tuohy EL: A case of splenomegaly with polymorphonuclear neutrophil hyperleukocytosis. *Am J Med Sci* 160:18–25, 1920.

Turz T, Flandrin G, Brouet JC, et al: Coexistence d'une myeloma et d'une leucémie granuleuse en l'absence de tout traitment. Étude de quatre observations. *Nouv Rev Fr Hématol* 14:693, 1974.

Vorobiof DA, Benjamin J, Kaplan H, et al: Chronic granulocytic leukaemia, neutrophilic type with paraproteinemia (IgA type K). *Acta Haematol* 60:316–320, 1978.

Watanbe A, Yoshida G, Yamamoto H, et al: A case of chronic neutrophilic leukemia with paraproteinemia (IgG lambda and IgA kappa). *Jpn J Med* 23:39–44, 1984.

Zoumbos NC, Chrysanthopoulos C, Starakis J, et al: Kappa light chain myeloma developing in a patient with chronic neutrophilic leukaemia. *Br J Haematol* 65:504–505, 1987.

Zoumbos NC, Symeonidis A, Kourakli-Symeonidis A: Chronic neutrophilic leukemia with dysplastic features. A new variant of the myelodysplastic syndromes? *Acta Haematol* 82:156–160, 1989.

Review Articles:

Minura AB, Takahashi T, Nishinari T: Chronic neutrophilic leukemia. *Rinsho Ketsueki* 28:505–512, 1987.

Yamaya T, Kamata Y, Nasai K, et al: An autopsy case of chronic neutrophilic leukemia and review of Japanese literature. *Rinsho Ketsueki* 23:1808–1810, 1982.

You W, Weisbrot IM: Chronic neutrophilic leukemia. Report of two cases and review of the literature. *Am J Clin Pathol* 72:233–242, 1979.

CASE 5

PATIENT: 72-year-old male.

CHIEF COMPLAINT: Abdominal fullness and fatigue for 2 weeks.

MEDICAL HISTORY: Patient in good health until onset of chief complaint.

PHYSICAL EXAMINATION: Mild mucosal pallor present. No splenomegaly, hepatomegaly, or lymphadenopathy present.

LABORATORY RESULTS:

A. *Screening Procedure*
   WBC of 14.0 × 10^9/L with a differential of segmented neutrophils 21%, metamyelocytes 1%, eosinophils 4%, basophils 1%, monocytes 2%, lymphocytes 12%, atypical lymphocytes 59%. NRBC 1/100 WBC. HGB 12.7 g/dL. HCT 0.39 L/L, MCV 90.5 fL, MCH 30.0 pg, MCHC 33.1 g/dL, RDW 13.2. Platelets 75 × 10^9/L.

HOSPITAL COURSE: The atypical lymphocytes (Case 5.1) observed in the peripheral blood film revealed relatively round to oval nuclei, with one to two indistinct nucleoli, delicate chromatin, abundant gray-blue cytoplasm and occasional cytoplasmic projection. The bone marrow aspirate consisted of sinusoidal blood. However, the biopsy (Case 5.2) was hypercellular, revealing a decrease in all normal

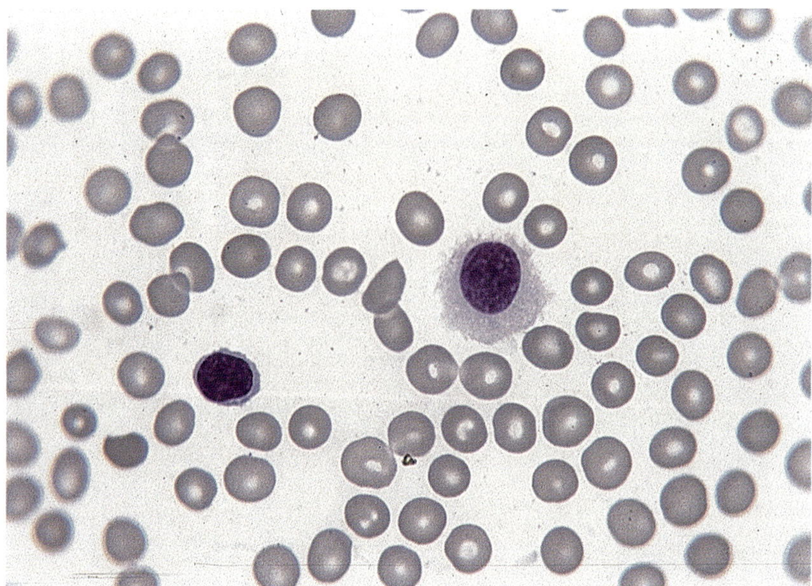

Case 5-1 Peripheral blood film showing a hairy cell, with abundant pale cytoplasm, irregular cytoplasmic membrane, oval nucleus, and inconspicuous nucleoli. Compare with adjacent small lymphocyte. (×600).

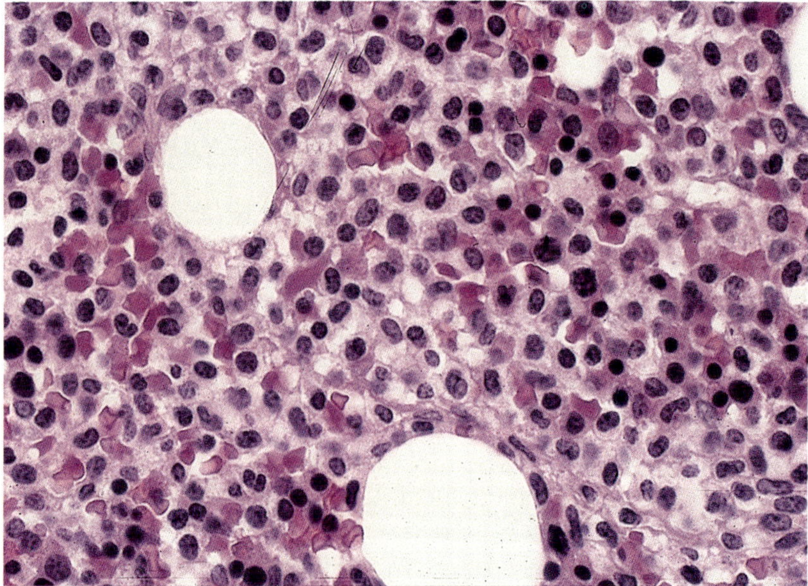

Case 5-2 Bone marrow biopsy. Note diffuse infiltration with small loosely cohesive hairy cells. (×400).

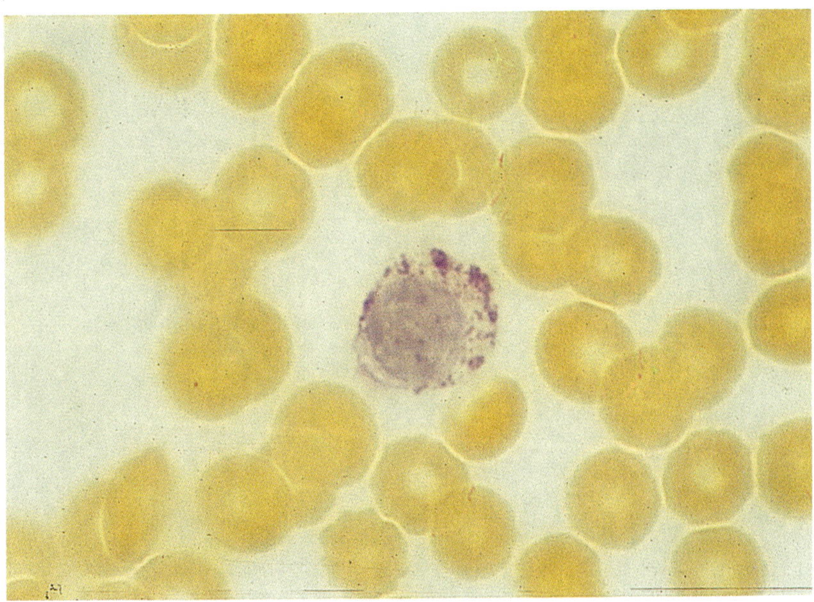

Case 5-3 TRAP+ hairy cell from peripheral blood. (×100).

hematopoietic elements and a marked increase in abnormal lymphoid forms. Spleen size evaluated by CT scan was reported as normal.

QUESTIONS:

1. Can the diagnosis be suspected from the available information?
2. What special stain should be considered?
3. Do immunophenotyping and electron microscopy have a role in making the diagnosis?

LABORATORY RESULTS:

B. *Confirmatory Results*

Cytochemistry and special stains: TRAP+ (Case 5.3) in buffy coat prep of peripheral blood. Pericellular reticulin noted around tumor cells in bone marrow biopsy (Case 5.4).

Immunophenotyping studies: Performed on lymphoid cells in buffy coat: CD19+, CD20+, CD25+, FMC7+, HLA-DR+, sIgM+, Tdt−.

Cytogenetics: Not performed.

Gene rearrangement studies: Both alleles of the IgH clonally rearranged. Both alleles of kappa IgL gene deleted. Lambda IgL

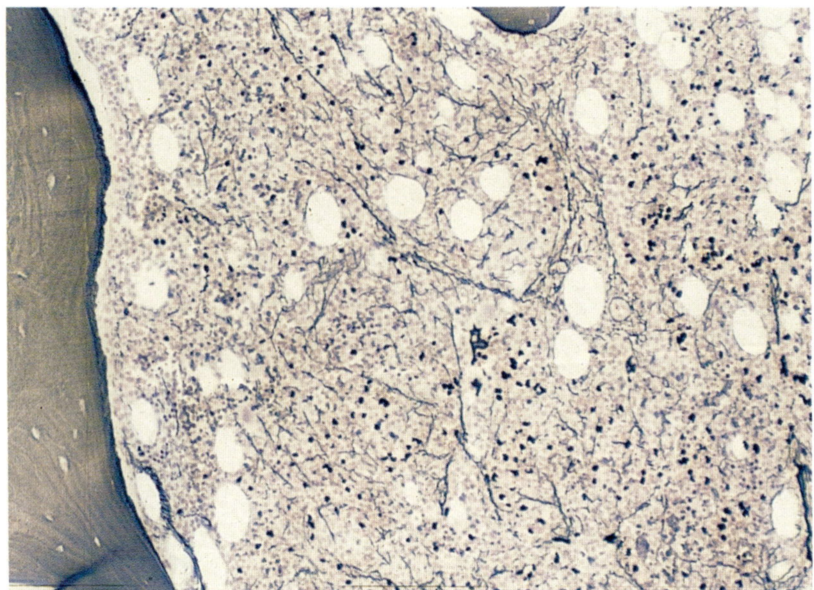

Case 5-4 Reticulin stain of bone marrow biopsy. Increased and focally pericellular reticulin proliferation is evident. (×100).

gene not assayed. Beta and gamma subunits of TCR in germline configuration. Patterns and intensities of rearranged bands indicated a clonal B-cell proliferation.

DIAGNOSIS: Hairy Cell Leukemia.

DISCUSSION: HCL is an unusual lymphoproliferative disease characterized by pancytopenia, cytologically distinctive tumor cells, splenomegaly, and myelofibrosis. This disease was designated leukemic reticuloendotheliosis by Bouroncle et al in 1958, and following the description of "hairy" leukemic cells in the peripheral blood, the name HCL gained general acceptance. In the majority of instances the diagnosis of HCL can be made without difficulty and errors averted if well-prepared material is examined and the differential diagnosis carefully considered.

HCL is a disease of middle-aged adults. A distinctive male predominance is evident (M/F 4.2:1). Most patients are over the age of 30. Presenting symptoms usually relate to pancytopenia and include fatigue, infections, and easy bruisability. Splenomegaly at initial examination is present in 80% of patients, and hepatomegaly in less than 50%. Peripheral adenopoathy is uncommon, but retroperitoneal, abdominal, and mediastinal adenopathy eventually develop.

At presentation, pancytopenia is observed in greater than 50% of cases. Moderate, normocytic, normochromic anemia is usually evident. Thrombocytopenia under 100 × 10^9/L and leukopenia with neutrophil counts below 1.5 × 10^9/L are present in 70% of cases. Hairy cells (HCs) in the peripheral blood are present in about 90% of cases, but a leukemic presentation with greater than 5000 HCs/μL is observed in less than 20%. Monocytopenia is invariably present, and the neutrophil alkaline phosphatase score is generally elevated. A polyclonal gammopathy is observed in about 30% of patients. HCs preferentially express IgG_3 subclass and in contrast to other B-cell neoplasms are known to simultaneously express multiple IgH isotypes.

In Wright-Giemsa preparations, HCs characteristically reveal a round to oval centrally or eccentrically placed nucleus with evenly distributed lacy chromatin and one or two inconspicuous nucleoli. Occasionally bilobed, multilobated, and ring-shaped nuclei have been reported. The cytoplasm is generally pale blue-gray and abundant. Rarely, rod-shaped inclusions may be observed and correspond to ribosome-lamella complexes (RLCs). A ruffled or "hairy" cell membrane is usually present and although distinctive, must be evaluated in concert with other cytologic and cytochemical features, since irregularities of the cell membrane may be observed in other lymphoid lesions, or result from preparation artifact.

In 1971, Yam et al. drew attention to the presence of TRAP activity in HCL. This correlates with isoenzyme-5 on polyacrylamide gel electrophoresis. Enzyme activity is localized in cytoplasmic vesicles and the Golgi area. Variation in the intensity of staining and the number of positive cells is usual from case to case. Activity declines with progressive disease and may be absent following interferon therapy. In less than 5% of cases, TRAP activity may be absent de novo. Since TRAP activity has been reported in some cases of CLL, malignant lymphoma (small lymphocytic), large cell lymphoma, the SS, ATLL, WM, PLL, and certain other nonlymphoid leukemias, careful clinical and cytologic correlation is invaluable.

The outcome of bone marrow aspiration in greater than 90% of cases is a dry tap, secondary to reticulum fibrosis. However, some HCs are usually identifiable in smears of sinusoidal blood. In an adequate bone marrow biopsy, focal or diffuse involvement is usually evident. The lesion may be hypercellular at dignosis and is characteristically monomorphic. Nuclei are round to oval or spindle-shaped and surrounded by abundant clear cytoplasm. Hairy changes are normally not apparent in paraffin sections. However, pericellular reticulin fibrosis is usually present at diagnosis and characteristically does not evolve into collagen fibrosis. The cellularity of residual hematopoietic tissue is usually decreased. When greater than 85% of the marrow space is replaced by tumor, splenectomy does not appear to result in long-term clinical benefit. Bone marrow biopsy remains a most reliable means of establishing the diagnosis of HCL. Appearances are quite distinctive and lack the paratrabecular localization and close apposition patterns of tumor cells as in other small B-cell lymphoid neoplasms. Extravasated red cells may be found among tumor cells, and dilated vascular sinuses have been observed. Plasma cells and mast cells may be increased.

On electron microscopy, the surface of tumor cells reveal broad ruffles and clusters of fingerlike microvilli. The latter reveal surface cytoplasm covered by cell membrane. A second striking feature of HCL is the presence of the RLC, a cylindrical cytoplasmic inclusion of undetermined function, present in about 50% of cases. These inclusions are composed of concentric lamellae studded with ribosomes. No preferential cytoplasmic localization is evident, and the RLC is not unique to HCL. Zucker-Franklin first described RLCs in CLL. Subsequently, they have been described in lymphosarcoma cell leukemia, Sézary cells, WM, multiple myeloma, monoblastic leukemia and other nonhematopoietic cells. Lysosomal bodies and pinocytic activity are virtually absent in HCs.

Following the demonstration of endogenous sIg production and the presence of IgH and IgL gene rearrangement, the origin of HCL from late B lymphocytes or pre-plasma cells has been established in most instances. However, the presence of an unusual biphenotype with additional myeloid, monocytic, T-lymphoid, and plasma cell markers remains perplexing. Using monoclonal antibodies, the following pattern of immune reactivity has been observed in HCL: CDC11c+, CD13+, CD19+, CD20+, CD22+, CD25+(interleukin-2 receptor), CD33+, HLA-DR+, FMC7+, HCL-1+, HCL-2+, HCL-3+, PCA-1+, and B-ly7+. The latter, along with the monoclonal antibodies HML-1, LF61, and Ber-Act8, appears to identify the HC-associated trimeric protein t-GP and when tested with CD22, using dual immunofluorescence, reveal as few as 1% of HCs in the peripheral blood. Similar results may be obtained by using a combination of CD20 and CD11c. In bone marrow biopsies, CD20 and CD45 have been similarly utilized to detect residual disease. Recently, soluble IL-2 receptor (sIL-2R) levels in the blood have been found to drop following treatment with 2-deoxycoformycin (DCF) and alpha interferon, and holds promise as a noninvasive means of evaluating response to treatment and tumor burden. HCs have also been found to express S-100 protein and stain for vimentin. Occasional reports of Tdt and CD3 activity in some cases has led to the belief that a small percentage of HCL patients are of T phenotype. Etiologic association with HTLV-II has been linked with this latter group. However, the majority of patients with HCL are seronegative for HTLV-II. The recent detection of Epstein-Barr virus mRNA by in situ hybridization in some patients with HCL, and the high incidence of seropositivity in such cases, do suggest a role in the pathogenesis. The nature of the dyspoiesis resulting in monocytopenia remains unresolved. Likewise, the physiological counterpart of the HC is uncertain. It is believed however that an sIg-bearing B cell, the monocytoid B cell, or splenic marginal zone lymphocytes are likely candidates.

The differential diagnosis of HCL includes CLL, lymphosarcoma cell leukemia, PLL, and SLVL, a rare neoplasm with circulating villous lymphocytes with variable TRAP activity and negative reactivity with anti-HC2 and anti-Tac. HCs may be observed in unusual locations such as the cerebrospinal fluid, and a group of "variant" HCLs need to be differentiated from the more classic form described above. In the blastic variant, tumor cells reveal large nuclei and prominent nucleoli. TRAP activity is present, and cells are CD20+. Reticulin fibrosis is present. Patients with the Japanese variant present with leukocytosis and lack TRAP activity, but unlike classic HCL patients are CD10+, CD5+ and HC-1− and HC-2−. Similarities exist between this latter variant and the hybrid HCL-CLL variant recently reported by Hanson et al (1990). In this group, tumor cells expressed CD5 and CD11c activity. There also appear to be some overlapping features between the variants of HCL described by Cawley et al., Catovsky et al., and Lampert et al. In this group, tumor cells appear to reveal hybrid features between HCL and B-PLL and in some instances do not respond to conventional therapy.

A 14q+ clonal abnormality involving breakpoint q32 has been found in some cases of HCL. Specific translocations include t(14;18)(q32;q21), t(9;14)(q34;q32), and t(14;22)(q32;q11). Abnormalities of the short arm of chromosome 12 have also been observed. In this case, cytogenetic analysis was not considered necessary to make the diagnosis. However, gene rearrangement studies performed did support the observed immunophenotypic profile of a B-cell neoplasm.

SUMMARY

Morphology	**Lymphocytes, hairy cytoplasmic projections**
Cytochemistry	**TRAP+, Tdt−**

Immunophenotyping	**CD19+, CD20+, CD25+, HLA-DR+, sIgM+, FMC7+**
Cytogenetics	**Not performed**
Molecular Genetics	**Clonal pattern consistent with B-cell neoplasm**
Diagnosis	**Hairy cell leukemia**

ANSWERS:

1. Yes. Although splenomegaly was not evident, cytologic appearances of leukemic cells, monocytopenia, and the dry bone marrow tap make the diagnosis of HCL highly likely.
2. The acid phosphatase stain with tartrate.
3. Yes. The unusual biphenotypic immunologic profile of HCs and the presence of RLCs can be valuable adjuncts in establishing the diagnosis.

BIBLIOGRAPHY

Articles:

Brito-Babapulle V, Pittman S, Melo JV, et al: The 14q+ marker in hairy cell leukemia. A cytogenetic study of 15 cases. *Leuk Res* 10: 131–138, 1986.

Burke JS, Rappaport H: The diagnosis and differential diagnosis of hairy cell leukemia in bone marrow and spleen. *Semin Oncol* 11: 334–346, 1984.

Burke JS, Sheibani K: Hairy cells and monocytoid B lymphocytes: Are they related? *Leukemia* 1:298–300, 1987.

Catovsky D, O'Brien M, Melo JV, et al: Hairy cell leukemia (HCL) variant: An intermediate disease between HCL and B prolymphocytic leukemia. *Semin Oncol* 11:362–369, 1984.

Cawley JC, Burns GF, Hayhoe FGJ: A chronic lymphoproliferative disorder with distinctive features. A distinct variant of hairy cell leukemia. *Leuk Res* 4:547–559, 1980.

Chadburn A, Inghirami G, Knowles DM: Hairy cell leukemia-associated antigen Leu M5(CD11c) is preferentially expressed by benign activated and neoplastic CD8 T cells. *Am J Pathol* 136:29–37, 1990.

Cotelingam JD, Knop RH, Garvin DF, et al: Hairy cells in the cerebrospinal fluid. *N Engl J Med* 308:47, 1983.

Diez Martin JL, Li C-Y, Banks PM: Blastic variant of hairy-cell leukemia. *Am J Clin Pathol* 87:576–583, 1987.

Falini B, Pileri SA, Flenghi L, et al: Selection of a panel of monoclonal antibodies for monitoring residual disease in peripheral blood and bone marrow of interferon-treated hairy cell leukemia patients. *Br J Haematol* 76:460–468, 1990.

Flenghi, L, Spinozzi F, Stein H, et al: LF 61: A new monoclonal antibody directed against a trimeric molecule (150 kDa, 125 kDa, 105 kDa) associated with hairy cell leukemia. *Br J Haematol* 76:451–459, 1990.

Genot E, Valentine MA, Degos L, et al: Hyperphosphorylation of CD20 in hairy cells. Alteration by low molecular weight B cell growth factor and IFN-alpha. *J Immunol* 146:870–878, 1991.

Golomb HM, Braylan R, Polliack A: "Hairy" cell leukemia (leukemic reticuloendotheliosis): A scanning electron microscopic study of 8 cases. *Br J Haematol* 29:455–460, 1975.

Haegart DG, Furlong MD, Smith JL: Co-expression of surface immunoglobulin and T3 on hairy cells. *Scand J Haematol* 37:196–202, 1986.

Hanson CA, Ward PC, Schnitzer B: A multilobular variant of hairy cell leukemia with morphologic similarities to T-cell lymphoma. *Am J Surg Pathol* 13:671–679, 1989.

Hanson CA, Gribbin TE, Schnitzer B, et al: CD11c (Leu-M5) expression characterizes a B-cell chronic lymphoproliferative disorder with features of both chronic lymphocytic leukemia and hairy cell leukemia. *Blood* 76:2360–2367, 1990.

Hassan IB, Hagberg H, Sundström C: Immunophenotype of hairy cell leukemia. *Eur J Haematol* 45:172–176, 1990.

Heirman C, Vaeremans E, Carels D, et al: Isotype switch and idiotype variation in hairy cell leukemia. *Leukemia* 4:856–862, 1990.

Hsu S-M, Yang K, Jaffe ES: Hairy cell leukemia: A B-cell neoplasm with a unique antigenic phenotype. *Am J Pathol* 80:421–428, 1983.

Janckila AJ, Wallace JH, Yam LT: Generalized monocyte deficiency in leukemic reticuloendotheliosis. *Scand J Haematol* 29:153–160, 1982.

Katayama I: Bone marrow in hairy cell leukemia. *Haematol Oncol Clin North Am* 2:585:602, 1988.

Katayama I, Yang JPS: JPS: Reassessment of cytochemical test for differential diagnosis of leukemic reticuloendotheliosis. *Am J Clin Pathol* 68:268–272, 1977.

Katayama I, Hirashima K, Maruyama K, et al: Hairy cell leukemia in Japanese patients: A study with monoclonal antibodies. *Leukemia* 1:301–305, 1987.

Kluin-Nelemans HC, Krouwels MM, Jansen JH, et al: Hairy cell leukemia preferentially expresses the IgG3-subclass. *Blood* 15:972–975, 1990.

Korsmeyer SJ, Greene WC, Cossman J, et al: Rearrangement and expression of immunoglobulin genes and expression of Tac antigen in hairy cell leukemia. *Proc Natl Acad Sci USA* 80:4522–4526, 1983.

Kritensen JS, Ellegaard J, Hokland P: A two-color flow cytometry assay for detection of hairy cells using monoclonal antibodies. *Blood* 70:1063–1068, 1987.

Leměz P, Friedmann B, Váňasek J, et al: Hairy cell leukemia with ring-shaped nuclei. *Blut* 61:251, 1990.

Machii T, Tokumine Y, Inoue R, et al: A unique variant of hairy cell leukemia in Japan. *Jpn J Med* 29:379–383, 1990.

Martin JLD, Li C-Y, Banks PM: Blastic variant of hairy cell leukemia. *Am J Clin Pathol* 87:576–583, 1987.

Melo JV, Robinson DS, Gregory C, et al: Splenic B cell lymphoma with "villous" lymphocytes in the peripheral blood: A disorder distinct from hairy cell leukemia. *Leukemia* 1:294–298, 1987.

Möller P, Mielke B, Moldenhauer G: Monoclonal antibody HML-1, a marker for intra epithelial T cells and lymphomas derived thereof, also recognizes hairy cell leukemia and some B-cell lymphomas. *Am J Pathol* 136:509–512, 1990.

Mulligan SP, Travade P, Matutes E, et al: B-ly-7, a monoclonal antibody reactive with hairy cell leukemia, also defines an activation antigen on normal CD8+ T cells. *Blood* 76:959–964, 1990.

Naeim F, Jacobs AD: Bone marrow changes in patients with hairy cell leukemia treated by recombinant alpha 2-interferon. *Hum Pathol* 16:1200–1205, 1985.

Naeim F, Capostagno VJ, Johnson CE, et al: Sézary syndrome: Tartrate-resistant acid phosphatase in neoplastic cells. *Am J Clin Pathol* 71:528–531, 1975.

Naeim F, Hoon DS, Cheng L, et al: Reactivity of neoplastic cells of hairy cell leukemia with antisera to S-100 protein. *Am J Clin Pathol* 88:86–91, 1987.

Ng JP, Hogg RB, Cumming RL, et al: Primary splenic hairy cell leukemia: A case report and review of the literature. *Eur J Haematol* 39:349–352, 1987.

Posnett DN, Duggan A, McGrath H: Hairy cell leukemia-associated antigen (HC2) is an activation antigen of several hemopoietic cell lineages, inducible on monocytes by IFN-gamma. *J Immunol* 144: 929–933, 1990.

Ratain MJ, Vardiman JW, Baker CM, et al: Prognostic variables in hairy cell leukemia after splenectomy as initial therapy. *Cancer* 62:2420–2424, 1988.

Richards JM, Mick R, Latta JM, et al: Serum soluble interleukin-2 receptor is associated with clinical and pathologic disease status in hairy cell leukemia. *Blood* 76:1941–1945, 1990.

Rosenblatt JD, Golde DW, Wachsman W, et al: A second isolate of HTLV-II associated with atypical hairy cell leukemia. *N Engl J Med* 315:372–377, 1986.

Rosenblatt JD, Gasson JC, Glaspy J, et al: Relationship between human T cell leukemia virus-II and atypical hairy cell leukemia: A serological study of hairy cell leukemia patients. *Leukemia* 1:397–401, 1987.

Sainati L, Matutes E, Mulligan S, et al: A variant form of hairy cell leukemia resistant to alpha-interferon: Clinical and phenotypic characterization of 17 patients. *Blood* 76:157–162, 1990.

Schwarting R, Stein H, Wang CY: The monoclonal antibodies αS-HCL 1(Leu-14) αS-HCL-3(α-LeuM5) allow the diagnosis of hairy cell leukemia. *Blood* 65:974–983, 1985.

Screck R, Donnelly WJ: "Hairy" cell in blood in lymphoreticular neoplastic disease and "flagellated" cells of normal lymph nodes. *Blood* 27:199–211, 1966.

Silingardi V, Davolio-Marani S, Federico M, et al: Bone marrow infiltration in hairy cell leukemia after interferon therapy detected by magnetic resonance imaging. *Eur J Cancer Clin Oncol* 25:209–213, 1989.

Strickler JG, Schmidt CM, Wick MR: Methods in pathology: Immunophenotype of hairy cell leukemia in paraffin sections. *Mod Pathol* 3:518–523, 1990.

Sun T, Susin M, Shevde N, et al: Hybrid form of hairy cell leukemia and chronic lymphocytic leukemia. *Hematol Oncol* 8:283–294, 1990.

Thaler J, Dietze O, Faber V, et al: Monoclonal antibody B-ly7: A sensitive marker for detection of minimal residual disease in hairy cell leukemia. *Leukemia* 4:170–176, 1990.

Usui T, Konishi H, Sawada H, et al: Existence of tartrate-resistant acid phosphatase activity in differentiated lymphoid leukemic cells. *Am J Hematol* 12:47–54, 1982.

van den Oord JJ, de Wolf-Peeters C, Desmet VJ: Hairy cell leukemia: A B-lymphocytic disorder derived from splenic marginal zone lymphocytes? *Blut* 50:191–194, 1985.

Vardiman JW, Golomb HM: Autopsy findings in hair cell leukemia. *Semin Oncol* 11:370–380, 1984.

Vardiman JW, Gilewski TA, Ratain MJ, et al: Evaluation of Leu-M5(CD11c) in hairy cell leukemia by alkaline phosphatase anti-alkaline phosphatase technique. *Am J Clin Pathol* 90:250–256, 1988.

Variakojis D, Vardiman JW, Golomb HM: Cytochemistry of hairy cells. *Cancer* 45:72–77, 1980.

Wolf BC, Martin AW, Neiman RS, et al: The detection of Epstein-Barr virus in hairy cell leukemia cells by in situ hybridization. *Am J Pathol* 136:717–723, 1990.

Yam LT, Janckila AJ, Li C-Y, et al: Tartrate-resistant acid phosphatase isoenzyme in the reticulum cells of leukemic reticuloendotheliosis. *N Engl J Med* 284:357–360, 1971.

Yam LT, Phyliky RL, Li C-Y: Benign and neoplastic disorders simulating hairy cell leukemia. *Semin Oncol* 11:353–361, 1984.

Zinzani PL, Lauria F, Buzzi H, et al: Hairy cell leukemia variant: A morphological, immunological and clinical study of 7 cases. *Haematologica* 75:54–57, 1990.

Zucker-Franklin D: Virus like particles in the lymphocytes of a patient with chronic lymphocytic leukemia. *Blood* 21:509–512, 1963.

Review Articles:

Bouroncle BA, Wiseman BK, Doan CA: Leukemic reticuloendotheliosis. *Blood* 13:609–630, 1958.

Doane LL, Ratain MJ, Golomb HM: Hairy cell leukemia: Current management. *Hematol Oncol Clin North Am* 4:489–502, 1990.

Katayama I, Li C-Y, Yam LT: Ultrastructural characteristics of the "hairy cells" of leukemic reticuloendotheliosis. *Am J Pathol* 67:361–366, 1972.

Paoletti M, Bitter MA, Vardiman JW: Hairy cell leukemia. Morphologic, cytochemical and immunologic features. *Clin Lab Med* 8:179–195, 1988.

Rosner MC, Golomb HM: Ribosome-lamella complex in hairy cell leukemia. Ultrastructure and distribution. *Lab Invest* 42:236–247, 1980.

Yam LT, Janckila AJ, Li C-Y, et al: Cytochemistry of tartrate-resistant acid phosphatase: 15 years' experience. *Leukemia* 1:285–288, 1987.

CASE 6

PATIENT: 74-year-old male.

CHIEF COMPLAINT: Patient being followed for idiopathic hypereosinophilia, returned with complaints of fatigue and weakness.

MEDICAL HISTORY: Eosinophilia was first detected during a routine checkup 4 years earlier. At that time the absolute eosinophil count (AEC) was 1100 × 10^9/L. Two years later he developed and survived an acute myocardial infarction. At that time the AEC had increased to 14,300 × 10^9/L.

PHYSICAL EXAMINATION: Afebrile. No organomegaly. Lung fields clear.

LABORATORY RESULTS:

A. *Screening Procedure*
WBC of 26.5 × 10^9/L with a differential of segmented neutrophils 35%, bands 9%, metamyelocytes 2%, eosinophils 36% (AEC 9.54 × 10^9/L), basophils 2%, monocytes 2%, and lymphocytes 14%. HGB 13.3 g/dL. HCT 0.41 L/L, MCV 90.0 fL, MCH 29.1 pg, MCHC 32.1 g/dL, RDW 15.7. Platelets 122 × 10^9/L.

HOSPITAL COURSE: The peripheral blood revealed marked eosinophilia (Case 6.1). The bone marrow was focally hypercellular (fat/

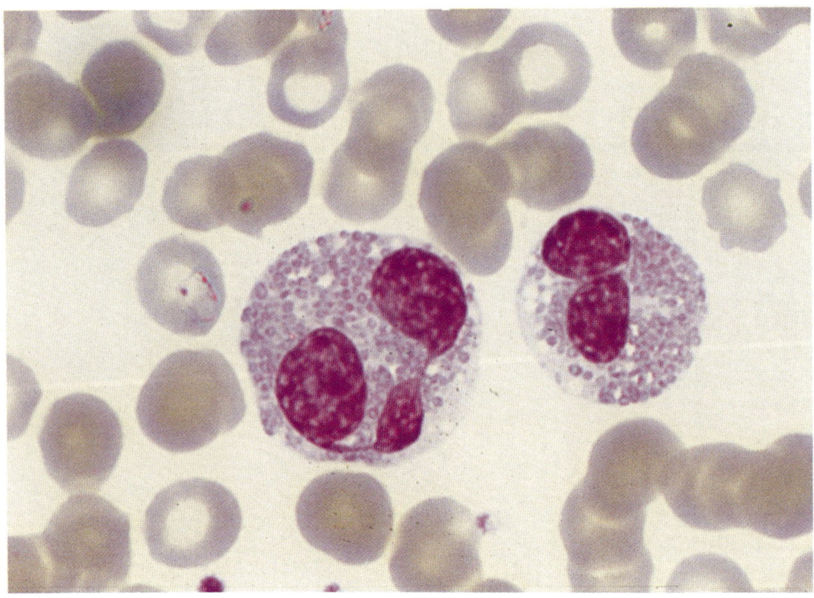

Case 6-1 Peripheral blood with eosinophils. Note abnormal nuclear segmentation. (×1000).

cell ratio 35:65) with increased eosinophilic myelocytes and eosinophils (Case 6.2). On subsequent evaluation 2 months later the WBC count had increased to 43.8 × 10^9/L with 14% eosinophils (AEC 6.76 × 10^9/L). Blast count in the bone marrow was 12%. A diagnosis of RAEB was added to that of idiopathic hypereosinophilia. On final admission 3 months later the bone marrow blast count was 90% (Case 6.3). Auer rods were absent. Based on the cytochemical profile, a diagnosis of AML (AML-M5a) was made. The patient expired on the thirteenth hospital day despite chemotherapy and supportive measures.

QUESTIONS:

1. How best could the process be classified during the initial phase of hospitalization?
2. Was a diagnosis of RAEB appropriate during the subsequent evaluation?
3. Does chronic idiopathic hypereosinophilia usually terminate in EL?

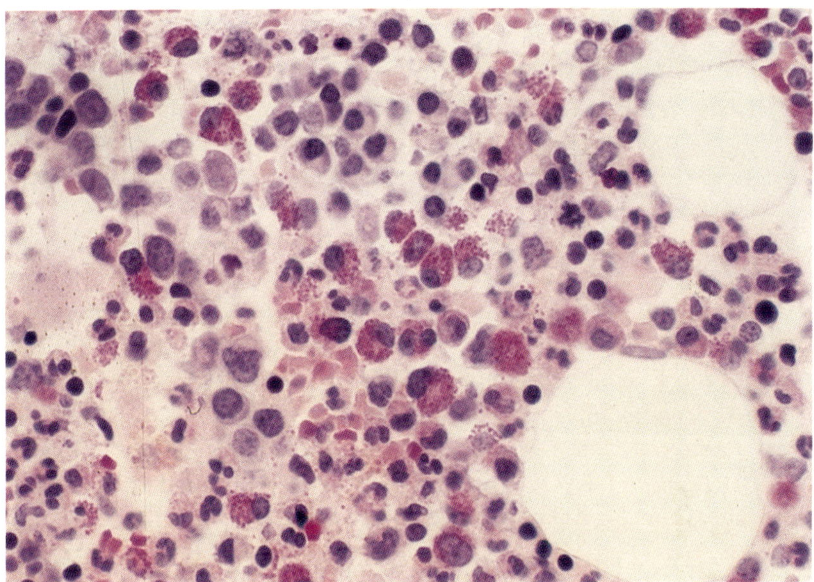

Case 6-2 Bone marrow biopsy demonstrating focally increased eosinophils and eosinophilic myelocytes. (×400).

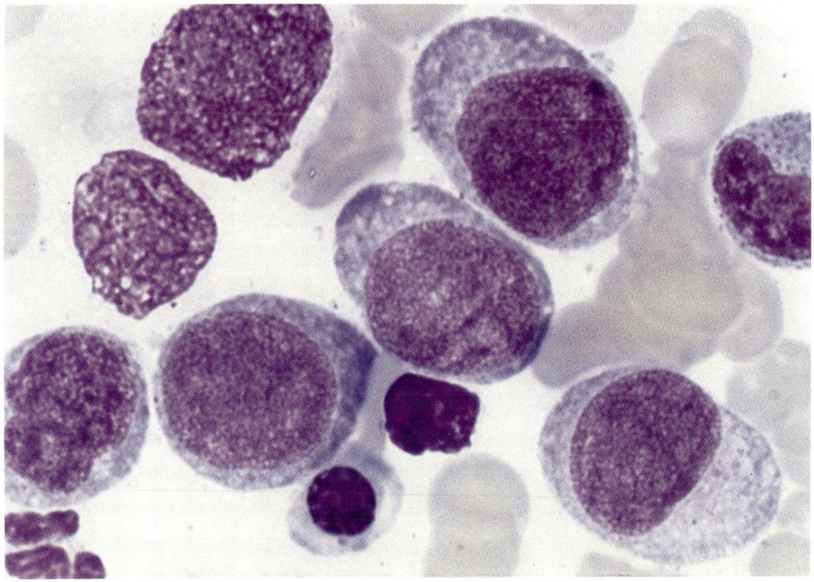

Case 6-3 Bone marrow aspirate showing increased blast forms with multiple nucleoli and abundant cytoplasm. (×1000).

LABORATORY RESULTS:

B. Confirmatory Results

Cytologic examination of eosinophils: Dysmorphic nuclear features, i.e., hypersegmentation and mononuclear forms noted.

Electron microscopy of eosinophils: No abnormality of internal crystalloids observed.

Stool and blood examination for parasites: Negative on repeated studies.

Cytochemistry: Blast forms during the myelodysplastic and leukemic phases were nonspecific esterase, i.e., A-EST and B-EST+, specific esterase (Leder)−, MPEX−, and Tdt−.

Immunophenotyping studies: Leukemic blasts were CD13+, CD14+, CD33+, CD2−, and CD7−.

Cytogenetics: 46 XY. The Y chromosome was deleted in 2 of 9 metaphase preparations from the bone marrow.

DIAGNOSIS: Hypereosinophilic syndrome terminating in monocytic leukemia (AML-M5a).

DISCUSSION: This case serves to illustrate the problem of hypereosinophilia, and the remarkable heterogeneity of disorders that enter into the differential diagnosis.

Since 1879, when Paul Ehrlich announced the discovery of the eosinophil at a meeting of the Physiological Society of Berlin, investigators have been fascinated and perplexed by the structure and function of this cell. From that time, eosinophilia of the blood and parenchymal tissues has been associated with an ever-widening spectrum of disorders. In some, the eosinophilia, although protracted, is an essentially benign and reactive host response. In others, it is an integral component of a malignant and fatal process.

Eosinophils constitute between 1 and 6% of circulating white cells, and an absolute eosinophil count ranging from 40 to 600/mm^3 of blood is considered normal. For the purpose of simplicity and clarity, we have grouped patients with eosinophilia into three broad categories: first, those cases associated with a prevailing nonneoplastic condition; second, an idiopathic category, where eosinophilia may be protracted and unexplained; and finally a third and heterogeneous group where eosinophilia either precedes, succeeds, or is part of a malignant process.

In the first group of patients, benign reactive eosinophilia is observed in association with allergies, putative hypersensitivity disorders, drug reactions, parasitic infestation, immunologic disorders, and collagen vascular diseases, involving virtually every organ system in the body. Eosinophilia is frequently transient and either abates or disappears with appropriate therapy. An exhaustive list of specific disease entities is present in each aforementioned category, and they are well outlined in several reviews including that by Wykoff. Eosinophilia in these patients is reactive and cytologically and karyotypically normal.

It is for the second idiopathic group of patients that Hardy and Anderson in 1968 appropriately proposed the designation *hypereosinophilic syndrome.* Their intent was to encompass within this spectrum both localized and generalized forms of disease. Eosinophilia and widespread organ involvement frequently coexist, and since the outcome in untreated patients is often fatal, confusion with EL has been a problem. To meet the criteria for diagnosis of the hypereosinophilic syndrome, the absolute eosinophil count should be greater than 1.5 $\times$ 10^9/L, remain sustained for at least 6 months, or be preceded by death. In most patients, multisystem lesions characterized by marked eosinophilia develop and involve the bone marrow, spleen, liver, heart, and nervous system. Some have argued that the process is actually an eosinophilic leukemoid reaction and that in its most severe clinicopathologic form the breakdown products of eosinophils discussed below are responsible for tissue damage resulting in death. Others believe that the hypereosinophilia is in itself a MPD. The cytologic appearance of eosinophils from these patients has variously been reported as either normal or dysmorphic with cytoplasmic vacuolization, increased or decreased nuclear lobulation, with "ring" nuclei and nuclear pockets on electron microscopy. No such nuclear pockets were present in our case. Cytogenetic abnormalities described in the literature are essentially confined to those patients with associated hematopoietic neoplasms and are hence summarized below.

In the third category of patients the eosinophilia is either reactive and precedes, succeeds, or accompanies a malignant tumor, or is neoplastic and an integral part of the neoplasm. Based on the types of tumors reported, it is our view that these cases are amenable to further subclassification into lymphoid, myeloid, and a miscellaneous group.

Within the lymphoid subtype are examples of both malignant lymphoma and leukemia. Most frequently encountered is mixed cellularity Hodgkin's disease, where it is well known that eosinophils are a prominent component of the pathologic infiltrate. There is also a less-frequent though well-established association between eosinophilia and MF, T-cell lymphoma, HTLV-I–associated T-cell lymphoma-leukemia, and ALL. The eosinophilia in these disorders is believed to be reactive, although ultrastructural alterations of the inner crystalline core within eosinophil granules has been observed in Hodgkin's disease; and in some cases of ALL, hypogranular eosinophils have been identified. Of interest is an exceptional case of T-ALL reported by Preis et al. which underwent a lineage switch following therapy and resulted in the resurgence of a malignant clone of eosinophils considered to be leukemic. In a review of 26 patients with ALL, Hogan et al observed that hypereosinophilia preceded the ALL by 1–9 months in 13 patients, was concurrent in 1 patient, and developed subsequent to the diagnosis of ALL in 12 others. Although invariably all lymphoid neoplasms associated with eosinophilia are of T-lineage, no specific phenotypic profile has been identified, and the results of CD3, CD4, and CD8 analysis have been variously reported as positive and negative. Cytogenetic abnormalities reported in the literature include 44XY, −8, −2; 46XY,t(5;14)(q?;q32); and trisomy for chromosomes 4, 11, 14, and 21. However, it remains doubtful whether these abnormalities were present in eosinophilic or lymphoid elements.

The association of myeloid lesions with eosinophilia was first observed by Virchow in the last century. It is noteworthy that considerable diversity also exists in this subtype of neoplasms. Included herein are examples of AML, myelomonocytic leukemia, myelodysplasia, CML, and true EL. The AML cases in this group were specifically designated M2Eo at the Fourth International Workshop on Chromosomes and Leukemia. Eosinophilia appears confined to the bone marrow, and these cells have been reported as either cytologically normal, dysmorphic with abnormalities of nuclear lobulation and granule distribution, or frankly malignant with Auer rods. No cytogenetic abnormality was found in eosinophils obtained from colony culture in one case. In others, an 8–21 translocation and trisomy 1 have been reported, attesting further to the diversity of the eosinophilia in AML.

Since the identification of a unique subtype of AML(FAB-M4Eo) by Arthur and Bloomfield in 1983, numerous reports have confirmed the presence of abnormal bone marrow eosinophils in some patients with AML, with abnormalities of chromosome 16 (deletion of the long arm, pericentric inversion, and translocation between homologous chromosomes) and a relatively favorable prognosis. The eosinophils observed are characterized by a component of large basophilic granules, which, unlike normal eosinophil granules, are PAS and CAE positive and frequently fail to reveal well-defined internal crystalloids. Whether these dysmorphic features indicate that the cell is neoplastic remains uncertain. It is of interest, however, that such eosinophils have also be observed in Ph[1]-positive AMML with inversion of chromosome 16, myelodysplasia, AML-M5b, and EL. In contrast, the dysmorphic eosinophils observed in the present case of AML-M5a and in another report of M5b and AML-M2Eo were devoid of basophil granules.

While the association of eosinophilia with CML is well known, it is only recently that the Ph[1] chromosome has been identified within such eosinophils. Also, glucose-G-phosphate dehydrogenase isoenzyme studies have revealed the clonal identity of these eosinophils and other leukemic elements, thereby confirming their malignant nature. In reports preceding the era of BCR technology, a case of Ph[1]-negative CML with chloroma and chronic hypereosinophilia was reported by Huang et al. The authors believed this to be an example of chronic EL. In yet another report, Goh et al. (1985) describe a patient with multiple chromosomal abnormalities, eosinophilic chloroma, and EL.

Since the description of EL by Stillman in 1912, both acute and chronic forms have been observed. However, although more than 100 cases have been documented in adults and children, the diagnosis of this unusual form of leukemia has remained a problem. This is because large enough numbers of immature elements have not been present and putative blasts have not been fully characterized. Moreover, the association of hypereosinophilia with the numerous entities discussed above have frequently detracted against its existence in pure form. Furthermore, although a variety of chromosomal abnormalities, including the Ph[1] chromosome, trisomy 7, 8, 9, and 10, 9q−, translocation abnormalities of chromosome 12p13, t(10;11), t(5;11), t(8;21), a short Y chromosome, and isochromosome 17 have been observed and catalogued by Keene et al., no specific marker appears to be present. Absolute eosinophil counts have varied considerably. Cytologic examination of eosinophils has demonstrated nuclear hypo- and hypersegmentation with pseudo-Pelger eosinophils and numerous eosinophilic promyelocytes in the bone marrow of some cases. Specific granules have frequently been decreased in number and varied in size. Cytoplasmic vacuoles, albeit of a nonspecific nature, have been variably present. Cytochemical examination has revealed PAS activity, ascribed to glycogen and located outside Luxol fast blue–positive specific granules. Also, a strong positive reaction with arylsulphatase, acid phosphatase, and perixodase (Udritz modification) has been observed. Peroxidase activity has been located in the endoplasmic reticulum, nuclear envelope, and Golgi region. Specific eosinophil granules (potassium pyroantimonate–positive) have been observed in eosinophilic promyelocytes and are devoid of internal crystalloids, although these appear at later stages of maturation. In a cell line established from a case of EL, Saito et al. found surface Ia antigen, the myeloid antigens IF10 and My9, and membrane receptors for IL-2 and the Tac antigen. This conundrum of information prompted the belief that EL does in fact exist as a distinct entity. Recently, Keene et al. have demonstrated translocation abnormalities of chromosome 12p13 in cases of acute EL, Ph^1-negative myeloproliferative disease, and ALL and speculate that a gene regulating eosinophil production may be located at this site, which is in proximity to the oncogene c-Ki *ras* 2. The only well-documented case of acute secondary EL is reported by Maeda et al, and developed 8 years after melphalan treatment for multiple myeloma in a 71-year-old woman. The cytogenetic abnormalities included a 5q− and monosomy 7, being similar to those observed in other patients with chemotherapy-induced secondary ANLL.

Within the miscellaneous subtype of the third category are reports of reactive eosinophilia associated with nonhematopoietic neoplasms including carcinomas of the cervix, pancreas, and colon; malignant fibrous histiocytoma; malignant histiocytosis; and non–small cell carcinoma of the lung. Eosinophilia in these patients has been either within the neoplasms, in the peripheral blood, or in both sites and in some instances has been associated with metastases. Of interest is the report by Dincsoy et al. of hypereosinophilia associated with a malignant melanoma and circulating Charcot-Leyden crystals.

Since the conditions associated with eosinophilia are often unrelated, it appears that a complex interplay of hematopoietic, immunologic, and chemotactic factors are responsible for bringing eosinophils within the proximity of foreign antigens and neoantigens. Eosinophils are end-stage effector cells, and usually several hundred times as many are present in the tissue as in the blood. The development and maturation of eosinophils in the bone marrow and in vitro has been shown to be regulated by a synergism between several cytokines including GM-CSF, IL-1, IL-2, IL-3, and IL-5. T lymphocytes from patients with hypereosinophilia produce soluble eosinopoietic factors including IL-5, which appears to be primarily responsible for the eosinophilia. Eosinophils are functionally equipped with primary cytoplasmic granules, secondary crystalloid-containing granules, small arylsulphatase and acid phosphatase containing granules, tubular vesicular structures (microgranules), and arachidonic acid–containing lipid bodies. The orange color of the large refractile granules is apparently due to a high content of major basic protein (MBP), which appears concentrated within the crystalline core of the secondary granules. Peroxidase activity has also been located within the granule matrix and is capable of generating hypohalous acids. Internal dissolution of the crystalline core results in a vacuolar cytoplasmic appearance, and fusion results in the development of protein-rich dipyrimidal structures (Charcot-Leyden crystals) with lysophospholipase activity. Additionally, an eosinophil-derived neurotoxin and an eosinophilic cationic protein have also been isolated. Eosinophils are known to release superoxide and H_2O_2, and to express receptors for IgG, IgE, IgA, C1q, C3b/C4b (CR1), iC3b(CR3), C5a, IL-3, IL-5, GM-CSF, platelet-activating factor, leukotriene B4, estrogens, and glucocorticoids. Additionally, eosinophils express the leukocyte adhesion glycoproteins LFA-1(CD11a), CR3(CD11b) and gp150/95(CD11c); and the common beta chain (CD18). Mature eosinophils retain the ability to synthesize CD4 and HLA-DR, and may hence form new proteins relevant to immunologic demands. However, the precise mechanism involved in the interaction of eosinophils with neoantigens remains to be elucidated.

In the present case, it is uncertain whether the eosinophilia observed was reactive or malignant. Although a Y-chromosomal deletion was identified in some metaphase preparations, we are doubtful of its significance, since this has been observed as a sequela of cellular senescence. Furthermore, c-N-*ras* activation, which has been observed in some cases of hypereosinophilia with myeloproliferative disease, was not studied. Irrespective of its nature, however, the eosinophilia was completely effaced by the evolving monocytic leukemia and was virtually absent in all organs at autopsy. We believe, therefore, that the eosinophilia observed in this case was reactive and an epiphenomenon.

SUMMARY

Morphology	**Dysmorphic eosinophils; monoblasts**
Electron Microscopy	**Unremarkable crystalloids in eosinophils**
Cytochemistry	**Blasts A-EST+, B-EST+, Leder−, MPEX−**
Immunophenotyping	**Blasts CD13+, CD14+, CD33+**
Cytogenetics	**46XY; missing Y chromosome in two metaphase preparations**
Diagnosis	**Hypereosinophilic syndrome terminating in monocytic leukemia (AML-M5a)**

ANSWERS:

1. Since the eosinophilia was idiopathic, blast forms in the marrow not increased, and AEC greater than $1.5 \times 10^9/L$ for over 6

months, the designation *Hypereosinophilic syndrome* was appropriate during the early phase of hospitalization.

2. Yes. Based on the observed blast count in the bone marrow (12%). A diagnosis of EL was not considered since eosinophilic promyelocytes were not increased.
3. No. Studies on the natural history of the hypereosinophilic syndrome indicate that cardiovascular morbidity is the leading cause of death.

BIBLIOGRAPHY

Articles:

Abbondanzo SL, Gray RG, Whang-Peng J, et al: A myelodysplastic syndrome with marrow eosinophilia terminating in acute nonlymphocytic leukemia, associated with an abnormal chromosome 16. *Arch Pathol Lab Med* 111:330–332, 1987.

Bennett JM, Catovsky D, Daniel MT, et al: Proposed revised criteria for the classification of acute leukemia. *Ann Intern Med* 103:626–629, 1985.

Bentley HP Jr., Reardon AE, Knoedler JP, et al: Eosinophilic leukemia. Report of a case with review and classification. *Am J Med* 30:310–322, 1961.

Benvenisti DS, Ultmann JE: Eosinophilic leukemia. Report of five cases and review of literature. *Ann Intern Med* 71:731–745, 1969.

Binder C, Granditsch G: Zur Frage einer Eosinophilie während der präleukämischen Phase einer akuten myeloischen Leukämie. *Pädiatrie und Pädologe* 11:234–239, 1976.

Bitter MA, LeBeau MM, Larson RA, et al: A morphologic and cytochemical study of acute myelomonocytic leukemia with abnormal marrow eosinophils associated with Inv(16)(p13q22). *Am J Clin Pathol* 81:733–741, 1984.

Brandt L, Mitelman F, Beckman G, et al: Different composition of the eosinophilic bone marrow pool in reactive eosinophilia and eosinophilic leukemia. *Acta Med Scand* 201:177–180, 1977.

Broustet A, Bernard Ph, Dachary D, et al: Acute eosinophilic leukemia with translocation (10p+;11q−). *Cancer Genet Cytogenet* 21: 327–333, 1986.

Carbol C: Chromosomal anomaly in eosinophilic leukemia. *N Engl J Med* 301:439, 1979.

Catovsky D, Bernasconi C, Verdonck PJ, et al: The association of eosinophilia with lymphoblastic leukemia or lymphoma. A study of seven patients. *Br J Haematol* 45:523–534, 1980.

Chen KTK, Marsh HH: Philadelphia chromosome–negative chronic myelogenous leukemia with prominent eosinophilic component. *Am J Clin Pathol* 81:789–791, 1984.

Chusid MJ, Dale DC, West BC, et al: The hypereosinophilic syndrome: Analysis of fourteen cases with review of the literature. *Medicine* 54:1–27, 1975.

Dincsoy HP, Burton TJ, vander Bel-Kahn JM: Circulating Charcot-Leyden crystals in the hypereosinophilic syndrome: *Am J Clin Pathol* 75:236–243, 1981.

Dvilansky A, Alkan ML, Ho W, et al: Chronic eosinophilic leukemia complicated by epidural myoblastoma. *Acta Haematol* 53:356–361, 1975.

Ellman L, Hammond D, Atkins L: Eosinophilia, chloromas and a chromosomal abnormality in a patient with a myeloproliferative syndrome. *Cancer* 43:2410–2413, 1979.

Fischkoff SA, Test JR, Schiffer CA: Acute eosinophilic leukemia with a (10;11) chromosomal translocation. *Leukemia* 2:394–397, 1988.

Flannery EP, Dillon DE, Freeman MVR, et al: Eosinophilic leukemia with fibrosing endocarditis and short Y chromosome. *Ann Intern Med* 77:223–228, 1972.

Fourth International Workshop on Chromosomes in Leukemia. *Cancer Genet Cytogenet* 11:275–360, 1984.

Ghadially FN: Lysosomes in eosinophil leucocytes. In *Ultrastructural Pathology of the Cell and Matrix*, vol 2. London, Butteworths, 1988, pp 658–663.

Gleich GJ: Current understanding of eosinophil function. *Hosp Pract* 23:137–160, 1988.

Gleich GJ, Adolphson CR: The eosinophilic leukocyte. Structure and function. *Adv Immunol* 39:177–253, 1986.

Gleich GJ, Frigas E, Loegering DA, et al: Cytotoxic properties of the eosinophil major basic protein. *J Immunol* 123:2925–2927, 1979.

Goh K, Swisher SN, Rosenberg CA: Cytogenetic studies in eosinophilic leukemia. The relationship of eosinophilic leukemia and chronic myeloid leukemia. *Ann Intern Med* 62:80–86, 1965.

Goh KO, Ho FSC, Tso SC, et al: Is hypereosinophilia a malignant disease? *Cancer* 55:2395–2399, 1985.

Goldman JM, Najfeld V, Th'ng KH: Agar culture and chromosome analysis of eosinophilic leukemia. *J Clin Pathol* 28:956–961, 1975.

Gruenwald H, Kissoglou, Mitus W, et al: Philadelphia chromosome in eosinophilic leukemia. *Am J Med* 39:1003–1010, 1965.

Hardy WR, Anderson RE: The hypereosinophilic syndromes. *Ann Intern Med* 68:1220–1229, 1968.

Harrington DS, Peterson C, Ness M, et al: Acute myelogenous leukemia with eosinophilic differentiation and trisomy-1. *Am J Clin Pathol* 90:464–469, 1988.

Henderson DW, Sage RE: Malignant histiocytosis with eosinophilia. *Cancer* 32:1421–1428, 1973.

Hogan TF, Koss W, Murgo AJ, et al: Acute lymphoblastic leukemia with chromosomal 5;14 translocation and hypereosinophilia: Case report and literature review. *J Clin Oncol* 5:382–390, 1987.

Holahan KP: Hypereosinophilic syndrome. *ASCP Check Sample* 32: No 90–7 (H-222), 1990.

Huang CS, Gomez GA, Kohno S, et al: Chromosomes and causation of human cancer and leukemia. 34. A case of "hypereosinophilic syndrome" with unusual cytogenetic findings in a chloroma, terminating in blastic transformation and CNS leukemia. *Cancer* 44:1284–1289, 1979.

Ishibashi T, Kimura H, Abe R, et al: Involvement of eosinophils in leukemia. Cytogenetic study of eosinophilic colonies from acute myelogenous leukemia associated with translocation (8;21). *Cancer Genet Cytogenet* 22:189–194, 1986.

Isoda M, Yasumoto S: Eosinophilic chemotactic factor derived from a malignant fibrous histiocytoma. *Clin Exp Dermatol* 11:253–259, 1986.

Kaneko Y, Kimpara H, Kawai S, et al: 8;21 chromosome translocation in eosinophilic leukemia. *Cancer Genet Cytogenet* 9:181–183, 1983.

Kauer GL, Engle RL, Jr.: Eosinophilic leukaemia with Ph^1-positive cells. *Lancet* 2:1340, 1964.

Kimura H, Abe R, Shiga Y, et al: A case of acute myelogenous leukemia associated with eosinophilia. Cytogenetic study of eosinophilic colonies showing the origin of the normal clone. *Acta Haematol* 77:15–19, 1987.

Kim CH, Park SH, Chi JG: Idiopathic hypereosinophilic syndrome terminating as disseminated T-cell lymphoma. *Cancer* 67:1064–1069. 1991.

Koeffler PH, Levine AM, Sparkes M, et al: Chronic myeloid leukemia. Eosinophils in malignant clone. *Blood* 55:1063–1065, 1980.

Larson RA, Williams SF, LeBeau MM, et al: Acute myelomonocytic leukemia with abnormal eosinophils and inv(16) or t(16;16) has a favorable prognosis. *Blood* 68:1242–1249, 1986.

LeBeau MM, Larson RA, Bitter MA, et al: Association of an inversion of chromosome 16 with abnormal marrow eosinophils in acute myelomonocytic leukemia. A unique cytogenetic-clinicopathologic association. *N Engl J Med* 309:630–636, 1983.

Liao KT, Rosai J, Daneshbod K: Malignant histiocytosis with cutaneous involvement and eosinophilia. *Am J Clin Pathol* 57:438–448, 1972.

Liso V, Troccol G, Specchia G, et al: Cytochemical 'normal' and 'abnormal' eosinophils in acute leukemia. *Am J Hematol* 2:123–131, 1977.

Lonnquist B, Gahrton G, Ericksson P, et al: Isochromosome 17 in a patient with a myeloproliferative disorder terminating in eosinophilic leukemia. *Acta Med Scand* 206:321–325, 1979.

Maeda K, VanSlyck E, VanDyke D: Multiple myeloma terminating in acute eosinophilic leukemia. *Cancer Genet Cytogenet* 16:81–89, 1985.

Marshall GM, White L: Effective therapy for a severe case of the idiopathic hypereosinophilic syndrome. *Am J Ped Hematol/Oncol* 11:178–183, 1989.

Matsurra Y, Sato N, Kimura F, et al: An increase in basophils in a case of acute myelomonocytic leukaemia associated with marrow eosinophilia and inversion of the chromosome 16. *Eur J Haematol* 39:457–461, 1987.

Maubach PA, Bauchinger M, Emmerich B, et al: Trisomy 7 and 8 in Ph-negative chronic eosinophilic leukemia. *Cancer Genet Cytogenet* 17:159–164, 1985.

Mecucci C, Noens L, Aventin A, et al: Philadelphia-positive acute myelomonocytic leukemia with inversion of chromosome 16 and eosinobasophils. *Am J Hematol* 27:69–71, 1988.

Miller RR, Lewis JP, Knapp W: Acute eosinophilic leukemia associated with neutropenia. *West J Med* 123:399–404, 1975.

Mitelman F, Panani A, Brandt L: Isochromosome 17 in a case of eosinophilic leukemia: An abnormality common to eosinophilic and neutrophilic cells. *Scand J Haematol* 14:308–312, 1975.

Miyachi H, Toyama K: Hypereosinophilic syndrome. *Rinsho Ketsueki* 26:1729–1740, 1985.

Mori Y, Ebira H, Shindo Y, et al: Eosinophilic leukemia with trisomy of no. 8 and 9 chromosomes: Report of a case. *Rinsho Ketsueki* 27:565–569, 1968.

Needleman SW, Mane SM, Gutheil JC, et al: Hypereosinophilic syndrome with evolution to myeloproliferative disorder: Temporal relationship to Y chromosome deletion and c-N-*ras* activation. *Blood* 74(suppl. 1):237a, 1989.

Parillo JE, Fauci AS: Human eosinophils. Purification and cytotoxic capability of eosinophils from patients with the hypereosinophilic syndrome. *Blood* 51:457–473, 1978.

Parillo JE, Fauci AS, Wolff SM: Therapy of hypereosinophilic syndrome. *Ann Intern Med* 89: 167–172, 1978.

Preis PP, Zielinski CC, Linkesch W: Shift in phenotype of acute T-lymphocytic leukemia to eosinophilic leukemia. A case report. *Wien Klin Wochenschr* 13:331–336, 1988.

Rickles FR, Miller DR: Eosinophilic leukemoid reaction. Report of a case, its relationship to eosinophilic leukemia and review of the pediatric literature. *J Pediatr* 80:418–428, 1972.

Rohrbach MS, Wheatley CL, Slifman NR, et al: Activation of platelets by eosinophil granule proteins. *J Exp Med* 172:1271–1274, 1990.

Saito H, Bourinbaiar A, Ginsburg M, et al: Establishment and characterization of a new human eosinophilic leukemia cell line. *Blood* 66:1233–1240, 1985.

Schmitz N, Maubach PA, Godde-Salz E, et al: Acute eosinophilic leukemia: Characterization by cytochemistry, chromosomal analysis, and in vitro colony formation. *Klin Wochenschr* 63:133–137, 1985.

Siebenmann RE: Paraneoplastic eosinophilic leukemoid reaction with eosinophilic parietal thromboendocarditis in malignant melanoma. *Schweiz Med Wochenschr* 107:1247–1265, 1977.

Siering VH: Die eosinophile Leukämie als diagnostisches Problem. *Z. Gesamte Inn Med Jahrg* 42:363–365, 1987.

Sigaux E, Imbert M, Jouault, et al: Involvement of the eosinophilic series in t(8;21) acute myeloid leukemia (AML). *Blood* 60(suppl 1):482a, 1982.

Sjogren J: Bone marrow morphology in acute eosinophilic-monocytic leukaemia. *Acta Hematol* 62:17–19, 1979.

Spitzer G, Garson OM: Lymphoblastic leukemia with marked eosinophilic. A report of two cases. *Blood* 42:377–384, 1973.

Stillman RG: A case of myeloid leukemia with predominance of eosinophilic cells. *Med Rec* 81:594–595, 1912.

Swirsky DM, Li YS, Matthews JG, et al: 8;21 Translocation in acute granulocytic leukaemia: Cytological, cytochemical and clinical features. *Br J Haemat* 56:199–213, 1984.

Tai P-C, Spry CJF: The mechanisms which produce vacuolated and degranulated eosinophils. *Br J Haematol* 49:219–226, 1981.

Tai PC, Hayes DJ, Clark JB, et al: Toxic effects of human eosinophil secretion products on isolated heart cells in vitro. *Biochem J* 204:75–80, 1982.

Tantravahi R, Schwenn M, Henkle C, et al: A pericentric inversion of chromosome 16 is associated with dysplastic marrow eosinophils in acute myelomonocytic leukemia. *Blood* 63:800–802, 1984.

Troxell ML, Mills GM, Allen RC: The hypereosinophilic syndrome in acute lymphocytic leukemia. *Cancer* 54:1058–1061, 1984.

Weinfeld A, Westin J, Swolin B: Ph^1-negative eosinophilic leukaemia with trisomy 8. Case report and review of cytogenetic studies. *Scand J Haematol* 18:413–420, 1977.

Weinger RS, Andre-Schwartz J, Desforges JF, et al: Acute leukemia with eosinophilia or acute eosinophilic leukemia: A dilemma. *Br J Haematol* 30:65–70, 1975.

Xavier AM, Zebari D: Eosinophilia as a precursor of acute myelomonocytic leukemia. *Arch Pathol Lab Med* 112:577, 1988.

Yam LT, Li C-Y, Necheles TF, et al: Pseudoeosinophilia, eosinophilic endocarditis and eosinophilic leukemia. *Am J Med* 53:193–202, 1972.

Yamada K, Horiuchi N, Shintani Y, et al: Eosinophilic leukemia with myelofibrosis and dysplasia terminating in marked increase of blast cells: A report of an autopsied case. *Rinsho Ketsueki* 27:1964–1970, 1986.

Yoo TJ, Orman SV, Patil SR, et al: Evolution to eosinophilic leukemia with a t(5;11) translocation in a patient with idiopathic hypereosinophilic syndrome. *Cancer Genet Cytogenet* 11:389–394, 1984.

Review Articles:

Arthur DC, Bloomfield CD: Partial deletion of the long arm of chromosome 16 and bone marrow eosinophilia in acute nonlymphocytic leukemia. A new association. *Blood* 61:994–998, 1983.

Fauci AS, Harley JB, Roberts WC, et al: The idiopathic hypereosinophilic syndrome. *Ann Intern Med* 97:78–92, 1982.

Keene P, Mendelow B, Pinto MR, et al: Abnormalities of chromosome 12p13 and malignant proliferation of eosinophils: A nonrandom association. *Br J Haematol* 67:25–31, 1987.

Presentey B, Jerushalmy Z, Mintz U: Eosinophilic leukemia. Morphological, cytochemical and electronmicroscopic studies. *J Clin Pathol* 32:261–271, 1979.

Weller PF: The immunobiology of eosinophils. *N Engl J Med* 324:1110–1118, 1991.

Wykoff RF: Eosinophilia. *South Med J* 79:608–612, 1986.

CASE 7

PATIENT: 59-year-old female.

CHIEF COMPLAINT: Fever and heaviness in the abdomen of 6 weeks' duration.

MEDICAL HISTORY: The patient was a former postal employee and enjoyed good health until she experienced febrile episodes and a dragging left upper abdominal sensation.

PHYSICAL EXAMINATION: Temperature 99.3°F. Mild mucosal pallor was observed. The spleen was nontender and enlarged 10.0 cm below the left costal margin. Adenopathy and hepatomegaly were absent.

LABORATORY RESULTS:

A. *Screening Procedure*
   WBC of 9.2×10^9/L with a differential count of segmented neutrophils 55%, band forms 2%, eosinophils 2%, basophils 1%, monocytes 8%, and lymphocytes 32%. HGB 11.9 g/dL. HCT 0.36 L/L. MCV 97.0 fL, MCH 32.1 pg, MCHC 33.4 g/dL, RDW 13.6. Platelets 112×10^9/L.

HOSPITAL COURSE: Following clinical and radiologic evaluation, the cause of splenomegaly remained unresolved. A bone marrow biopsy was performed. Appearances were normocellular and devoid

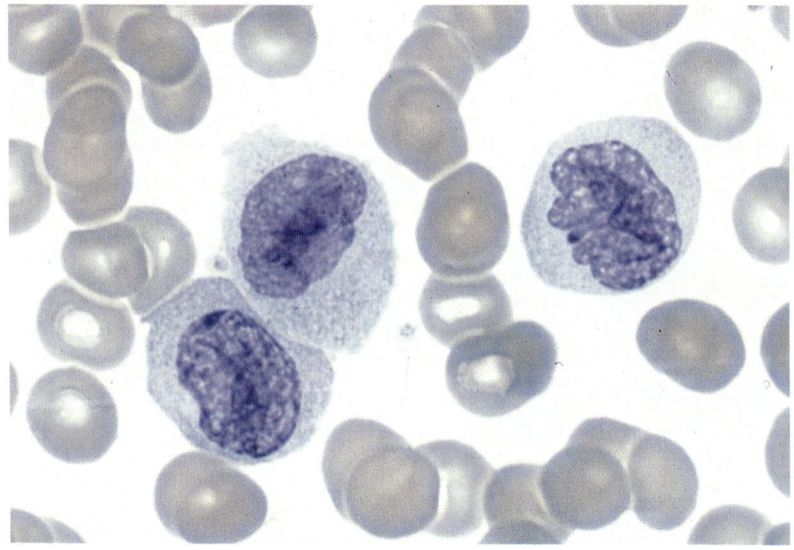

Case 7-1 Monocytes in peripheral blood at 6 weeks postsplenectomy. Note irregular nuclear membranes. ($\times$1000).

of any abnormal infiltrate. Splenectomy was therefore considered and performed on the eleventh hospital day. Subsequently, the platelet count rose to 140 $\times$ 10^9/L. Six weeks following splenectomy, the total white blood count increased to 15.4 $\times$ 10^9/L and was accompanied by a monocytosis of 14% (Case 7.1). A second bone marrow biopsy was obtained and material submitted for cytogenetic evaluation. Following establishment of the diagnosis, the patient was started on combination chemotherapy with busulfan and 6-mercaptopurine. Complete remission was achieved. Two months thereafter, the patient was injured in an automobile accident and died.

QUESTIONS:

1. Does a normal total and differential WBC at presentation exclude a diagnosis of leukemia?
2. What conditions enter into the differential diagnosis?
3. Is there a role for cytochemical analysis?

LABORATORY RESULTS:

B. Confirmatory Results

Pathology of the spleen: The spleen was enlarged and weighed 980.0 g. Cross-section revealed a diffuse process. On mi-

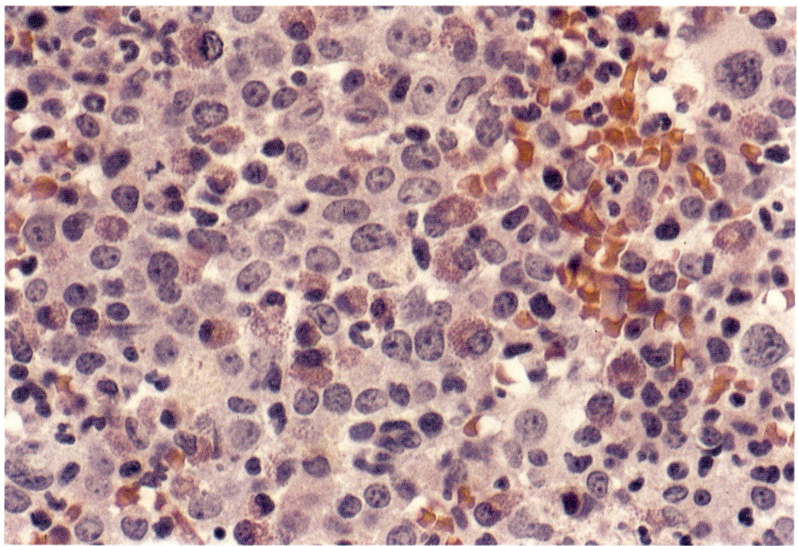

Case 7-2 Hypercellular bone marrow biopsy at 6 weeks postsplenectomy, with monocytic infiltrate. (×400).

croscopy, the red pulp was found to be infiltrated by mature monocytes with round, oval, or folded nuclei, occasional inconspicuous nuclei, and rare erythrophagocytosis. Leukemic cells expanded the Billroth cords, obliterated sinuses, and encroached on and destroyed the white pulp. Occasionally, sinuses were dilated and contained leukemic cells.

Peripheral blood: At 6 weeks postsplenectomy, circulating monocytes were cytologically indistinguishable from those observed at presentation and revealed minimal irregularity of nuclear membranes.

Bone marrow analysis: At 6 weeks postsplenectomy, the bone marrow was hypercellular with a fat/cell ratio of 15:85 and revealed an interstitial and focal leukemic monocytic infiltrate (Case 7.2) constituting 65% of marrow cellularity. Other hematopoietic tissues were decreased and maturing. Leukemic cells were cytologically similar to those observed in the postsplenectomy blood films and spleen. Myelofibrosis was absent.

Cytochemistry: Leukemic cells from the bone marrow aspirate were A-EST+ (Case 7.3), B-EST+, MPEX−, SBB+, PAS+ (blush and finely granular), specific esterase (Leder) negative.

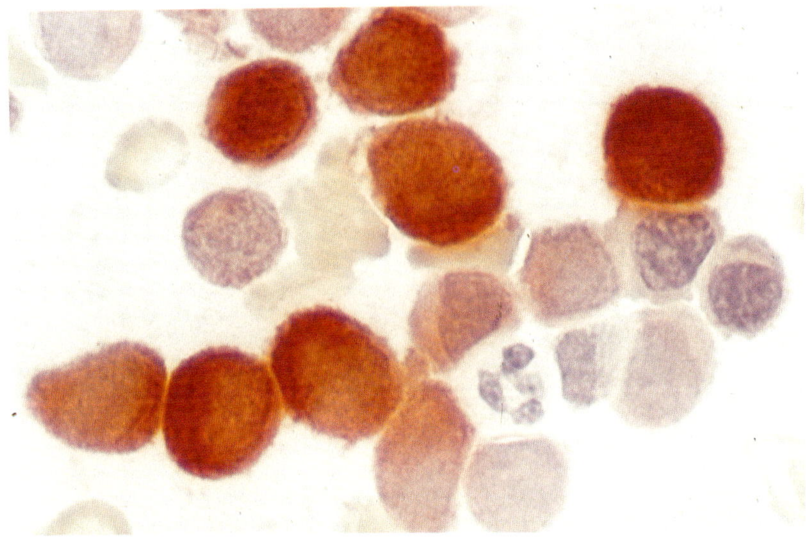

Case 7-3 Bone marrow aspirate with prominent A-EST+ leukemic cells. (×1000).

Immunophenotyping studies: CD9+, CD14+, CD23+, CD64+, and CD74+.

Cytogenetics: 46XX. No Ph^1 chromosome present.

DIAGNOSIS: Chronic monocytic leukemia.

DISCUSSION: CMoL is a very rare and poorly documented disease. Since 1913, when the first case was reported by Reschad and Schilling-Torgau, a variety of other conditions believed to be of monocytic origin have been confused with CMoL. Included herein are cases that would be interpreted at this time as CMML, AML-M4, AML-M5, HCL, and the chronic form of malignant histiocytosis. It is clear from a review of these reports that bona fide CMoL is among the rarest of these lesions and is seldom encountered in clinical practice. Hence, no universal criteria for the diagnosis have been established, and several contemporary works dedicated to the subject of leukemia do not mention this entity.

In 1981, Bearman et al. published a critical review of CMoL and, based on the existing literature and five of their own cases, developed the first clear set of guidelines for establishing the diagnosis. Males appear to be more frequently affected than females. Most patients are adults, and in the pediatric age group, CMoL is considered rare enough to be a curiosity. Clinical presentation is most often with weakness, fever, and pain in the left upper quadrant of the abdomen. Splenomegaly has been a consistent finding, and hepatomegaly has also been frequently manifest.

Mild normocytic and normochromic anemia is generally present. At diagnosis, the total WBC has been reported to be either normal, decreased, or increased as high as 27.1×10^9/L. In most cases, the differential leukocyte count has been within normal limits at presentation. However, in one case reported by Bearman et al. (1981), monocytosis was an initial manifestation. Thrombocytopenia at diagnosis is reported in about 50% of patients.

Absolute monocytosis may develop immediately following splenectomy or may manifest up to 24 months later. Monocytes in the peripheral blood reveal abundant slate-gray cytoplasm with delicate magenta granules and vacuoles. Nuclei are of variable shape, ranging from reniform and oval to round, often with a folded and relatively transparent delicate chromatin through which underlying nuclear folds may be seen. Nucleoli are normally absent or small and inconspicuous but may be more prominent in accompanying promonocytic forms. Monoblasts and Auer rods are absent. Erythropoiesis and platelet phagocytosis may be observed. No myelodysplastic hypogranular or "Pelgeroid" changes are reported in accompanying granulocytes. On cytochemical analysis, circulating monocytes are fluoride-sensitive A-EST+, B-EST+, finely granular and blush PAS+, tartrate-sensitive acid phosphatase–positive, and variably SBB+ and MPEX+.

The bone marrow may be either normocellular or hypocellular, and, in presplenectomy samples, a monocytic infiltrate may be absent. Following splenectomy, however, a focal or diffuse monocytic infiltrate develops and progressively replaces normal hematopoietic tissues. Monocytes in the bone marrow may appear slightly more immature than those in the peripheral blood, and phagocytosis of erythroid platelet and other leukocytic elements may occasionally feature prominently. Megaloblastoid erythropoiesis may be present, and megakaryocyte numbers are invariably decreased. Fibrosis does not appear to be a feature of CMoL.

Cytogenetic abnormalities have not been well established in CMoL. However, the Ph^1 chromosome is absent, and, in one case reported by Wahlin et al. (1986) that developed blastic transformation, an extra chromosome 20 was observed.

The immunophenotypic features and molecular genetics of CMoL have not been clearly characterized. As in the present case, however, leukemic cells may be expected to be variably CD9+, CD14+, CD23+, CD64+, CD74+, and CDw78+.

Parenchymal leukemic infiltrates in CMoL have been observed in the spleen, liver, lymph nodes, lungs, kidneys, testes, bladder, gastrointestinal tract, and skin. In histologic sections, leukemic cells demonstrate indented nuclei with delicate evenly distributed chromatin, inconspicuous nucleoli, and amphophilic cytoplasm.

The differential diagnosis of CMoL includes CMML, AML-M4, AML-M5, HCL, the chronic form of malignant histiocytosis, and other poorly classified histiomonocytic infiltrates. Since no myelodysplastic features are present in CMoL, as often seen in CMML, this latter entity can be excluded. Additional distinguishing features of CMML are outlined in the discussion for Case 11. The blastic cytologic features and Auer rods that characterize acute monocytic (AML-M5) and acute myelomonocytic (AML-M4) leukemia are absent in CMoL, and the absence of TRAP activity and the characteristic cytologic and bone marrow biopsy appearances of HCL exclude this diagnosis. The chronic form of malignant histiocytosis is another rare entity that may be confused with CMoL. In this condition, tumor cells are mitotically active, with bizarre cytologic forms and hyperchromatic nuclei.

The etiology and pathogenesis of CMoL are not understood. However, despite its rarity, CMoL is believed to be a distinct clinicopathologic entity. The development of splenomegaly before the presence of marrow involvement has prompted consideration that CMoL originates in the spleen. Additionally, the pronounced splenomegaly, with splenic weights reported as high as 2160.0 g, supports the concept that the cytopenias in this disease are primarily a manifestation of hypersplenism. Therefore, despite splenectomy for diagnostic or therapeutic reasons, no long-term curative outcome is reported.

SUMMARY

Morphology	**Increased monocytes in blood and marrow**
Spleen	**Splenomegaly with destructive monocytic infiltrate**
Cytochemistry	**A-EST+, B-EST+, specific esterase (Leder) negative, MPEX−**
Immunophenotyping	**CD9+, CD14+, CD23+, CD64+, CD74+**
Cytogenetics	**Ph^1 chromosome–negative**
Diagnosis	**Chronic monocytic leukemia**

ANSWERS:

1. No. CMoL is the only chronic leukemia that may present prior to splenectomy with uninvolved blood and marrow.

2. Reactive monocytosis, CML with monocytosis, CMML, and other infiltrative and malignant causes of splenomegaly.
3. Yes. Both nonspecific esterase stains A-EST and B-EST are positive, while the granulocyte–specific stains, specific esterase (Leder) and MPEX, are negative.

BIBLIOGRAPHY

Articles:

Amir J, Djaldetti M: Chronic monocytic leukaemia. A prolonged survival. *Scand J Haematol* 18:337–342, 1977.

Beattie JW, Seal RME, Crowther KV: Chronic monocytic leukemia. *Q J Med* 20:131–139, 1951.

DiGuglielmo G, Morelli A, Maurea C: Istioleucemia cronica. *Haematol Arch* 37:1–60, 1953.

Doan CA, Wiseman BK: The monocyte, monocytosis and monocytic leukosis: A clinical and pathologic study. *Ann Intern Med* 8:383–416, 1934.

Iavorkovskivi LL, Iavorkovskivi LI: Chromosomal aberrations in monocytic leukaemias. *Eksp Onkol* 90:3–8, 1987.

Jacobsen KM: Reticuloendotheliose-monoztenleukose. *Acta Med Scand* 11:30–56, 1942.

Marchal G, Lemoine J, Bloch-Michel R: Leucémie chronique à monocytes, sans splénomégalie, ni adenomégalie. *Sang* 8:694–700, 1934.

Meuret G, Bundschu-Lay A, Senn HJ, et al: Functional characteristics of chronic monocytic "leukemia." *Acta Haematol* 52:95–106, 1974.

Mischinger-Porzsolt A, Schauder S, Schauer A: Chronische Monozytenleukämie. *Hautarzt* 37:230–233, 1986.

Moraes M, Wilkes J, Lowder JN: Monocytic leukemoid reaction, glucocortocoid therapy and myelodysplastic syndrome. *Clev Clin J Med* 57:571–574, 1990.

Mufti GL, Oscier DG, Hamblin TJ, et al: Serous effusions in monocytic leukaemias. *Br J Haematol* 58:547–552, 1984.

Orr JW, Belf MD: Monocytic leukaemia: Two cases. *Lancet* 1:403–407,1933.

Osgood EE: Monocytic leukemia. Report of six cases, and review of one hundred and twenty seven cases. *Arch Intern Med* 59:931–951, 1937.

Pearson HA, Diamond LK: Chronic monocytic leukemia in childhood. *J Pediatr* 53:259–270, 1958.

Rappaport AE, Kugel VH: Monocytic leukemia. A case report illustrating variations in the clinical picture. *Blood* 2:332–355, 1947.

Reschad H, Schilling-Torgau V: Ueber eine neue Leukämie durch echte Uebergangsformen (Splenozytenleukämie) und ihre Bedeutung für die Selbständigkeit dieser Zellen. *München Med Wchnschr* 60:1981–1984, 1913.

Richter W, Fleischer J, Irmscher J: Zytochemische Befunde bei chronischen monozytären Leukosen. *Folia Haematol* 102:524–529, 1975.

Rodgers GM, Carrera CJ, Ries CA, et al: Blastic transformation of a well differentiated monocytic leukemia. Changes in cytochemical and cell surface markers. *Leuk Res* 6:613–622, 1982.

Ryder RJW: Chronic monocytic leukaemia. *Blut* 14:47–50, 1966.

Seligsohn U, Ramot B: Chronic monocytic leukemia: A case with an eight year survival. *Israel J Med Sci* 3:868–874, 1967.

Sinn CM, Dick FW: Monocytic leukemia. *Am J Med* 20:588–602, 1956.

Vardiman JW, Byrne GE, Rappaport H: Malignant histiocytosis with massive splenomegaly in asymptomatic patients. A possible chronic form of disease. *Cancer* 36:419–427, 1986.

Wahlin A, Nordenson I, Roos G: Chronic monocytic leukemia terminating in blastic transformation. *Blut* 53:405–409, 1986.

Review Article:

Bearman RM, Kjeldsberg CR, Panagalis GA, et al: Chronic monocytic leukemia in adults. *Cancer* 48:2239–2255, 1981.

CASE 8

PATIENT: 62-year-old white male.

CHIEF COMPLAINT: Fatigue, night sweats, and left calf pain of 3 weeks' duration.

MEDICAL HISTORY: Good health until onset of chief complaint.

PHYSICAL EXAMINATION: Afebrile patient. Left calf tenderness. Spleen enlarged 4.0 cm below left costal margin. Moderate cervical and inguinal adenopathy present.

LABORATORY RESULTS:

A. *Screening Procedure*
WBC of 426 × 10^9/L with a differential of segmented neutrophils 5.0%, monocytes 1%, and lymphocytes 94%. The majority of the lymphocytes were large and nucleolated. HGB 10.9 g/dL. HCT 0.32 L/L, MCV 103 fL, MCH 34.9 pg, MCHC 33.8 g/dL, RDW 13.8%. Platelets 59 × 10^9/L, MPV 6.3 fL.

HOSPITAL COURSE: Appearances of the peripheral blood film (Case 8.1) at admission were considered compatible with CLL. On examination of the bone marrow aspirate and biopsy, lymphocytes were found to constitute 85% of cellular elements. In some microscopic fields, greater than 50% of the lymphocytes were nucleolated. Those lacking nucleoli were small and occasionally plasmacytoid. Pat-

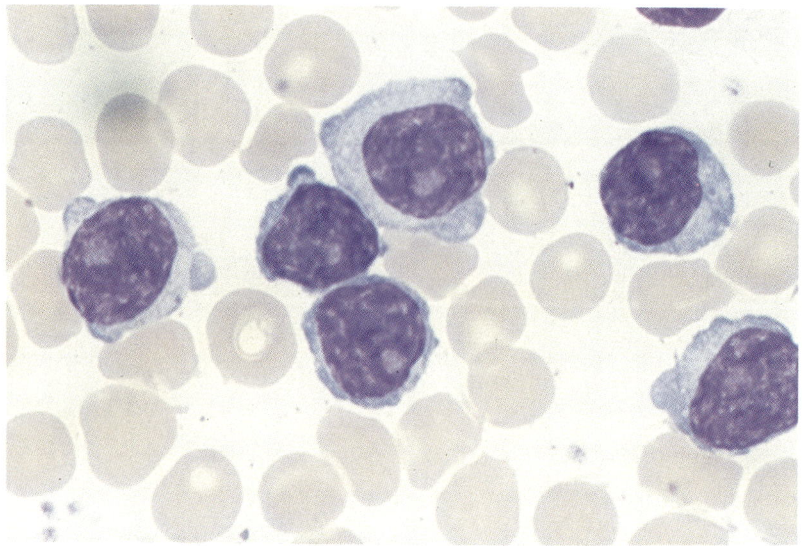

Case 8-1 Peripheral blood film. Note prominent nucleoli and varying amount of cytoplasm. (×1000).

tern of infiltration in the biopsy was interstitial and diffuse. Reticulin fibrosis was absent. A diagnosis of prolymphocytic transformation (PLT) of CLL (mixed CLL-PLL of the FAB group) was made. Tc 99m sulfur colloid scan revealed splenomegaly (15.0 cm), and transaxial scans revealed multiple enlarged mesenteric and femoral lymph nodes (1–3 cm). Duplex Doppler studies identified bilateral deep venous thrombosis from the popliteal to midthigh areas, which responded well to heparin and coumadin therapy. Combination chemotherapy with chlorambucil and prednisone was ineffective. Following the analysis of marker data, treatment with 2′-deoxycoformycin (Pentostatin) was commenced, with an excellent clinical response and drop in the absolute lymphocyte count. The patient has been stable for 16 months.

QUESTIONS:

1. Are the blood and marrow findings adequate to establish diagnosis?
2. How would immunophenotyping help?
3. Is the ribosome-lamella complex observed in this form of chronic leukemia?

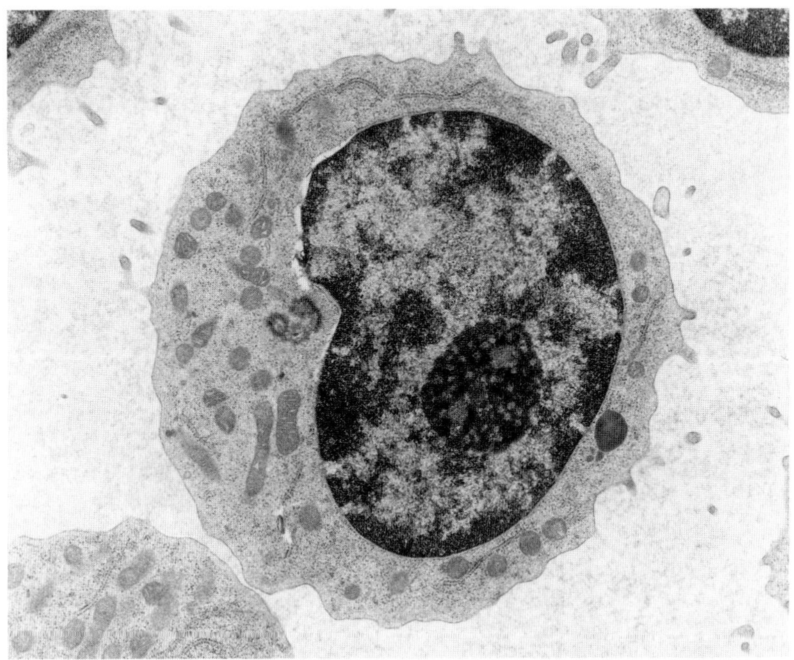

Case 8-2 Electron micrograph of a circulating leukemic PL. The large nucleolus is noteworthy. (×22,000). Courtesy of Gavin P. Riordan.

LABORATORY RESULTS:

B. Confirmatory Results

Cytochemistry: Lymphoid cells were beta-glucuronidase negative, acid phosphatase positive (punctate, perinuclear, and tartrate-sensitive), AEST+, beta-glucuronidase negative and PAS−.

Immunophenotyping studies: Lymphoid cells from the peripheral blood were CD4+, CD5+, CD7+, CD25+, and CD45+ and CD3−, CD8−, CD19−, CD20−, and CD22−. No surface Ig was identified.

Electron microscopy: Well-defined nucleoli were present in most tumor cells (Case 8.2). Occasional long profiles of endoplasmic reticulum were evident, as were scant osmophilic granules. No ribosome-lamella complexes were observed.

Cytogenetics: Performed on leukemic cells from peripheral blood. 46XY. Inversion of both chromosomes 14 with breakpoints at 14q11 and q32.

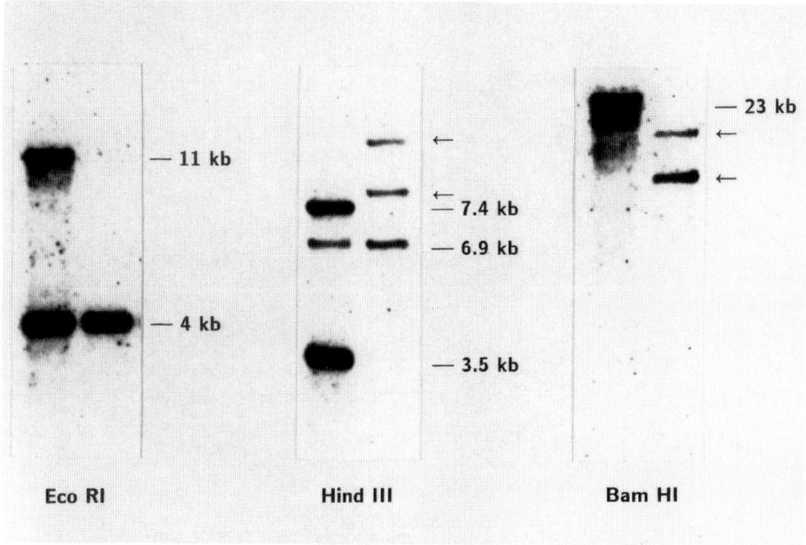

Case 8-3 Restriction fragment analysis (Southern blot) of the TCR-β gene. Peripheral blood. Genomic DNA was digested with restriction enzymes Eco R1, Hind III, and Bam H1, and hybridized with a Cβ probe. Germline configuration of DNA from a nonlymphoid cell line (left panels); and the molecular size is indicated by dashes. Rearranged DNA in patient's sample (right panels) is indicated by arrows. The Eco R1 digest reveals biallelic deletion of Cβ1. In the Hind III digest, biallelic rearrangement of Cβ2 is present, and the Bam H1 digest confirms the biallelic rearrangement of the TCRβ locus. Courtesy of Jay Lynch, Francine Foss, and Lynne V. Abruzzo.

Molecular genetics: Performed on leukemic cells from bone marrow. Biallelic rearrangement of β-TCR gene on Southern blot analysis (Case 8.3).

DIAGNOSIS: T-prolymphocytic leukemia.

DISCUSSION: The concept of PLL as an unusual variant of CLL was initially proposed by Galton et al. in 1963. Thereafter, Catovsky et al. published the first report of T-PLL in the *Lancet,* and PLL became recognized as a distinct disease entity with characteristic morphologic, immunologic, and cytogenetic features. More recently, the differences between the T and B phenotypic subtypes of PLL have become more clearly defined and have led to further refinements of diagnostic criteria.

Each year in the United States it is estimated that between 600 and 1,000 new cases of PLL are diagnosed. The overall frequency of PLL in relation to CLL is about 1:9. A slight male predominance is evident and is 2:1 in T-PLL. Fifty percent of patients are over 70 years of age at diagnosis, and the ratio of T/B phenotypes is estimated at around 1:3.

The cardinal manifestations of PLL include splenomegaly, hyperleukocytosis, bone marrow infiltration, and minimal lymphadenopathy. T-PLL is a more aggressive disease than B-PLL and has a higher incidence of leukocytosis, adenopathy, hepatomegaly, skin infiltration, and malignant effusions. Splenomegaly is more frequently observed in B-PLL and is not always massive. Hyperleukocytosis with counts greater than 100×10^9/L are present in over 65% of all patients with PLL and may result in fatal microvascular obstruction. The recognition of prolymphocytic elements in a peripheral blood film, and their enumeration as greater than 55% of circulating lymphocytes, is the single most important clue to the diagnosis. Prolymphocytes under 10% may be observed in CLL, and counts ranging between 11 and 55% are present in the PLT of CLL. However, as exemplified in the present case, definition of the immunophenotypic profile can be invaluable.

About 33% of patients with B-PLL reveal a monoclonal gammopathy, and sIg with or without IgD is demonstrable in most cases. Occasionally, cytoplasmic IgG has also been present. It is of interest that in contrast to B-CLL, B-PLL cells only rarely form rosettes with mouse erythrocytes (Table C8.1). This, despite the paradoxical connotation of the term *prolymphocyte,* suggests derivation of B-PLL from an immunologically more mature cell than the B-CLL lymphocyte. Serum IgGs are normal in T-PLL, and this disease is apparently not associated with HTLV-I infection.

In a well-prepared peripheral blood film, prolymphocytes are distinguished by their size, which is larger than normal and CLL lymphocytes. Cell size may, however, vary, and Matutes et al. have described the coexistence of large and small types of prolymphocytes. The cytoplasm is moderately abundant, light blue, and PAS−. The nucleus occupies about 3/4 to 7/8 of the cell volume, may be central or eccentric, focally abuts against the cell membrane, and often contains a large solitary nucleolus. Using the modalities of light microscopy, cytochemistry, and electron microscopy, it is considered possible to differentiate between T- and B-PLL. However, no difference in N/C ratios are apparent by either light or electron microscopy, and large nucleoli are present in up to 90% of T and B prolymphocytes.

The nuclei of B-PLL cells are usually round or oval with a smooth contour, although occasional superficial clefts may be present. In contrast, the nuclei of T-PLL are frequently irregular, folded, or clefted.

Table C8-1 Differentiating Features between B-PLL and PLT-(B)CLL

	B-PLL	*PLT-(B)CLL*	
Clinical			
Initial spleen size	+ + +	+ + to + + +	
Initial lymph node size	+	+ + +	
Median survival	6–24 months	12 months	
Laboratory			
Peripheral blood	>55% PLs	11–55% PLs	
Monoclonal spike	33%	5%	
Phenotype (T/B ratio)	25:75	virtually 100% B	
		*PLs***	*SmLc's**
Density of sIg	+ + +	+ + +	+
FMC7 reactivity	+ + +	−	+
MRBC receptors	±	−	+ + +
CD5 reactivity	−	−	+
Bone marrow biopsy	Diffuse, interstitital, and mixed patterns reported	Diffuse (with admixed SmLc and PLs and focal (aggregates of PLs with surrounding SmLc cells)	
	Mixed nodular-interstitial pattern most frequent	Mixed nodular-interstitial infiltrate in 25–30% of CLL	
	Purely nodular infiltrates not observed	Purely nodular infiltrates may be present	
	Reticulin fibrosis in most cases	Reticulin fibrosis in 30% CLL cases; not reported in PLT-CLL	
Cytogenetics	14q+(q32) t(6;12) t(11;14)(q13;32) trisomy 12	trisomy 12 When associated with t(6;12) suggests PLT-(B)CLL	

*SmLc = small CLL lymphocyte.
**PLs = prolymphocytes.

However, these features are less accentuated than those observed in Sézary cells and those of HTLV-I-associated lymphoma-leukemia and as in the present case may not be a striking feature. Perinuclear chromatin clearing with margination under the nuclear membrane may be present in both phenotypes. In the small cell variant with eccentric nuclei and attenuated nucleoli, a superficial resemblance to the plasmacytoid lymphocytes of Waldenström's macroglobulinemia may be apparent by light microscopy.

In the cytoplasm of both T- and B-PLL cells, large homogenous membrane-bound inclusions (Gall bodies) may be present. In T-PLL, such lysosomal bodies may not be azurophilic and hence not easily visible with Romanowsky stains. However, most are granular AEST+ and beta-glucuronidase positive, and variably TRAP+. The cytoplasm of B-PLL cells may occasionally reveal azurophilic crystalline inclusions that appear to be Ig in origin and are PAS and acid phosphatase negative. Small nonlysosomal azurophilic granules may also be present. Ribosome-lamella complexes are absent in PLL. However, long and short profiles of endoplasmic reticulum may be observed in both phenotypes.

Four patterns of bone marrow involvement by PLL were observed in biopsies by Nieto et al. (Table 8.1) and include interstitial, diffuse, mixed (interstitial-diffuse), and mixed (interstitial-nodular) types, the last of which was most frequently encountered. In their study of 30 cases, these observers found that PLL differed from CLL by lacking a pure nodular pattern and by revealing a mixed interstitial-diffuse type. No significant histologic differences existed between the infiltrates of T- and B-PLL. Reticulin fibrosis was common and was more intense in diffuse T-PLL. In bone marrow aspirates, the cytologic appearance of tumor cells is similar to those observed in the peripheral blood.

In lymph nodes, architectural landmarks are usually obliterated by tumor cells in pseudofollicular configuration. Rarely, the infiltrate may be diffuse. Splenic lesions are characterized by extensive infiltration of the Malpighian follicles and Billroth cords in both T and B phenotypes. Cytologic features of tumor cells in lymph nodes, spleen, and bone marrow biopsies are better appreciated in Wright-Giemsa-stained touch preparations and B-5-fixed paraffin sections.

Since T-PLL cells are postthymic, they are Tdt− and CD1a−. Greater than 90% of cases studied are CD7+. In Catovsky's series, 70% of cases were CD4+/CD8−, 11% CD4−/CD8+, and 19% expressed both antigens. This latter group, however, appeared to be devoid of both helper and suppressor activity, implying derivation from a less mature phenotype, comparable to that of lymphoblastic lymphoma. About 50% of T-PLL patients are CD38+, and others have occasionally been OKT17+. In this case, CD3 reactivity was negative. This is acceptable, since a positive pattern is present in 73% of patients. In the case of T-PLL reported by Volk et al., 98% of circulating PLs had G_1DNA content and thus lacked S-phase activity.

Cytogenetic changes in T-PLL include loss of chromosomes 8, 12, and 22. Other abnormalities include 6−(q21 or q15), trisomy 7q and 8q, and 14q+. However, the tandem translocation or inversion involving 14q11, where the gene coding for the alpha chains of the T-cell receptor is located, and 14q32, which is located in the proximity of the IgH gene, appears to be unique to patients with T-PLL and only rarely is observed in other mature T-cell leukemias. In B-PLL, the cytogenetic abnormalities reported include 14+(q32), t(11;14)(q13;32), t(6;12), and trisomy 12. It is apparent therefore that the different karyotypic patterns of these phenotypic variants of PLL reflect fundamental differences and are useful in distinguishing these two disorders from each other. In this patient, both chromosomes 14 revealed inversion with breakpoints at 14q11 and q32.

The presence of both IgH and IgL gene rearrangement has been confirmed in B-PLL. More recently, β-TCR gene rearrangement has been observed in T-PLL, establishing the monoclonal nature of these disorders. In this patient, the presence of biallelic rearrangement of the TCR-β locus on Southern blot analysis (Case 8.3) additionally supported the diagnosis of T-PLL.

The differential diagnosis of PLL primarily includes the PLT of CLL. Additionally, HCL, lymphosarcoma cell leukemia, TGLD, HTLV-I-associated lymphoma-leukemia, and SS should be considered. Since each of these conditions is discussed elsewhere in the case studies, only the relevant immunophenotypic differences among the T-cell lesions are detailed here in Table C8.2. In this case, prior to immunophenotyping, a preliminary diagnosis of PLT transformation of CLL (mixed CLL/PLL) was considered. However, the presence of a relatively monomorphic prolymphocytic population of tumor cells (>55% of lymphocytes) in the peripheral blood, positive CD7 reactivity, and the karyotypic and molecular genetic patterns observed prompted exclusion of this possibility. To our knowledge, PLT of T-CLL has not been well documented. Furthermore, the lack of response to conventional CLL therapy and excellent response to 2′-deoxycoformycin are of additional interest. Whether the failure of response to conventional therapy is due to an mdr[3]-encoded transmembrane glycoprotein, as has been recently suggested by Nooter et al. in B-PLL, awaits further elucidation. Current studies suggest

Table C8-2 Usual Immunophenotypic Pattern of T-Cell Lesions in Differential Diagnosis of T-PLL

	CD Antigens				
*Disease Entity**	*CD4*	*CD5*	*CD7*	*CD8*	*CD25*
T-PLL	±	+	+	±	±
T-CLL	+	±	−	−	−
TGLD	−	−	+	+	−
HTLV-I-associated lymphoma-leukemia	+	+	−	−	+
SS	+	+	−	−	+
T-HCL	+	−	−	−	−

Source: Modified from Sibler R, Stahl R: Phenotype of cells in CLL and related diseases. In *Hematology*, ed 4. Williams WJ, Bentler E, Erslev AJ, et al (eds): New York, McGraw-Hill, 1990, p. 1015.
*All disorders listed are usually CD2+ and CD3+, and Tdt−.

that in contrast to CLL, which originates in the bone marrow, PLL originates primarily in the spleen.

SUMMARY

Morphology	**Greater than 55% PLs in peripheral blood**
Bone Marrow	**Interstitial and diffuse infiltrate**
Cytochemistry	**β-glucuronidase negative, AP+ (tartrate sensitive), AEST+**
Immunophenotyping	**CD4+, CD5+, CD7+, CD8−, CD25+**
Cytogenetics	**46XY; inversion of both chromosomes 14 with breakpoints at 14q11 and q32**
Molecular Genetics	**TCR-β gene rearranged**
Electron Microscopy	**Well-defined nucleoli; minimally irregular nuclear membranes; no ribosome-lamella complexes**
Diagnosis	**T-prolymphocytic leukemia**

ANSWERS:

1. The diagnosis can be suspected from the peripheral smear and marrow findings. Nevertheless, to firmly establish a diagnosis of PLL, a complete workup including enumeration of the PL count, cytochemistry, immunophenotyping, cytogenetic analysis, and electron microscopy is usually necessary.
2. Immunophenotyping enables the classification of PLL into either T or B phenotypes and excludes other entities included in the differential diagnosis.

3. No. Ribosome-lamella complexes are not a characteristic feature of PLL.

BIBLIOGRAPHY

Articles:

Bennett JM, Catovsky D, Daniel M-T, et al: Proposals for the classification of chronic (mature) B and T lymphoid leukaemias. *J Clin Pathol* 42:567–584, 1989.

Brito-Babapulle B, Melo JV, Foroni L, et al: Neoplastic kappa and lambda cells in a B-PLL with chromosome translocations of both light chain gene regions. *Int J Cancer* 34:769–773, 1984.

Brito-Babapulle V, Pomfret M, Matutes E, et al: Cytogenetic studies on prolymphocytic leukemia: II. T-cell prolymphocytic leukemia. *Blood* 70:926–931, 1987.

Brynes RK: Prolymphocytic leukemia. Personal communication, 1991.

Caligaris-Cappio F, Janossy G: Surface markers in chronic lymphoid leukemias of B cell type. *Semin Hematol* 22:1–2, 1985.

Catovsky D: Prolymphocytic leukemia. *Nouv Rev Fr Hematol* 24:343–347, 1982.

Catovsky D: Prolymphocytic and hairy cell leukemias. In *Leukemia*, ed 5. Philadelphia, W.B. Saunders, 1990, pp 639–660.

Catovsky D, Matutes E, Crockard AD, et al: Prolymphocytic leukemia of B and T cell types. Morphological differences by light and electron microscopy. In *Human Leukemia*. Boston, Martinus Nijhoff, 1984, pp 251–259.

Catovsky D, Okos A, Wiltshaw E, et al: Prolymphocytic leukemia of B and T cell types. *Lancet* 2:232–234, 1973.

Chan CSP, Soehnlen F, Schecter GP: Differential response of malignant human B-cells to anti-IgM Immunoglobulin (anti-μ) and B-cell growth factor: Unique direct cytotoxicity of anti-μ on prolymphocytic leukemia cells. *Blood* 76:1601–1606, 1990.

Chan WC, Check IJ, Heffner LT, et al: Prolymphocytic leukemia of helper cell phenotype. *Am J Clin Pathol* 77:643–647, 1982.

Corwin DJ, Kadin ME, Andres TL: T-cell prolymphocytic leukemia. Two cases having a post thymic helper phenotype with complement receptors and 14q+ chromosome abnormality. *Acta Haematol* 70:43–49, 1983.

Foa R, Pelicci PG, Migone N, et al: Analysis of T-cell receptor beta chain (Tβ) gene rearrangements demonstrates the monoclonal nature of T-cell chronic lymphoproliferative disorders. *Blood* 67:247–250, 1986.

Galton DAG, Wiltshaw E, Boesen E, et al: *Rep Br Emp Cancer Campn* 41:55, 1963.

Ghani AM, Krause JR, Brody JP: Prolymphocytic transformation of chronic lymphocytic leukemia. *Cancer* 57:75–80, 1986.

Kluin-Nelemans HC, Gmelig-Meyling FHJ, Kootte AMM, et al: T-cell prolymphocytic leukemia with an unusual phenotype CD4+, CD8+. *Cancer* 60:794–803, 1987.

Lauria F, Foa R, Raspadori D, et al: T-cell prolymphocytic leukemia. A clinical and immunological study. *Scand J Haematol* 35:319–324, 1985.

Megaludis AM, Winkelstein A, Zeigler ZR, et al: Leukostasis: A phenomenon of prolymphocytic leukemia. *Am J Hematol* 32:146–147, 1989.

Melo JV, Brito-Babapulle V, Foroni L, et al: Two new cell lines from B-prolymphocytic leukemia: Characterization by morphology, immunological markers, karyotype and lg gene rearrangement. *Int J Cancer* 38:531–538, 1986.

Nieto LH, Lampert IA, Catovsky D: Bone marrow histological patterns of B-cell and T-cell prolymphocytic leukemia. *Hematol Pathol* 3:79–84, 1989.

Nooter K, Sonneveld P, Janssen A, et al: Expression of the *mdr*3 gene in prolymphocytic leukemia: Association with cyclosporin-A induced increase in drug accumulation. *Int J Cancer* 45:626–631, 1990.

Pittman S, Morilla R, Catovsky D: Chronic T-cell leukemia: II. Cytogenetic studies. *Leuk Res* 6:33–42, 1982.

Roberts JD, Tindale BH, MacPherson BR: Prolymphocytic transformation of chronic lymphocytic leukemia. A case report of lengthy survival after intensive chemotherapy. *Am J Hematol* 31:131–132, 1989.

Robinson DSF, Melo JV, Andrews C, et al: Intracytoplasmic inclusions in B-prolymphocytic leukemia. Ultrastructural, cytochemical and immunologic studies. *J Clin Pathol* 38:897–903, 1985.

Sibler R, Stahl R: Phenotype of cells in CLL and related diseases (Table 114-5). In *Hematology*, ed 4. New York, McGraw-Hill, 1990, p. 1015.

Stone RM: Prolymphocytic leukemia. *Hematol/Oncol Clin North Am* 4:457–471, 1990.

Tsai LMC, Tsai CC, Hyde TP, et al: T-cell prolymphocytic leukemia with helper-cell phenotype and a review of the literature. *Cancer* 54:463–470, 1984.

Turco MC, DeFelice M, Alfinito F, et al: Proliferative pathways in CD1−, CD3+, CD4+, CD8+, T-prolymphocytic leukemic cells:

Analysis with monoclonal antibodies and cytokines. *Blood* 74:1651–1657, 1989.

Volk JR, Kjeldsberg CR, Eyre HJ, et al: T-cell prolymphocytic leukemia. *Cancer* 52:2049–2054, 1983.

Weiss LM, Bindl JM, Picozzi VJ, et al: Lymphoblastic lymphoma: An immunophenotypic study of 26 cases with comparison to T cell acute lymphoblastic leukemia. *Blood* 67:474–478, 1986.

Review Articles:

Costello C, Catovsky D, O'Brien M, et al: Prolymphocytic leukemia: An ultrastructural study of 22 cases. *Br J Haematol* 44:389–394, 1980.

Galton DAG, Goldman JM, Wiltshaw E, et al: Prolymphocytic leukemia. *Br J Haematol* 27:7–23, 1974.

Kjeldsberg CR, Marty J: Prolymphocytic transformation of chronic lymphocytic leukemia. *Cancer* 48:2447–2457, 1981.

Matutes E, Talavera JG, O'Brien M, et al: The morphological spectrum T-prolymphocytic leukemia. *Br J Haematol* 64:111–124, 1986.

Melo JV, Catovsky D, Galton DAG: The relationship between chronic lymphocytic leukemia and prolymphocytic leukemia. *Br J Haematol* 63:377–387, 1986.

CASE 9

PATIENT: 52-year-old female.*

CHIEF COMPLAINT: Referred to the hospital for workup of fever and a 4.5 kg weight loss.

MEDICAL HISTORY: Eight months prior to admission, a diagnosis of chronic duodenal ulcer was made. Symptoms responded to antacid therapy. Three months prior to admission, intermittent fever, diarrhea, nausea, fatigue, and weight loss developed.

PHYSICAL EXAMINATION: The patient was afebrile. Tachycardia was present with a pulse rate of 100/min. The spleen was enlarged 9.0 cm below the left costal margin.

LABORATORY RESULTS:

A. *Screening Procedure*
WBC of 6.5 $\times$ 10^9/L with a differential of segmented neutrophils 54.5%, metamyelocytes 0.5%, myelocytes 1.0%, eosinophils 0.5%, mast cells 10.5%, monocytes 2.5%, and lymphocytes 30.5%. HGB 9.5 g/dL. Platelets 82 $\times$ 10^9/L.

*This case was previously reported by Travis WD et al: *Mayo Clin Proc* 61:957–966, 1986. Selected materials are reproduced here with permission.

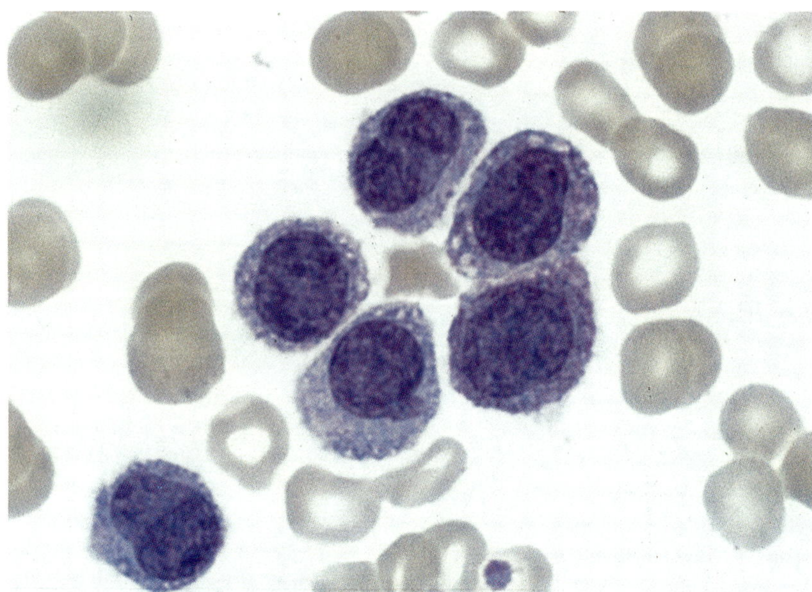

Case 9-1 Leukemic mast cells in peripheral blood film. Note round to oval nuclei and finely granular cytoplasm. (×1000).

HOSPITAL COURSE: Peripheral blood examination revealed numerous hypogranular mast cells (Case 9.1), with extensive and diffuse replacement of the bone marrow (Case 9.2). Splenectomy was performed, and the diarrhea and flushing subsided. About a week later she developed perforation of her duodenal ulcer and underwent emergency surgery. Subsequently, she developed evidence of DIC, respiratory failure, and fatal upper-GI hemorrhage.

QUESTIONS:

1. Can the diagnosis be made from the clinical and screening laboratory data provided?
2. How do the mast cells differ from basophils?
3. Does the presence of a mast cell infiltrate in the marrow signify leukemia?

LABORATORY RESULTS:

B. *Confirmatory Results*

Cytochemistry: Tumor cells stained with toluidine blue and were CAE+, aminocaproate esterase+, and TRAP+ but were MPEX- and B-EST−.

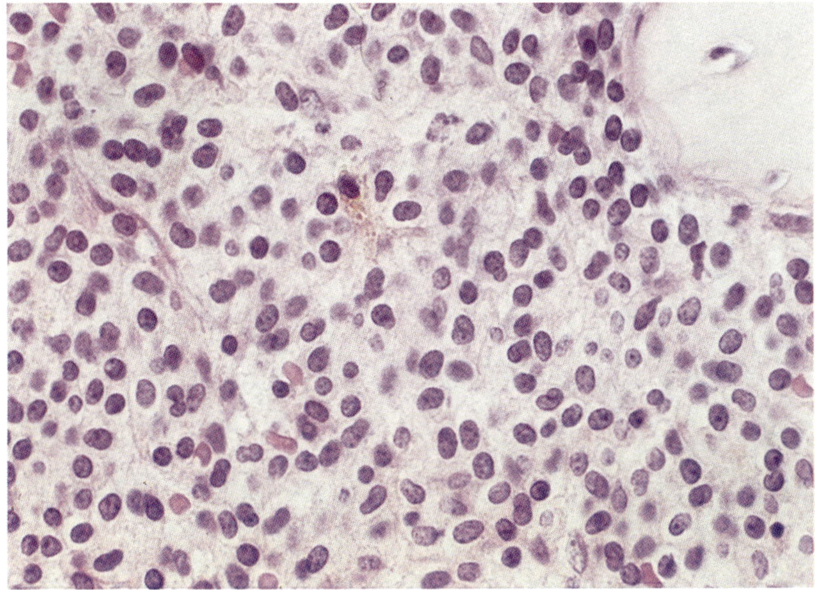

Case 9-2 Bone marrow biopsy with diffuse leukemic mast cell infiltrate. Appearances are reminiscent of those observed in HCL. (×400).

Immunophenotyping studies: Tumor cells were CD5−, CD11b−, CD19−, CD20−, Lyt3−, and HP1-1D− (Mayo Clinic platelet-megakaryocyte marker).

Electron microscopy: Numerous cytoplasmic villi and varying numbers of sharply demarcated membrane-bound granules with a dark core (Case 9.3) were present.

Cytogenetics: An insertion-translocation—46,XX,dir ins (10;16) (q2?2;q13q22) abnormality was demonstrated in a cell line from peripheral blood.

DIAGNOSIS: Mast cell leukemia.

DISCUSSION: Mast cell leukemia (MCL) is among the rarest and most unusual of human leukemias, and in our review only 10 well-documented cases were located in the literature. Additionally, criteria to differentiate this entity from systemic mastocytosis (SM) with circulating tumor cells are imperfect, making the diagnosis difficult. In most cases, however, as in the present case, the clinical presentation includes some features of mastocytosis. Hence, the diagnosis may be suspected on examination of the peripheral blood film. However, other forms of acute nonlymphocytic leukemia, and CML have been

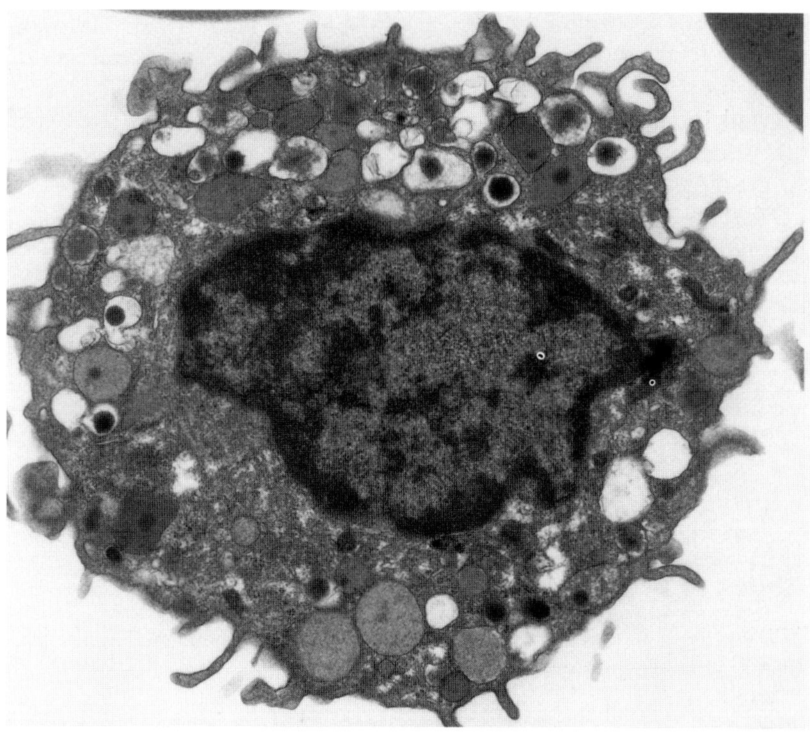

Case 9-3 Electron micrograph of leukemic mast cell from bone marrow aspirate. Cytoplasmic villi and numerous granules are present, some with a dark central core and surrounding halo. (×10,000). From Travis WD, et al: *Mayo Clin Proc* 61:957–966, 1986. Reproduced with permission.

reported in patients with mastocytosis, prompting the need for a thorough multiparameter hematologic analysis in each suspected case.

At the present time, proliferative disorders of mast cells are classified into indolent, aggressive, and leukemic forms. Although indolent disease is often primarily cutaneous, and the latter two systemic, some overlap of manifestations may exist. Appropriately so, the term *malignant mastocytosis* (MM) has been applied to the aggressive and leukemic forms.

Most cases of SM are sporadic. Albeit, rare familial cases have been recognized. Symptoms may first manifest in infancy, childhood, adolescence, or adult life and are due to the abnormal proliferation of mast cells in the skin, bone marrow, lymph nodes, spleen, and liver. Patterns of clinical presentation and the principal sites of tumor burden vary considerably. The clinical effects of mastocytosis are due to the effects of tissue infiltration and the release of histamine and other mediators of mast cell proliferation. As in this case, an increased incidence of peptic ulcer disease has been reported. Also, urticaria, flushing, palpitation, diarrhea, and hypotensive episodes are among other frequently reported clinical problems.

Mastocytosis arising in infancy and childhood has a tendency to improve or resolve at puberty. Disease is frequently dominated by cutaneous manifestations in the form of maculopapular, erythrodermic, and nodular-focal infiltrates that urticate on rubbing. In contrast, adult-onset mastocytosis may remain indolent or pursue an aggressive course. Urticaria pigmentation (UP), hepatosplenomegaly, and constitutional symptoms are often worse in aggressive mastocytosis (AM).

Under physiological circumstances, and in patients with indolent mastocytosis (IM), mast cells do not circulate in the peripheral blood. In cases of AM, however, mast cells may be present and identified in routine peripheral blood smears. This situation is therefore analogous to that observed in the NHLs, multiple myeloma, and MF, where the presence of a few circulating tumor cells indicates peripheralization but not necessarily leukemic transformation of these disorders.

MCL is the least common and most rapidly progressive form of SM. Constitutional symptoms are frequently present and usually associated with severe peptic ulcer disease. UP and histamine-related manifestations are uncommon and may be absent. Moderate anemia and thrombocytopenia are frequently present at diagnosis. Total WBCs have varied between 8500 and 66,300/mm^3 of blood, and absolute counts of circulating mast cells have ranged between 650 and 47,736. Following assessment of the problem, Travis et al. (1986) recommended that mast cells constitute a minimum of 10% of the circulating white cell mass to qualify for diagnosis of MCL. In a recent study of MCL, however, Torrey et al (1990) indicated that the number of circulating mast cells did not directly correlate with either tumor burden or survival and therefore caution against using this yardstick as the sole parameter in classification or initiation of therapy. Caution is also recommended in establishing a diagnosis by total reliance on Wright-Giemsa-stained smears of the peripheral blood alone, since patients with the blast crisis of CML may present with cytologically transitional blast forms with features of both basophils and mast cells.

The bone marrow is the most frequently documented site of extracutaneous disease in patients with SM, and in a recent study by Lawrence et al. 32 of 46 patients (74.4%) revealed bone marrow disease. However, since the bone marrow is often involved in the indolent and nonleukemic forms of SM, the concept of tumor burden in the bone marrow as evidence of leukemia is not readily applicable.

In aspirate preparations of the bone marrow, variable numbers of atypical mast cells are present in IM and are far more numerous than observed in the reactive mastocytosis that often accompanies the bone marrow infiltrates of CML and WM. In AM and MCL, however, neoplastic mast cells form the predominant cellular element and are readily identified by their blue-black granules that characteristically pack their cytoplasm and minimally overlie a centrally located nucleus.

In their review of mast cells and mast cell neoplasms, Lennert and Parwaresh indicate that mast cells in MM have larger nuclei than normal mast cells. Mitotic activity is, however, very uncommon. In AM, erythrophagocytosis and bizarre megakaryocytic changes have been reported, and the latter are ascribed to the effects of histamine mediators.

Bone marrow biopsies from patients with IM generally reveal focal lesions, while diffuse and extensive involvement is the usual pattern of infiltration in AM and MCL. Focal lesions may be monomorphic and primarily composed of mast cells or polymorphic with varying numbers of mast cells, eosinophils, neutrophils, histocytes, fibroblasts, and endothelial cells in haphazard configuration. Occasionally, eosinophils are scattered among the mast cells, which either surround or are surrounded by well-differentiated lymphocytes. Resemblance to the eosinophilic fibrohistiocytic lesion is striking, and it is believed now that this entity is actually a manifestation of SM. The intervening marrow may be unremarkable or reveal granulocytic hyperplasia with eosinophilia. Tumor cells are usually spindle-shaped with round or oval nuclei, occasional nucleoli, and faintly eosinophilic granular cytoplasm. Mitotic activity is inconspicuous. Varying degrees of fibrosis may be present, and trabeculae in the vicinity of tumor deposits may be sclerotic or rendered atrophic and eroded with associated osteoclastic activity.

While correlating prognosis with histologic appearances in the bone marrow, Horny et al. observed three patterns in patients with mastocytosis. The type 1 pattern was observed in the best prognostic group and was characterized by focal paratrabecular and perivascular polymorphic infiltrates with reticulin fibrosis and intervening normocellular marrow. These patients primarily had cutaneous manifestations and an indolent clinical course. In the type 2 pattern, sheets of mast cells were present in a perivascular and paratrabecular location and were associated with myelofibrosis and osteosclerosis. The intervening marrow revealed granulocytic hyperplasia. Patients in this group had either concomitant CML, AMML, or AML. The type 3 pattern was characterized by diffuse lesions in the bone marrow, and all patients in this worst prognostic category had MCL.

The differential diagnosis of lesions in a bone marrow biopsy include HCL, idiopathic myelofibrosis, Hodgkin's disease, eosinophilic fibrohistiocytic lesion, hypergranular promyelocytic leukemia, other forms of acute nonlymphocytic leukemia arising in the milieu of systemic mast cell disease, the bone marrow changes of angioimmunoblastic lymphadenopathy with dysproteinemia, and the blast crisis of CML with basophil and mast cell precursors.

Cytochemical analysis of tumor cells in suspected cases is of great value. Metachromasia with the toluidine blue stain is invariably present. Normal mast cells and those from lesions of UP appear to stain best at pH 4.0. In contrast, tumor cells from MM are believed by some observers to exhibit maximum staining at a pH range between 5.0 and 6.0. Positive staining reactions are also reported with the PAS, SBB, histamine (Cubas alcian blue), TRAP, and CAE (Leder) stains.

Immunophenotyping studies have been variously reported in neoplastic mast cells as CD2+, CD4+, CD11b+, CD33+, and CD45+; and CD8−, CD19−, CD7(WT1)−, Tdt−, and HLA-DR−. The presence of CD33 activity supports a bone marrow and myeloid origin of tumor cells and the E-rosetting T-cell antigen CD2 raises the question of some connection with a T-cell lineage. However, in the case reported by Dalton et al., there was rearrangement neither of the beta TCR gene nor of the IgH gene.

Ever since mast cells were described by Ehrlich in 1877, considerable interest has centered around their origin and a possible relationship to basophils. Under physiological circumstances, these cells reveal distinctive biochemical and ultrastructural characteristics. However, in some patients with myeloproliferative disease including the blast crisis of CML, blast forms have revealed overlapping ultrastructural features, with both theta granules (normally present only in basophil precursors) and the characteristic lamellar scroll- and ropelike material ordinarily found only in mast cell granules. Additionally the patterns of myeloperoxidase and platelet peroxidase activity in mast cells and basophils further suggests a relationship, and Merger et al have recently described a Ph^1-negative acute hematopoietic neoplasm with ultrastructural cytochemical and immunocytochemical evidence of basophil and mast cell differentiation. No consistent chromosomal abnormality has so far been identified in MCL. However, an autonomously growing cell line was established from the peripheral blood of this case, and revealed an insertion-translocation: 46, XX, dir ins(10;16)(q2?;q13q22) abnormality. Subsequently, a neutral tryptase has been purified and sequenced from these cells. In another case of MM, near-haploid, near-diploid and polyploid cells have been identified in the bone marrow. In Ph^1 positive cases the possibility of concomitant CML and SM, or blast crisis of CML with circulating basophils and mast cells should be considered, and studies for BCR/ABL rearrangement pursued in the Ph^1 negative cases where this diagnosis is suspected.

SUMMARY

Morphology	**Numerous granulated white cells resembling mast cells and basophils. (Granules are small, and often few or absent in some cases.)**
Bone Marrow	**Heavily infiltrated by small tumor cells with granular cytoplasm.**
Cytochemistry	**Toluidine Blue +, CAE +, TRAP +**
Immunophenotyping	**Negative results**
Cytogenetics	**10;16 translocation**
Electron Microscopy	**Membrane bound granules with halo**
Diagnosis	**Mast Cell Leukemia**

ANSWERS:

1. The combination of chronic peptic ulcer disease with splenomegaly and mast cells in the peripheral blood is suspicious for SM. However, since circulating basophils and mast cells are observed in other circumstances, the diagnosis of MCL cannot be made with certainty from the clinical and screening laboratory data alone.
2. Basophils normally comprise up to 2% of circulating WBC. They contain segmented nuclei and on Wright-Giemsa stain reveal a sparse component of violet-blue granules. These are CAE (Leder) negative, and optimally metachromatic at pH 2.8. Reactivity with the granulocyte specific marker Ki-M5 is observed. On electron microscopy basophil granules contain membranelike myelinic figures or finely-particulate material which contains heparin, histamine, eosinophilic major basic protein (MBP) and Charcot-Leyden Crystal protein. In some patients with CML, scroll-like and crystalloid inclusions may be present in circulating basophils, making ultrastructural distinction from mast cells virtually impossible.

   Mast cells do not normally circulate in the peripheral blood. They contain nonsegmented nuclei, and are heavily packed with blue-black granules. Mast cell granules are CAE (Leder) positive, and optimally metachromatic at pH 3.5. Reactivity with the monoclonal antibody KiMC1 is present. Mast cell granules contain histamine, and ultrastructurally scroll-like ropy or amorphous material with a central core. As in this case of MCL, scroll-like inclusions may be absent.

3. No. Although the presence of a nodular or diffuse mast cell infiltrate excludes a diagnosis of reactive mastocytosis in a bone marrow biopsy, and a diffuse infiltrate is invariably present in MCL, diffuse bone marrow disease may be evident in the absence of MCL.

BIBLIOGRAPHY

Bauchinger M, Mezger J: A case of malignant mastocytosis with near haploid, near-diploid and polyploid cells in the bone marrow. *Cancer Cytogenetics* 48:13–21, 1990.

Butterfield JH, Weiler D, Dewald G, et al: Establishment of an immature mast cell line from a patient with mast cell leukemia. *Leukemia Research* 12:345–355, 1988.

Butterfield JH, Weiler DA, Hunt LW, et al: Purification of tryptase from a human mast cell line. *J Leukocyte Biol* 47:409–419, 1990.

Dalton R, Chan L, Batten E, et al: Mast cell leukemia: Evidence for bone marrow origin of the pathological clone. *Br J Haematol* 64:397–406, 1986.

Lawrence JB, Friedman BS, Travis WD, et al: Hematologic manifestations of systemic mast cell disease. A prospective study of laboratory and morphologic features and their relation to prognosis. *Am J Med* 91:612–624, 1991.

Loomis LJ, Vardiman JW: Mast cell leukemia. *ASCP Check Sample* No. 90–10 (H-225), 1990.

Mezger J, Permanetter H, Gerhartz H, et al: Philadelphia chromosome-negative acute hematopoietic malignancy: Ultrastructural cytochemical and immunocytochemical evidence of mast cell and basophil differentiation. *Leukemia Research* 14:169–175, 1990.

Schmiegelow K, Pluczynska MJ: Philadelphia chromosome-negative acute hematopoietic malignancy: Ultrastructural cytochemical and immunocytochemical evidence of mast cell and basophil differentiation. *Europ J Hematol* 44:74–77, 1990.

Soler J, O'Brien M, DeCastro JT, et al: Blast crisis of chronic granulocytic leukemia with mast cell and basophilic precursors. *Am J Clin Pathol* 83:254–259, 1985.

Torrey E, Simpson K, Wilbur S, et al: Malignant mastocytosis with circulating mast cells. *Am J Hematol* 34:283–286, 1990.

Travis WD, Li C-Y Su WPD: Adult onset urticaria pigmentosa and systemic mast cell disease. *Am J Clin Pathol* 84:710–714, 1985.

Travis WD, Li C-Y: Pathology of the lymph nodes and spleen in systemic mast cell disease. *Modern Pathol* 1:4–14, 1988.

Travis WD, Li C-Y, Yam LT, et al: Significance of systemic mast cell disease with associated hematologic disorders. *Cancer* 62:965–972, 1988.

Travis WD, Li C-Y, Bergstrath MS: Solid and hematologic malignancies in 60 patients with systemic mast cell disease. *Arch Pathol Lab Med* 113:365–368, 1989.

Udoji WC, Razvi SA: Mast cells and myelofibrosis. *Am J Clin Pathol* 63:203–209, 1975.

Zucker-Franklin D: Basophils. In *Atlas of Blood Cells.* Zucker-Franklin D (ed): Philadelphia, Lea & Febiger, 1988, pp 287–320.

Review Articles:

Brunning RD, McKenna RW, Rosai J, et al: Systemic mastocytosis. *Am J Surg Pathol* 7:425–438, 1983.

Horny HP, Parwaresch MR, Lennert K: Bone marrow finding in systemic mastocytosis. *Hum Pathol* 16:808–814, 1985.

Lennert K, Parwaresch MR: Mast cells and mast cell neoplasia: A review *Histopathology* 3:349–365, 1979.

Travis WD, Li C-Y, Hoagland HC, et al: Mast cell leukemia: Report of a case and review of the literature. *Mayo Clin Proc* 61:957–966, 1986.

Travis WD, Li C-Y, Bergstralh EJ, et al: Systemic mast cell disease. *Medicine* 67:345–368, 1988.

CASE 10

PATIENT: 41-year-old native Jamaican male.*

CHIEF COMPLAINT: Skin rash of several weeks' duration.

MEDICAL HISTORY: The patient presented to his physician in Florida with a generalized rash. Skin biopsy was initially interpeted as mycosis fungoides, and treatment with petrolatum and PUVA was initiated. Following 15 months of irregular therapeutic compliance, he presented to another medical center with a 4-week history of malaise and weight loss. The serum calcium level was 16.3 mg/dL. Clinical examination and peripheral blood findings were considered compatible with ATLL. Following the control of hypercalcemia, the patient was transferred to the National Cancer Institute at Bethesda.

PHYSICAL EXAMINATION: A generalized dry and scaly skin rash was present. Cervical adenopathy and hepatomegaly were noted, and the spleen was palpable 3.0 cm below the left costal margin. Bilateral pleural effusions were detected.

LABORATORY RESULTS:

A. *Screening Procedure*
WBC of 84.8 $\times$ 10^9/L with a differential of segmented neutrophils 9%, lymphocytes 12%, and atypical lymphocytes (Case 10.1) with

*Contributed by Elaine S. Jaffe, M.D., and Jacqueline Whang-Peng, M.D. Aspects previously published in *Am J Surg Pathol* 8:263–275, 1984, and *JNCI* 74:357–369, 1985. Selected data reproduced with permission.

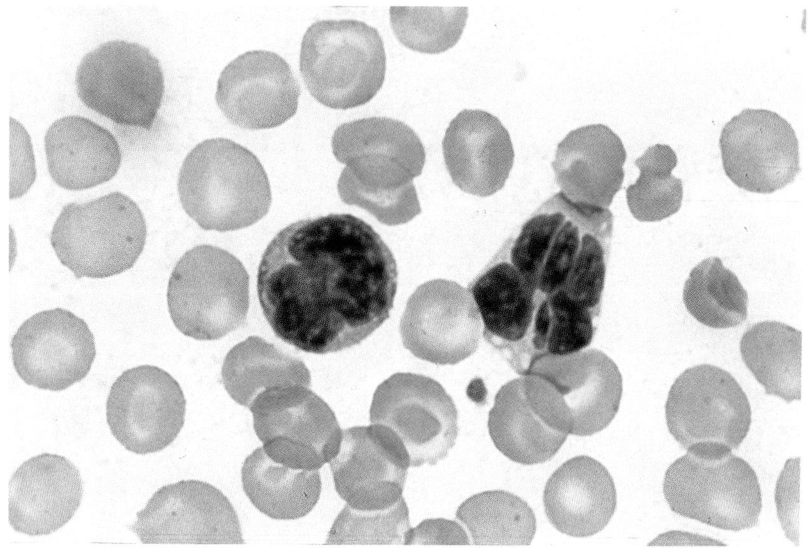

Case 10-1 Atypical and multifoliate nuclear configuration of lymphocytes in peripheral blood. (×1000).

highly convoluted nuclei 79%. HGB 9.6 g/dL. HCT 0.29 L/L. MCV 88 fL, MCH 28.9 pg, MCHC 32.0 g/dL, RDW 14.0. Platelets 228 $\times$ 10^9/L.

HOSPITAL COURSE: Thoracentesis revealed numerous highly atypical lymphocytes, cytologically similar to those in the peripheral blood. Biopsies of a cervical lymph node, bone marrow, and skin were performed and showed an atypical lymphocytic infiltrate compatible with ATLL. Blood samples for immunophenotyping and cytogenetics were drawn. Hypercalcemia was controlled with mithramycin and saline hydration. Combination chemotherapy with Pro-MACE/MOPP and the monoclonal antibody anti-TAC were initiated. Subsequently, vincristine, L-asparaginase, prednisone, and daunomycin were added to the regimen. Ten weeks following admission, the patient died. Total course of disease was about 17 months.

QUESTIONS:

1. Can the diagnosis be made from examination of the peripheral blood?
2. What is the differential diagnosis?
3. How is the hypercalcemia explained?

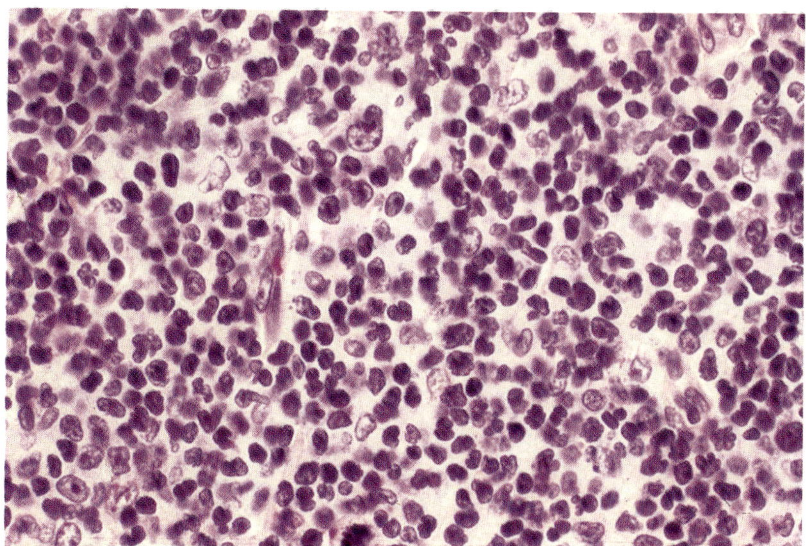

Case 10-2 Diffuse architectural obliteration of cervical lymph node, and replacement by an atypical mixed small and large cell lymphocytic infiltrate. (×400).

LABORATORY RESULTS:

B. Confirmatory Results

Cytochemistry: TRAP+.

Immunophenotyping studies: E-rosette (CD2)+, CD4+, CD25+, CD7−, CD8−, Tdt−.

Lymph node biopsy: Focal architectural effacement present. A leukemic pattern of infiltration with markedly atypical lymphocytes with convoluted nuclei observed, with variation in cell size and interspersed larger forms (Case 10.2). The lesion could not be readily classified into the Rappaport scheme or Working Formulation and was considered to be compatible with ATLL.

Bone marrow biospy: The marrow was diffusely replaced by an atypical and highly pleomorphic lymphocytic infiltrate. Appearances were similar to those observed in the lymph node biopsy.

Skin biopsy: A diffuse and atypical subepidermal lymphoid infiltrate, consisting of small and large cell forms, was observed. Pautrier's abscesses were not identified. Appearances did not support a diagnosis of MF, and the diagnosis of ATLL was favored.

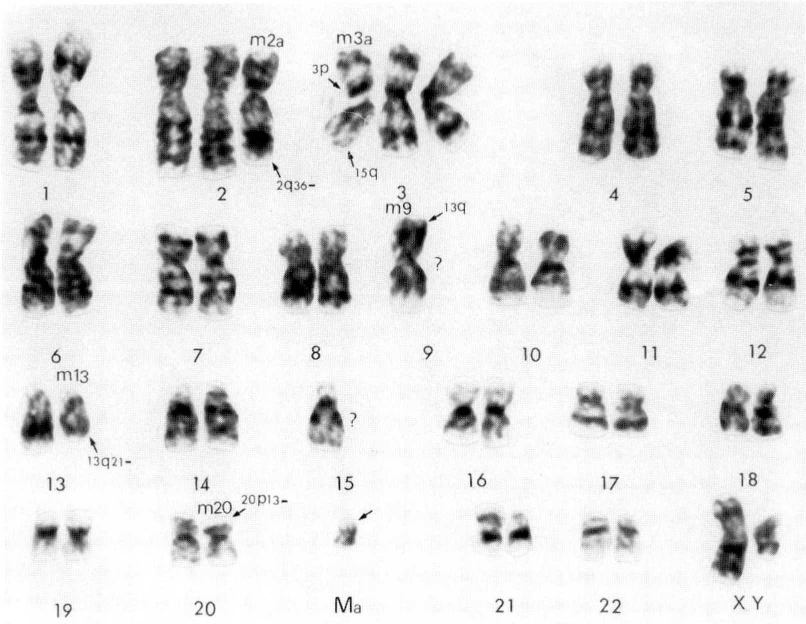

Case 10-3 Karyotype from a 6-day peripheral blood culture (sample 1). 47XY. Other details outlined in laboratory results. From Jacqueline Whang-Peng.

Cytogenetics: Two samples of peripheral blood were studied and rendered different cytogenetic profiles. In the first sample (Case 10.3) the pattern was 47XY, −9, −5, −15, +del(2)(q36), +t(3p;15q), rcp(9;13)(p22;q21), del(20)(p13), 21p+, +metacentric minute. In the second sample the pattern observed was 80XXYY, +4, +11, −15, +16, +16, +17, +18, +19, −21, −21, −22, −22, t(2;3)(q37;q21), t(3p;15q), del(3)(q22), +del(3)(q22), del(6)(q22 q24), +del(6)(q22 q24), rcp(9;13)(p22;q21), rcp(9;13)(p22;q21), del(13)(q21), +del(13)(q21), del(20)(p13), +del(20)(p13), +3 small markers.

Molecular genetics: Southern blot analysis (Case 10.4) of genomic DNA from leukemic cells revealed rearrangement of the β-TCR gene.

Serologic testing: Positive for HTLV-I-associated antibodies.

DIAGNOSIS: Adult T-cell lymphoma-leukemia.

DISCUSSION: ATLL is a distinct clinicopathologic entity, first described in the southwestern Japanese province of Kyoto by Uchiyama and Takatsuki et al. in 1977. Less prevalent areas include the Carib-

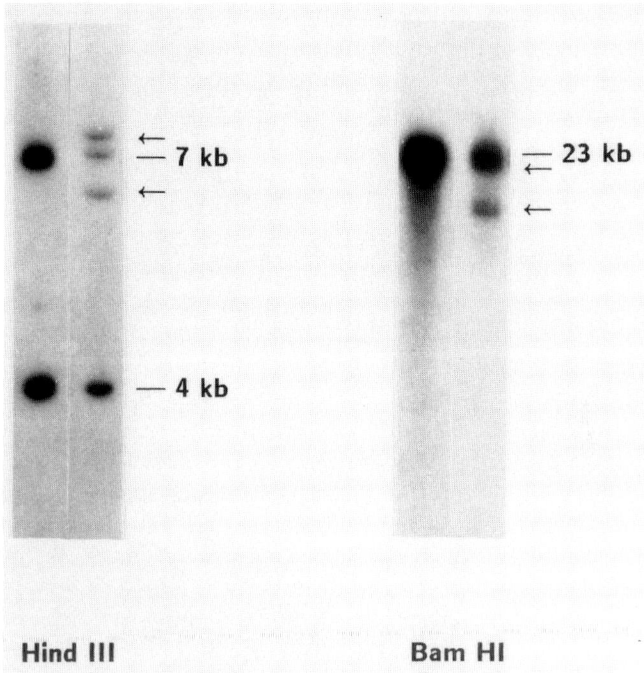

Case 10-4 Restriction fragment (Southern blot) analysis of the β-TCR gene. Genomic DNA from leukemic cells was digested with the restriction enzymes Hind III and Bam HI, and hybridized with a Cβ probe. The rearranged β-TCR gene in the patient's sample (right panel) is contrasted with germline placental DNA (left panels). Courtesy of Mark Raffeld, and Lynne V. Abruzzo.

bean basin, southeastern United States, and parts of southern Italy, South America, and Africa. Following the isolation and characterization by Poiesz et al. of the human T-cell lymphotropic virus type 1 (HTLV-I) from a patient with cutaneous T-cell lymphoma in 1980, the role of this virus in the pathogenesis of ATLL has become firmly established.

Onset of disease is in adult life, and chronic, smoldering, and acute forms are recognized. Clinical manifestations include adenopathy, skin rash, hepatosplenomegaly, and hypercalcemia. Highly pleomorphic lobulated lymphocytes (flower cells) are present in the peripheral blood, and the bone marrow is involved in most cases. Although ATLL shows some features of the SS, most cases can be readily distinguished after careful clinical and pathologic evaluation. Among the 187 patients studied by Takatsuki et al. in Kyushu, a male preponderance was observed, with a male/female ratio of 1.5:1. Median age at onset was 55 years and ranged between 27 and 82 years. Peripheral lymphadenopathy was present in 72% of patients, skin lesions in 53%, heptomegaly in 47%, splenomegaly in 25%, and hypercalcemia in 28%. Less frequent manifestations at diagnosis included abdominal pain, diarrhea, ascites, cough with expectoration, pleural effusions, and abnormalities in the chest x-ray film.

Greater than 65% of patients have peripheral blood involvement at initial presentation. However, a leukemic phase develops eventually in virtually every case. Although leukocytosis with counts as high as 500×10^9/L have been reported, the leukocyte count may be normal, and in some cases of chronic and smoldering disease less than 3% of circulating white cells may be leukemic. In peripheral blood smears, leukemic cells demonstrate marked nuclear indentation and lobulation. In acute ATLL, some variation in cell size and degree of cytoplasmic basophilia is usually observed, and small vacuoles are often present within the cytoplasm. Nuclei are either bilobed or multifoliate with deep indentations. In contrast, the leukemic cells of chronic ATLL are smaller, relatively uniform in size, and only rarely display cytoplasmic vacuoles. Nuclear indentation is more frequently encountered, and lobulation is more likely to be bifoliate or trifoliate. Nuclear chromatin is usually coarsely stranded and stains more deeply than in acute ATLL. The size and N/C ratio of leukemic cells in both acute and chronic ATLL are larger than those of circulating small lymphocytes.

In the bone marrow aspirate, leukemic cells display cytologic appearances similar to those observed in the peripheral blood and on cytochemical analysis react positively for A-EST, B-EST, and AP, with partial tartrate inhibition in some cases. Although comprehensive descriptions of the bone marrow biopsy in ATLL are lacking, in their study, Jaffe et al. observed bone marrow involvement in 7 of 12 patients (58%). Infiltrates were nonparatrabecular, mainly interstitial, and generally sparse. In some patients with hypercalcemia, bony remodeling with marked osteoclastic activity has been observed. Such changes have been known to regress following therapy. Myelofibrosis has been documented in some cases.

Immunophenotyping studies in ATLL have revealed a heterogenicity of T-cell phenotypes. In most cases, leukemic cells demonstrate the helper lymphocyte phenotype CD4. However, in other instances, the profile has been CD4+/CD8+ or CD4−/CD8−. Additionally, ATLL cells are invariably CD25+, CD1−, CD7−, and Tdt−. CD2, CD3, and CD5 activity have been present in some cases. Rarely, Leu-M1 and Ki-1 activity have been reported in paraffin-embedded tissue; and reactivity against the antibody FTF-148 has also been observed.

On electron microscopy, tumor cells reveal variably convoluted and indented nuclear configuration, reminiscent of the small cell variant of the Sézary cell. Nuclear pockets have been described, and one or two inconspicuous nucleoli may be present. On immunoelectron microscopy, the cell membrane and Golgi apparatus react with the antibody FTF-148; and Type C virus-like particles have been observed at the plasma membrane of PHA-stimulated tumor cells cultured with 5-iodo-2′-deoxyuridine. Scant cytoplasmic organelles are present and include a moderate number of mitochondria, free ribosomes, a well-developed Golgi apparatus, and endoplasmic reticulum. Clustered lysosomal dense bodies, tubulorecticular and crystalline inclusions, and Gall bodies have been reported.

Adenopathy is present in greater than 70% of patients at diagnosis, and biopsy appearances have revealed a variable histologic appearance. Jaffe et al. observed mixed small and large cell, large cell immunoblastic, large cell, and small lymphocytic subtypes and found that some cases were not readily classifiable into either Rappaport's classification or the Working Formulation.

Skin lesions develop in >50% of patients and clinically present as plaques, nodules, vesicles, or perifollicular infiltrates. In 8 of the 13 patients studied by Jaffe et al., skin biopsies were positive at the time of initial presentation. Five patients had Pautrier's abscesses, and in 3 patients the infiltrate was exclusively dermal. Lesions have been variably perivascular, periadnexal, or diffuse, and a grenz zone between the infiltrate and the epidermis has been observed in some cases. Other sites of leukemic infiltration have included the liver, lungs, cerebrospinal fluid, brain, gastrointestinal tract, breast, nasopharynx, and kidneys.

Cytogenetic analyses performed on endogenous Japanese and Americans of varied ethnicity have revealed differing karyotypic profiles. In their review, Takatsuki et al. report that the most frequently encountered chromosomal abnormalities in Japanese patients were trisomy 3, trisomy 7, and loss of the X chromosome in women. These observations are corroborated by the reports of Sanada et al. and Ueshima et al. However, in their study of 11 patients from the United States, Whang-Peng et al. most frequently encountered structural abnormalities of chromosome 6. Included were deletions with breakpoints at q11, q13, q16q23, q21q23, q22q24, and q23q24. Of additional interest was the observation that patients with deletion abnormalities of chromosome 6 had an aggressive course and correlated with a large cell tumor type, high white cell counts, hypercalcemia, bone lesions, and a poor therapeutic response. Numerous other complex structural karyotypic abnormalities are frequently present in

ATLL and have been observed in virtually every chromosomal pair. For a comprehensive listing of these abnormalities, the reader is referred to the articles by Kamada et al. and Whang-Peng et al.

Molecular genetic studies in ATLL have revealed rearrangement of β- and γ-TCR genes. Immunoglobulin genes are usually not rearranged, and in this case, rearrangement of the β-TCR gene was observed on Southern blot analysis (Case 10.4). Deletion of the N-*RAS* gene, which is located on chromosome 1, has also been observed in some cases and is believed to be a step in the pathogenesis of this neoplasm. Additionally, mutation of the p53 gene is considered to be linked to the transformation of chronic ATLL to an acute and more rapidly progressive lesion.

At the present time, ATLL is the only chronic human leukemia with an established viral etiology, and virtually 100% of patients with ATLL have antibodies against HTLV-I. However, in the endemic areas of Japan, 6–37% of healthy persons above the age of 40 years are also antibody-positive. This attests to the widespread local prevalence of infection with HTLV-I and the apparent role of other factors in the pathogenesis of ATLL. Viral transmission is believed to occur via sexual or other intimate contact, transfusion of infected blood, intrauterine infection, and breast milk. A long latent period (20–30 years) between infection and neoplasia is believed to exist.

HTLV-I is a 100-nm-enveloped retrovirus that preferentially infects and replicates within T-helper lymphocytes. The single-stranded RNA genome has 8,000–10,000 nucleotides and is endowed with 3 genes between the 5′ and 3′ positions. The *gag* gene specifies viral core proteins, *pol* sequence encodes viral transcriptase, and *env* encodes for the glycoprotein viral envelope. In addition to these unusual structural genes, HTLV-I contains extra genes (*tax*-1 and *rex*) that provide regulating signals essential to the biological activity and replication of the virus. Following receptor-mediated entry into the cell, and despite the lack of a host-related oncogene, the genomic viral RNA is transcribed into double-stranded DNA by a viral DNA polymerase (revese transcriptase) within the cytoplasm of the infected cell. Subsequent integration into host DNA results in the formation of a "provirus" that duplicates with cell division, rendering the cell immortal and capable of controlling the replication of exact copies of the HTLV-I genome, which are enveloped and released by budding of the host cell membrane. Following infection by HTLV-I, T-helper lymphocytes express increased receptors for IL-2, and this phenomenon is believed to be due to the *tax* gene.

The differential diagnosis of ATLL includes the Sézary syndrome, and as in this case, differentiation may be difficult early in the course of disease. Although Pautrier's abscesses may be observed in the skin biopsies of both conditions, the cells of ATLL reveal more pronounced external nuclear convolutions in peripheral blood and tissue samples. Additionally, HTLV-I-associated antibodies, hypercalcemia, and osteoclastic activity in bone marrow biopsy samples are generally absent in the Sézary syndrome. Rare instances of coexistent ATLL and AIDS have been described, and the immunophenotypic features distinguishing ATLL from other postthymic T-cell leukemias are outlined in Table 8.2.

SUMMARY

Morphology	**Highly atypical and cleaved lymphocytes in peripheral blood, and biopsies of bone marrow, lymph node, and skin**
Cytochemistry	**TRAP+**
Clinical Chemistry	**Hypercalcemia**
Immunophenotyping	**CD2+, CD4+, CD25+, CD7−, CD8−, Tdt−**
Cytogenetics	**Complex; 47XY and 80XXYY with chromosome 6 deletion**
Serology	**HTLV-I-antibody-positive**
Molecular Genetics	**Rearranged β-TCR gene**
Diagnosis	**Adult T-cell lymphoma-leukemia**

ANSWERS:

1. A diagnosis of ATLL can be suspected from the convoluted and multifoliate clefting of lymphocyte nuclei in the peripheral blood. Additionally, the presence of hypercalcemia and other supportive data including TRAP activity, an appropriate immunophenotype, the presence of HTLV-I-associated antibodies, and positive lymph node, bone marrow, and skin biopsies are usually necessary to establish the diagnosis.
2. The primary consideration in the differential diagnosis is mycosis fungoides. Nevertheless, since the peripheral blood, bone marrow, lymph node, and skin biopsies may not be diagnosed by the same observer, other causes of an atypical lymphoid process in these organs would have to be considered.
3. Hypercalcemia is ascribed to the osteolytic effects of tumor-associated cytokines including an osteoclast-activating factor, similar to that identified in some cases of multiple myeloma. This occasionally results in a monolayered osteoclastic proliferation between the tumor and adjacent bone.

BIBLIOGRAPHY

Articles:

Blayney DW, Jaffe ES, Blattner WA, et al: The human T-cell leukemia/lymphoma virus (HTLV) associated with American adult T-cell leukemia/lymphoma (ATL). *Blood* 62:401–405, 1983.

Catovsky D, Rose M, Goolden AWG, et al: Adult T-cell lymphoma-leukemia in blacks from the West Indies. *Lancet* 1:639–643, 1982.

Chan HL, Su IJ, Kuo T, et al: Cutaneous manifestations in adult T-cell leukemia/lymphoma. Report of three different forms. *J Am Acad Dermatol* 13:213–219, 1985.

Cossman J, Uppenkamp M: T-cell rearrangements and the diagnosis of T-cell neoplasms. *Clin Lab Med* 8:31–44, 1988.

Ehrlich GD, Davey FR, Kirshner JJ, et al: A polyclonal CD4+ and CD8+ lymphocytosis in a patient doubly infected with HTLV-I and HIV-I: A clinical and molecular analysis. Am J Hematol 30:128–139, 1989.

Garret RI, Durie BGM, Nedwin GE, et al: Production of a lymphotoxin. A bone resorbing cytokine by cultured human myeloma cells. *New Engl J Med* 317:526–532, 1987.

Hattori T, Matsuoka M, Yamamoto S, et al: Role of T3–T cell receptor complex for leukemogenesis of adult T-cell leukemia. In Hanaoka M, Kadin ME, Mikata A, et al (eds): *Lymphoid Malignancy.* New York, Field & Wood, 1990, pp 33–39.

Hattori T, Uchiyama T, Toibana T, et al: Surface phenotype of Japanese adult T-cell leukemia cells characterized by monoclonal antibodies. *Blood* 58:645–647, 1981.

Hinuma Y, Nagata K, Hanaoka M, et al: Antigen in an adult T-cell leukemia cell line and detection of antibodies to the antigen in human sera. *Proc Natl Acad Sci USA* 78:6476–6480, 1981.

Kalyanaraman VS, Sarngadharan M, Bunn PA, et al: Antibodies in human sera reactive against an internal structural protein of human T-cell lymphoma virus. *Nature* 294:271–273, 1981.

Kalyanaraman VS, Sarngadharan MG, Nakao Y, et al: Natural antibodies to the structural core protein (p24) of the human T-cell leukemia (lymphoma) retrovirus found in sera of leukemia patients in Japan. *Proc Natl Acad Sci USA* 79:1653–1657, 1982.

Kalyanaraman VS, Sarngadharan MG, Robert-Guroff M, et al: A new subtype of human T-cell leukemia virus (HTLV-II) associated with a T-cell variant of hairy cell leukemia. *Science* 218:571–573, 1982.

Kamada N, Tanaka K, Sakatani K, et al: Chromosomal aberrations in lymphoid malignancies and transforming gene in adult T-cell leukemia. In Hanaoka M, Kadin ME, Mikata A, et al (eds): *Lymphoid Malignancy.* New York, Field & Wood, 1990, pp 57–66.

Kondo T, Kono H, Nonaka H, et al: Risk of adult T-cell leukemia/lymphoma in HTLV-I carriers. *Lancet* 2:159, 1987.

Kuo T-t, Shih L-Y: Surgical pathology of lymph node biopsy specimens in Taiwan with an update on adult T-cell leukemia/lymphoma. In Hanaoka M, Kadin ME, Mikata A, et al (eds): *Lymphoid Malignancy*. New York, Field & Wood, 1990, pp 109–115.

Michalovitz D, Halevy O, Oren M: p53 mutations: Gains or losses? *J Clin Biochem* 45:22–29, 1991.

Miller C, Mohandas T, Wolf D, et al: Human p53 localized to short arm of chromosome 17. *Nature* 319:783–784, 1986.

Miyamoto Y, Yamaguchi K, Nishimura H, et al: Familial adult T-cell leukemia. *Cancer* 55:181–185, 1985.

Miyoshi I, Kubonishi I, Sumida S, et al: A novel T-cell line derived from adult T-cell leukemia. *Gann* 71:155–156, 1980.

Nakano S, Ando Y, Saito K, et al: Primary infection of Japanese infants with adult T-cell leukemia–associated retrovirus (ATLV): Evidence for viral transmission from mothers to children. *J Infect* 12: 205–212, 1986.

Namba Y, Tsubai F, You-Li Z, et al: A novel antigen expressed in HTLV-I infected cells, detected with a monoclonal antibody (FTF-148). In Hanaoka M, Kadin ME, Mikata A, et al (eds): *Lymphoid Malignancy*. New York, Field & Wood, 1990, pp 25–32.

Okochi K, Sato H, Hinuma Y: A retrospective study on tranmission of adult T-cell leukemia virus by blood transfusion: Seroconversion in recipients. *Vox Sang* 46:245–253, 1984.

Robert-Guroff M, Nakao Y, Notake K, et al: Natural antibodies to human retrovirus HTLV in a cluster of paitents with adult T-cell leukemia. *Science* 215:975–978, 1982.

Rose RM, O-Hara CJ, Harbison MA, et al: Infiltration of the lower respiratory tract by helper/inducer T lymphocytes in HTLV-I associated adult T-cell leukemia/lymphoma. *Am J Med* 90:118–123, 1991.

Sakashita A, Hattori T, Miller CW, et al: Mutations of the p53 gene in adult T-cell leukemia. *Blood* 79:477–480, 1992.

Sanada I, Tanaka R, Kumagai E, et al: Chromosomal aberrations in adult T-cell leukemia: Relationship to the clinical severity. *Blood* 65:649–654, 1985.

Shamato M: Adult T-cell leukemia/lymphoma. Immunoelectron microscopy. In Hanaoka M, Kadin ME, Mikata A, et al (eds): *Lymphoid Malignancy*. New York, Field & Wood, 1990, pp 139–142.

Sodroski J, Rosen C, Goh WC, et al: A transcriptional activator protein encoded by the x-lor region of the human T-cell leukemia virus. *Science* 228:1430–1434, 1985.

Takatsuki K, Uchiyama T, Sagawa K, et al: Adult T-cell leukemia in

Japan. In *Topics in Hematology*. Amsterdam, Excerpta Medica, 1977, p 73.

Takatsuki K, Yamaguchi K, Hattori T: Adult T-cell leukemia. In Henderson ES, Lister TA, et al (eds): *Leukemia* ed 5. Philadelphia, W.B. Saunders, pp 661–667.

Tokudome S, Tokunaga O, Shimamoto Y, et al: Incidence of adult T-cell leukemia/lymphoma among human T-lymphotropic virus type 1 carriers in Saga, Japan. *Cancer Res* 49:226–228, 1989.

Tokunaga M, Tokudome T, Hasui K, et al: Immunohistopathology of adult T-cell leukemia/lymphoma. In Hanaoka M, Kadin ME, Mikata A, et al (eds): *Lymphoid Malignancy*. New York, Field & Wood, 1990, pp 117–124.

Ueshima Y, Fukuhara S, Hattori T, et al: Chromosomal studies in adult T-cell leukemia in Japan. Significance of trisomy 7. *Blood* 58:420–425, 1981.

Wong-Staal F, Gallo RC: Human T-lymphotropic retroviruses. *Nature* 317:395–403, 1985.

Yamaguchi K, Nishimura H, Kohrogi H, et al: A proposal for smouldering adult T-cell leukemia: A clincopathologic study of 5 cases. *Blood* 62:758–766, 1983.

Review Articles:

Erlich GD, Poiesz BJ: Clinical and molecular parameters of HTLV-I infection. *Clin Lab Med* 8:65–84, 1988.

Jaffee ES, Blattner WA, Blayney DW, et al: The pathologic spectrum of adult T-cell leukemia/lymphoma in the United States. *Am J Surg Pathol* 8:263–275, 1984.

Nerurkar LS, Wong-Staal F, Gallo R: Human retroviruses, leukemia and AIDS. In Henderson ES, Lister TA, et al (eds): *Leukemia* ed 5. Philadelphia, WB Saunders, 1990, pp 225–244.

Poiesz BJ, Ruscetti FW, Gazdar AF, et al: Detection and isolation of type C retrovirus particles from fresh and cultured lymphocytes of a patient with cutaneous T-cell lymphoma. *Proc Natl Acad Sci USA* 77:7415–7419, 1980.

Shamoto M: Ultrastructure of adult T-cell leukemia in Japan. In Polliack A (ed): *Human Leukemias*. Boston, Martinus-Nijhoff, 1984, pp 297–307.

Uchiyama T, Yodoi J, Sagawa K, et al: Adult T-cell leukemia: Clinical and hematologic features of 16 cases. *Blood* 50:481–492, 1977.

Whang-Peng J, Bunn PA, Knutsen T, et al: Cytogenetic studies in human T-cell lymphoma virus (HTLV)-positive leukemia-lymphoma in the United States. *JNCI* 74:357–369, 1985.

CASE 11

PATIENT: 65-year-old white male.

CHIEF COMPLAINT: Weakness, weight loss, and mild abdominal discomfort of 5 weeks' duration.

MEDICAL HISTORY: The patient was a retired government employee and had served in the Pacific, performing decontamination of supplies following the atomic bomb testing of 1946. He remained in good health until admission in June 1991.

PHYSICAL EXAMINATION: Cachectic patient with mild pitting edema of the ankles. The liver was enlarged, nontender, and palpable 8.0 cm below the costal margin in the right midclavicular line. The spleen was enlarged 4.0 cm below the left costal margin.

LABORATORY RESULTS:

A. *Screening Procedure*
   WBC of 28.0 $\times$ 10^9/L with a differential count of segmented neutrophils 41%, band forms 2%, blasts 3%, eosinophils 4%, basophils 1%, monocytes 26%, and lymphocytes 23%. A rare NRBC (1/100 WBC) and hypogranular "Pelgeroid" neutrophils were identified. HGB 9.2 g/dL. HCT 0.28 L/L. MCV 102 fL, MCH 36.0 pg, MCHC 33.9 g/dL, RDW 17.2. Platelets 135 $\times$ 10^9/L.

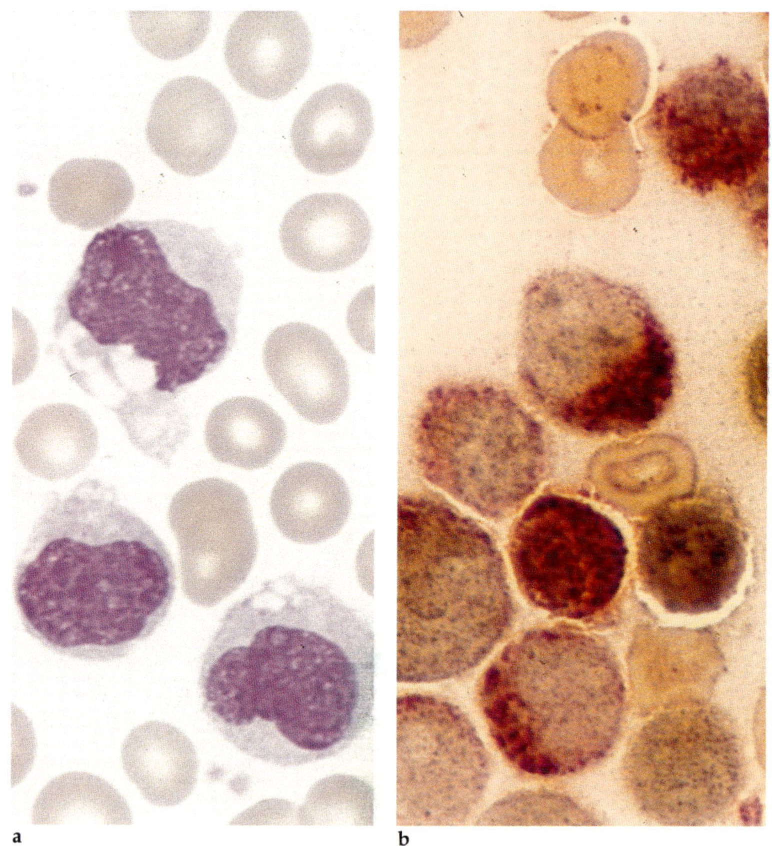

Case 11-1(a) Peripheral blood film with monocytosis (×1000). **(b)** Bone marrow aspirate with A-EST– and specific esterase (Leder)–staining cells. C-EST (×1000).

HOSPITAL COURSE: Appearances of the peripheral blood film (Case 11.1A) at admission were considered compatible with those of a chronic nonlymphocytic leukemia. The bone marrow was hypercellular (fat/cell ratio 25:75) and revealed 8% nucleolated blasts. Promonocytes numbered 6%, and numbers of myelomonocytic forms were increased. The M/E ratio was 9:1. Auer rods were absent. Megakarocyte numbers were decreased, and dysmegakaryopoiesis was present with occasional dwarf megakaryocytes. Erythropoiesis was decreased, and some megaloblastoid and dyskinetic changes were noted. Rare ringed sideroblasts were observed in the iron stain of the aspirate. Myelofibrosis was absent. Aliquots of the marrow were submitted for cytochemical, cell sorter, and cytogenetic studies. The patient was started on hydroxyurea. Following analysis of confirmatory laboratory studies and establishment of the diagnosis, the patient declined further therapy and left the hospital against medical advice.

QUESTIONS:

1. What is the differential diagnosis?
2. Should CMoL be a consideration?
3. Is it necessary to also obtain a bone marrow biopsy in such cases?

LABORATORY RESULTS:

B. *Confirmatory Results*

Cytochemistry: Blast forms, promonocytes and myelomonocytic cells from the bone marrow were mostly A-EST+, B-EST+, MPEX+, SBB+, PAS+ (blush and finely granular), and specific esterase (Leder)–positive. Dual staining (A-EST/Leder) was observed in 7% of cells in the C-EST preparation, and the ratio of A-EST/Leder staining cells was about 1:2 (Case 11.1B).

Immunophenotyping studies: Leukemic cells from the bone marrow were $CD11^c$+, CD13+, CD14+, CD16+, CD30+ and CD35+, CD64+, and CDw78+.

Cytogenetics: Karyotypic studies performed on bone marrow cells revealed a 45XY pattern with monosomy 7. The Ph^1 chromosome was absent.

Clinical chemistry: Serum lactate dehydrogenase (LDH), 1500 U/L.

DIAGNOSIS: Chronic myelomonocytic leukemia.

DISCUSSION: CMML is a progressive neoplastic disorder mostly developing in patients over the age of 50 years and terminating in either ANLL or the complications of cytopenia, such as infection or hemorrhage. A rarer juvenile form (JCMML) has also been identified.

It has long been recognized that a group of irreversible hematopoietic disorders with trilineage dysplasia variably terminate in acute leukemia. In 1982, the FAB working group classified these disorders into a family of MDSs. Included were refractory anemia, refractory anemia with ringed sideroblasts, refractory anemia with excess blasts, CMML, and refractory anemia with excess blasts in transformation. CMML is the rarest of the MDSs and has been reported to constitute between 5 and 25% of all cases. Excluded from the myelodysplastic lesions are the myeloproliferative disorders, which include polycythemia vera, agnogenic myeloid metaplasia, CML, and essential thrombocythemia, and also other constitutional chromosomal disturbances as in Fanconi's syndrome and Down's syndrome that predispose patients to an increased risk of developing acute leukemia.

Since CMML may clinically present either at an early and insidious stage of its evolution, when trilineage myelodysplasia predominates, or at a later time in its natural history when proliferative activity is dominant, there is some nosologic controversy as to whether this entity is best classified as a myelodysplastic or myeloproliferative disorder.

CMML more frequently develops in men, and >75% of patients are over 60 years of age at diagnosis. Onset is insidious, and weakness, infection, or bleeding complications usually prompt medical attention. Hepatomegaly and splenomegaly are present in about 40% of patients, and the criteria for diagnosis include peripheral blood monocytosis with <5% circulating blast forms, evidence of dysgranulopoiesis, dyserythropoiesis, dysmegakaryopoiesis, and no greater than 20% blast forms in the bone marrow. Increased levels of serum LDH have been reported in some patients, as has increased lysozyme activity in the serum and urine. Polyclonal hypergammaglobulinemia is observed in about a third of cases, and autoantibodies are present in greater than half. Hypogammaglobulinemia is also known to manifest in some cases.

In about 65% of patients with CMML, leukocytosis is present, and counts as high as 100×10^9/L have been reported. Monocytosis is often the dominant finding, and according to proposed criteria by the FAB working group, an absolute monocyte count of 1×10^9/L is considered necessary to establish the diagnosis. Recently, however, Storniolo et al. (1990) have recommended a lower threshold for monocytosis at 0.5×10^9/L. Cases with neutropenia and neutrophilia appear to be equally represented and either way factor into the modified Bournemouth prognostic scoring system described below. Granulocytes may reveal "Pelgeroid" changes, with reduced or absent cytoplasmic granules and decreased nuclear segmentation (Case 11.2A). Occasionally, circulating myelocytes and <5% blast forms may be observed. Neutrophils with ring-shaped nuclei have been noted in some cases. Thrombocytopenia is present at diagnosis in about 25% of patients. As with the other myelodysplastic syndromes, anemia is frequently manifest, with macroovalocytosis, elevated MCV, and other variable erythrocytic changes including anisocytes, stippling, polychromasia, and circulating NRBC.

The bone marrow aspirate in CMML reveals myeloid and monocytic predominance, with blast forms variably increased up to 20% and a decrease in other hematopoietic elements. When the blast

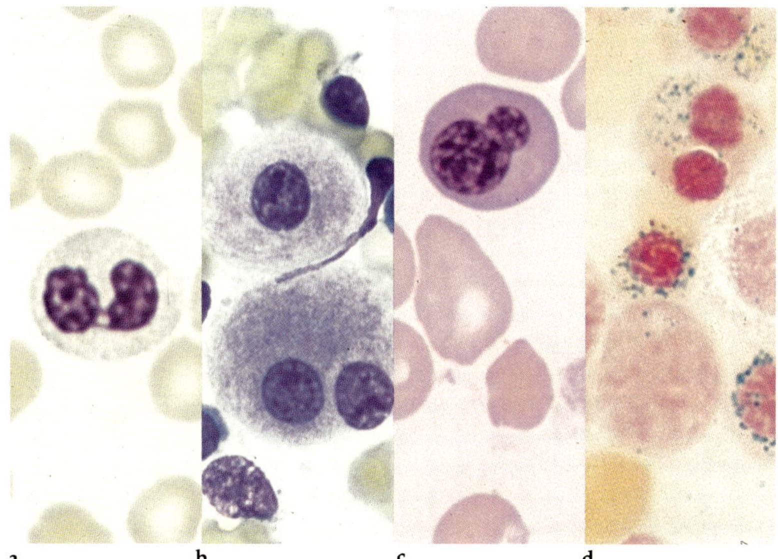

Case 11-2(a) "Pelgeroid" neutrophil. Peripheral blood (×1000). **(b)** Dysmegakaryopoiesis. Bone marrow aspirate. Notice small (dwarf) megakaryocytes with single and discrete nuclei. (×1000). **(c)** Dyskinetic normoblast. Bone marrow aspirate. (×1000). **(d)** Ring sideroblasts. Bone marrow aspirate. Prussian blue (×1000).

count is between 20 and 30% of the nucleated cells, the process is designated CMML in transformation, abbreviated CMML-T. As with the other myelodysplastic disorders, the cytologic designation of blast forms as types I and II is widely accepted. Accordingly, a type I blast has no granules, and a type II blast has <15 granules. The paramyeloid myelomonocytic nature of blastic and promonocytic forms and maturing myeloid elements is better delineated by the A-EST, B-EST, C-EST, and MPEX stains, and cells with dual cytoplasmic myelomonocytic properties may be observed. Since primary and secondary granules are variably decreased in CMML, the staining intensity for MPEX activity may be decreased. Dysmegakaryopoiesis with discrete megakaryocyte nuclei lacking lobation ("pawn ball" nuclei) and dwarf megakaryocytes (Case 11.2B) may be observed. Megaloblastoid erythropoiesis with dyskinesis (Case 11.2C) and ring sideroblasts (Case 11.2D) are also variably present. In bone marrow biopsies, hypercellularity is evident in most cases, and immature myeloid elements are often abnormally grouped away from bony trabeculae. Occasionally, nonparatrabecular benign lymphoid aggregates may be present, and in most instances, myelofibrosis does not develop.

On fluorescent activated cell sorter analysis, gated monocytes from the peripheral blood of patients with CMML are immunophenotypically identified as CD9+, CD14+, CD23+, CD64+, CD74+, and CDw78+; and myelomonocytic elements from the bone marrow are additionally $CD11^b$+, $CD11^c$+, CD12+, CD13+, CD15+, $CD16^a$+, CD31+, CD32+, CD33+, CD35+, and $CD67^a$+. Some overlap and variability of this immunologic profile is generally present.

Ultrastructural appearances of the paramyeloid leukemic cells in the marrow often reveal ruffed membranes with invaginations, pinocytic vesicles, indented nuclei, dysplastic cytoplasmic filaments, scant endoplasmic reticulum, nondescript mitochondria, a well-developed Golgi apparatus, lysosomal granules, phagocytic debris, and myelinic figures. Prominent nucleoli are present in promonocytic and blast forms.

Cytogenetic abnormalities are found in about 30% of patients at diagnosis. Monosomy 7 is the most frequently encountered defect, often occurring in younger patients and heralding a poor prognosis. Next in frequency are trisomy 8, iso(17q), and a 12p anomaly with breakpoints at p11 or p12. Patients with trisomy 8 are often elderly and are at high risk of evolution to AML-M4 or AML-M5. The ABL/BCR translocation abnormality does not occur in CMML. However, a t(5;12)(q31;12) defect has been observed and is associated with an overexpression of the K-*ras* oncogene. Additionally, terminal or interstitial deletions of the long arm of chromosome 11, trisomy 11, a 5q− abnormality with terminal or interstitial deletions at p11, and other rarer abnormalities have also been reported. None of the chromosomal abnormalities detailed above are specific for CMML.

With a view to prognostication and staging of patients with CMML, several scoring systems have been proposed. These include the Bournemouth score, which is based on the severity of the cytopenia and the percentage of marrow blasts; the Dusseldorf score, which additionally factors increases in levels of serum LDH; the Spanish score, which also considers the age of the patients; and the FAB score, which is the most complex. Since patients with CMML frequently have neutropenia, Worsley et al. (1988) have modified the original Bournemouth score to provide a practical and simple system. Accordingly, one point is assigned for each of the following: HGB $<$ 10.0 gm/dL; absolute neutrophil count $< 2.5 \times 10^9$/L or $> 16.0 \times 10^9$/L; platelets $< 100.0 \times 10^9$/L; and bone marrow blasts $>$ 5%. Median survival for CMML patients with a score of 0–1 is 32 months, and for those with a score of >2 is 9 months. All factors considered, the percentage of bone marrow blasts remains the most important prognostic factor.

JCMML is an indolent disease of monocyte-macrophage lineage

that mainly affects boys below the age of 4 years and eventuallly transforms to an acute growth phase with blast crisis. Clinical manifestations of JCMML include hepatosplenomegaly, facial rash, leukocytosis, thrombocytopenia, and increased numbers of mature and immature monocytes in the peripheral blood. Hypergammaglobulinemia and increased fetal hemoglobulin levels are frequently present. Cell culture studies of erythropoiesis in JCMML have shown a striking resemblance to erythropoiesis in the fetus and newborn, with an extremely high number of abnormal CFU-C colonies that are predominantly composed of monocytes and macrophages. A unique and unexplained finding in enlarged lymph nodes from patients with JCMML is the presence of an immature T-cell infiltrate in the paracortex. Such a phenomenon has also been reported in CMML. Efficacy of the Bournemouth score has not yet been fully evaluated in JCMML, but in children below 2 years of age with hepatomegaly, bleeding, thrombocytopenia, circulating NRBC, and an increased blast count, the prognosis is grave. Although the incidence is very low, there is an interesting association between JCMML and neurofibromatosis. In JCMML, as in CMML, the cytogenetic profile is ABL-BCR–negative, and the disease is thus distinguished from juvenile CML. Monosomy 7 may be observed in JCMML but is nonspecific and has also been observed in other forms of childhood AML and MDS.

Entities that should be considered in the differential diagnosis of CMML are the other myelodysplastic syndromes; "atypical CML," which appears to account for a very small number of Ph^1 chromosome–negative, BCR-ABL–negative patients and CML patients lacking basophilia and pronounced monocytosis; conditions such as brucellosis, which may be associated with monocytosis and myelomonocytic hyperplasia of the bone marrow; and CMML-T, which should be distinguished from AML-M4 and AML-M5. In these latter two conditions, myelodysplastic features are usually absent and Auer rods more frequently encountered. Extramedullary manifestations of CMML and CMML-T are well documented; have been observed in the skin, lymph nodes, and spleen; and are similar to granulocytic sarcoma. Transformation of CMML to acute leukemia in most instances is to AML-M4 or AML-M5. Rarely, CMML has coexisted with ALL, and cases of carcinoma observed in CMML patients do not appear to be any greater than expected by chance. In most instances, the cause of CMML remains obscure. However, about 10–20% of patients have a history of exposure to chemical carcinogens, chemotherapy, or irradiation. The role of *ras* mutation, which has been observed in 30–50% of patients, is uncertain and is in contrast to cases of "atypical CML," in which *ras* mutation is unusual.

SUMMARY

Peripheral Blood	**Absolute monocytosis; 3% blasts**
Bone Marrow	**Myelomonocytic predominance with 8% blasts and dysplastic erythroid and megakaryocytic changes**
Cytochemistry	**A-EST+, B-EST+, C-EST+, MPEX+, SBB+, PAS+**
Immunophenotyping	**CD11^c+, CD13+, CD14+, CD16+, CD30+, CD35+, CD64+, CDw78+**
Cytogenetics	**Monosomy 7**
Diagnosis	**Chronic myelomonocytic leukemia**

ANSWERS:

1. The differential diagnosis on review of the peripheral blood film includes CML with monocytosis, CMML, and leukemoid reaction.
2. Patients with CMoL lack the accompanying myelodysplastic features that frequently accompany CMML. Also, CMoL is a much rarer condition.
3. The bone marrow biopsy provides quantitative information in contrast to the aspirate, which is better suited to provide qualitative data. Both aspirate and biopsy should be examined to ensure complete evaluation.

BIBLIOGRAPHY

Articles:

Auger MJ, Ross FM, Mackie MJ: 8;21 translocation with the der(21) in a patient with myelomonocytic leukemia. *Cancer Genet Cytogenet* 51:139–141, 1991.

Bader JL, Miller RW: Neurofibromatosis and childhood leukemia. *J Pediatr* 92:925–929, 1978.

Barnaurd DL, Burns GF, Gordon J, et al: Chronic myelomonocytic leukemia with paraproteinemia but no detectable plasmacytosis. *Cancer* 44:927–936, 1979.

Bennett JM: Myelomonocytic leukemia. A historical review and perspectives. *Cancer* 27:1218–1220, 1971.

Bennett JM, Catovsky D, Daniel MT, et al: Proposals for the classification of the myelodysplastic syndromes. *Br J Haematol* 51:189–199, 1982.

Copplestone J, Oscier DG, Mufti GL, et al: Monocytic skin infiltration in chronic myelomonocytic leukemia. *Clin Lab Haematol* 8:115–119, 1986.

Dalton WT, Cork A, Stass SA, et al: Chronic myelomonocytic leukemia with trisomy 8 and a related clone with trisomy 8 and t(15;17). *Cancer Genet Cytogen* 32:287–292, 1988.

del Canizo MC, Sanz G, San Miguel JF, et al: Chronic myelomonocytic leukemia; clinicobiological characteristics. A multivariate analysis in a series of 70 cases. *Eur J Haematol* 42:466–473, 1989.

Diebold J, Audevin J: Peliosis of the spleen: Report of a case associated with chronic myelomonocytic leukemia, presenting with spontaneous splenic rupture. *Am J Pathol* 7:197–204, 1983.

Doll DC, Grogan TM, Greenberg BR: Chronic myelomonocytic leukemia terminating as malignant histiocytosis. *Hematol Pathol* 1:183–189, 1987.

Economopoulos T, Economidou J, Giannopoulos G, et al: Immune abnormalities in myelodysplastic syndromes. *J Clin Pathol* 38:908–911, 1985.

Facchetti F, De Wolf-Peeters C, Kennes C, et al: Leukemia associated lymph node infiltrates of plasmacytoid monocytes (so called plasmacytoid T-cells). Evidence for two distinct histological and immunophenotypical patterns. *Am J Surg Pathol* 14:101–112, 1990.

Fenaux P, Beuscart R, Lai JL, et al: Prognostic factors in adult chronic myelomonocytic leukemia: An analysis of 107 cases. *J Clin Oncol* 6:1417–1424, 1988.

Fiedler PN, Sussman J, McPhedran P: *Chronic Myelomonocytic Leukemia. ASCP Check Sample* 32:90-5 (H-220), 1990.

Freedman MH, Estrov Z, Chan HSL: Juvenile chronic myelogenous leukemia.*Am J Pediatr Hematol Oncol* 10:261–267, 1988.

Ganser A, Hoelzer D: Clinical course of myelodysplastic syndromes. *Hematol Oncol Clin North Am* 6:607–618, 1992.

Gardner H, Haas O: Experience in pediatric myelodysplastic syndromes. *Hematol Oncol Clin North Am* 6:655–672, 1992.

Geissler K, Hinterberger W, Bettelheim P, et al: Colony growth characteristics in chronic myelomonocytic leukemia. *Leuk Res* 12:373–377, 1988.

Gow J, Hughes D, Farr C, et al: Activation of Ha-*ras* in human chronic granulocytic and chronic myelomonocytic leukemia. *Leuk Res* 12: 805–810, 1988.

Haas OA, Zoubek A, Koller U, et al: Generalised lymphadenopathy in juvenile chronic myelomonocytic leukemia is due to lymph node infiltration with myelomonocytic cells and immature T-cells. In Schmalzl F, Mufti GJ (eds): *Myelodysplastic Syndromes.* Berlin, Springer-Verlag, 1992, p 146.

Hamblin T: Immunologic abnormalities in myelodysplastic syndromes. *Hematol Oncol Clin North Am* 6:571–586, 1992.

Hasegawa Y, Sakai N, Toyama M, et al: Chronic myelomonocytic leukemia transformed from refractory anemia with ring sideroblasts with a rare chromosome, inv(12). *Rinsho Ketsueki* 31:75–79, 1990.

Hirsch-Ginsberg C, LeMaistre AC, Kantarjian H, et al: *RAS* mutations are rare events in Ph chromosome–negative/*bcr* gene rearrangement–negative chronic myelogenous leukemia, but are prevalent in chronic myelomonocytic leukemia. *Blood* 76:1214–1219, 1990.

Hotta T, Utsumi M: Chronic myelomonocytic leukemia (CMML)-characterization of clinical features and prognosis. *Nippon Ketsueki Gakkai Zasshi* 51:1441–1447, 1988.

Iselius L, Hast R, Ost A, et al: Translocation t(1;3)(p36;q21) in chronic myelomonocytic leukemia. *Br J Haematol* 72:109–110, 1989.

Janssen JWG, Buschle M, Layton M, et al: Clonal analysis of myelodysplastic syndromes: Evidence for multipotential stem cell origin. *Blood* 73:248–254, 1989.

Kampmeier P, Anastasi J, Vardiman JW: Issues in the pathology of the myelodysplastic syndromes. *Hematol Oncol Clin North Am* 6: 501–522, 1992.

Kantarjian HP, Kurzrock R, Talpaz M: Philadelphia chromosome–negative chronic myelogenous leukemia and chronic myelomonocytic leukemia. *Hematol Oncol Clin North Am* 4:389–404, 1990.

Kojima S, Iwase K, Yamada H, et al: Chronic myelomonocytic leukemia in a 15-year-old boy. *Am J Pediatr Hematol Oncol* 9:23–26, 1987.

Kouides PA, Bennett JM: Morphology and classification of myelodysplastic syndromes. *Hematol Oncol Clin North Am* 6:485–499, 1992.

Kurata H, Miwa A, Kato Y, et al: Long survival of a patient with the blastic crisis of chronic myelomonocytic leukemia. *Rinsho Ketsueki* 31:41–45, 1990.

Lai JL, Zandecki M, Fenaux P, et al: Translocations (5;17) and (7;17) in patients with de novo or therapy related myelodysplastic syndromes or acute non-lymphocytic leukemia. A possible association with acquired pseudo-Pelger-Huet anomaly and small vacuolated granulocytes. *Cancer Genet Cytogenet* 46:173–184, 1990.

List AF, Gonzalez-Osete G, Kummet T, et al: Granulocytic sarcoma in myelodysplastic syndromes: Clinical marker of disease acceleration. *Am J Med* 90:274–276, 1991.

Lyons J, Janssen JWG, Bartram C, et al: Mutation of Ki-*ras* and N-*ras* oncogenes in myelodysplastic syndromes. *Blood* 71:1707–1712, 1988.

Mangi MH, Mufti GL: Primary myelodysplastic syndromes: Diagnostic and prognostic significance of immunohistochemical assessment of bone marrow biopsies. *Blood* 79:198–205, 1992.

Mangi MH, Mufti GL: Abnormal localization of abnormal precursors (ALIP) in the bone marrow of myelodysplastic syndromes: Current state of knowledge and future directions. *Leuk Res* 15:627–639, 1991.

Masaad L, Prieur M, Leonard C, et al: Biclonal chromosome evolution of chronic myelomonocytic leukemia in a child. *Cancer Genet Cytogenet* 44:131–137, 1990.

McKenna RW, Allison PM: Diagnosis, classification and course of myelodysplastic syndromes. *Clin Lab Med* 10:683–705, 1990.

Mecucci C, Vanden Berghe H: Myelodysplastic syndromes. Cytogenetics. *Hematol Oncol North Am* 6:523–541, 1992.

Molica S, Iannaccaro P, Alberti A: Chronic myelomonocytic leukemia. A test of a proposed staging system. *Am J Hematol* 35:129–130, 1990.

Mufti GL, Galton DAG: Myelodysplastic syndromes: Natural history and features of prognostic importance. *Clin Haematol* 15:953–971, 1986.

Mufti GL, Stevens JR, Oscier DG, et al: Myelodysplastic syndromes. A scoring system with prognostic significance. *Br J Haematol* 59: 425–433, 1985.

Polliack A, McKenzie S, Gee T, et al: A scanning electron microscopic study of 34 cases of acute granulocytic, myelomonocytic, monoblastic and histiocytic leukemia. *Am J Med* 59:308–315, 1975.

Pugh WC, Pearson M, Vardiman JW, et al: Philadelphia chromosome negative chronic myelogenous leukaemia: A morphological reassessment. *Br J Haematol* 60:457–467, 1985.

Ribera JM, Cervantes F, Reverter JC, et al: Acute transformation of chronic myelomonocytic leukemia: A multivariate study of predictive factors. *Eur J Haematol* 42:284–288, 1989.

Ribera JM, Cervantes F, Rozman C: A multivariate analysis of prognostic factors in chronic myelomonocytic leukemia according to the FAB criteria. *Br J Haematol* 65:307–311, 1987.

Rosenbloom B, Schreck R, Koeffler HP: Therapy related myelodysplastic syndromes. *Hematol Oncol Clin North Am* 6:707–722, 1992.

Sanz GF, Sanz MA, Vellespi T, et al: Two regression models and a scoring system for predicting survival and planning treatment in myelodysplastic syndromes. A multivariate analysis of prognostic features in 370 patients. *Blood* 74:395–408, 1989.

Solal-Celigny P, Desaint B, Herrera A, et al: Chronic myelomonocytic leukemia according to FAB classification: Analysis of 35 cases. *Blood* 63:634–638, 1984.

Srivastava A, Boswell HS, Heerema NA, et al: K-*ras*^{2} oncogene overexpression in myelodysplastic syndrome with translocation 5;12. *Cancer Genet Cytogenet* 36:61–71, 1988.

Stark AN, Thorogood J, Head C, et al: Prognostic factors and survival in chronic myelomonocytic leukemia. *Br J Cancer* 56:59–63, 1987.

Storniolo AM, Moloney WC, Rosenthal DS, et al: Chronic myelomonocytic leukemia. *Leukemia* 4:766–770, 1990.

Tefferi A, Hoagland HC, Therneau TM, et al: Chronic myelomonocytic leukemia. Natural history and prognostic determinants. *Mayo Clin Proc* 64:1246–1254, 1989.

Tricot G, De Wolf-Peeters C, Hendricks B, et al: Bone marrow histology in myelodysplastic syndromes: I. Histological findings in myelodysplastic syndromes and comparison with bone marrow smears. *Br J Haematol* 57:423–430, 1984.

Tricot G, De Wolf-Peeters C, Vlietinck R, et al: Bone marrow histology in myelodysplastic syndromes: II. Prognostic value of abnormal localization of immature precursors in MDS. *Br J Haematol* 58:217–225, 1984.

Varela GL, Chuang C, Woll JE, et al: Modifications in the classification of primary myelodysplastic syndromes. The addition of a scoring system. *Haematol Oncol* 3:55–63, 1985.

Verhoef G, De Wolf-Peeters C, Kerim S, et al: Update on the prognostic implications of morphology, histology and karyotype in primary myelodysplastic syndromes. *Hematol Pathol* 5:163–175, 1991.

Review Articles:

Bartram CR: Molecular genetic aspects of myelodysplastic syndromes. *Hematol Oncol Clin North Am* 6:557–570, 1992.

Castro-Malaspina H, Schaison G, Passe S, et al: Subacute and chronic myelomonocytic leukemia in children (juvenile CML). Clinical and hematologic observations and identification of prognostic factors. *Cancer* 54:675–686, 1984.

Groupe Français de Cytogenetique Hématologique: Cytogenetics of chronic myelomonocytic leukemia. *Cancer Genet Cytogenet* 21:11–30, 1986.

Harris NL, Demirjian Z: Plasmacytoid T-zone cell proliferation in a patient with chronic myelomonocytic leukemia. Histological and immunohistological characterization. *Am Surg Pathol* 15:87–95, 1991.

Martiat P, Michaux JL, Rodhain J, et al: Philadelphia-negative (Ph −) chronic myeloid leukemia (CML): Comparison with Ph + CML and chronic myelomonocytic leukemia. *Blood* 78:205–211, 1991.

Takasaki N, Kaneko Y, Maseki N, et al: Trisomy 11 in chronic myelomonocytic leukemia: Report of two cases and review of the literature. *Cancer Genet Cytogenet* 30:109–117, 1988.

Worsley A, Oscier DG, Stevens J, et al: Prognostic features of chronic myelomonocytic leukemia: A modified Bournemouth score gives the prediction of survival. *Br J Haematol* 68:17–21, 1988.

CASE 12

PATIENT: 67-year-old white female.

CHIEF COMPLAINT: Abdominal discomfort of 2 weeks' duration.

MEDICAL HISTORY: 20-year history of diabetes mellitus and hypertension.

PHYSICAL EXAMINATION: Bilateral axillary lymphadenopathy. Mild splenomegaly. No hepatomegaly.

LABORATORY RESULTS:

A. *Screening Procedure*
WBC of 89.8 × 10^9/L with a differential of segmented neutrophils 14%, eosinophils 2%, monocytes 3%, and atypical lymphocytes 81%. HGB 9.2 g/dL. HCT 27.5 L/L. MCV 99.1 fL, MCH 33.2 pg, MCHC 33.5 g/dL, RDW 17.7. Platelets 143 × 10^9/L.

HOSPITAL COURSE: A lymph node biopsy was performed, and a diagnosis of malignant lymphoma, follicular mixed small and large cell type (Case 12.1) was made. Review of the peripheral blood film revealed atypical lymphocytes, some with nuclear clefting (Case 12.2). Similar lymphoid cells were present in the bone marrow aspirate, and the biopsy was extensively replaced by a diffuse, interstitial, and paratrabecular lymphocytic infiltrate (Case 12.3) without fibro-

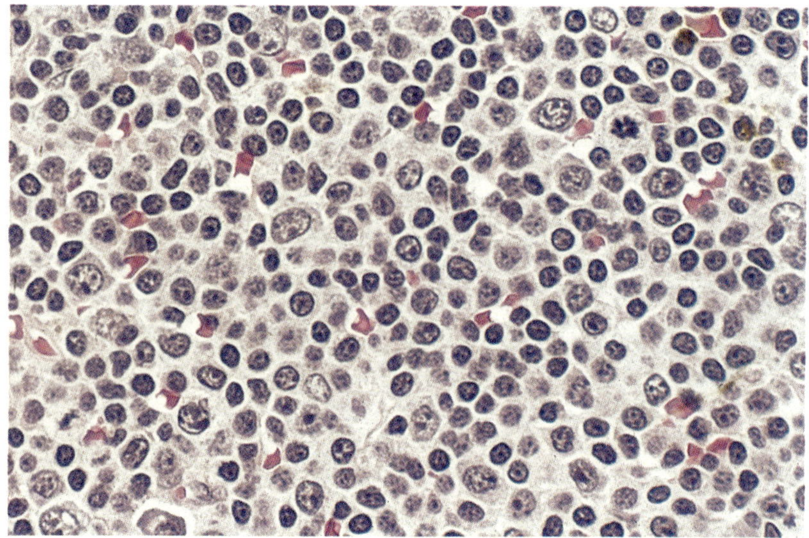

Case 12-1 Lymph node biopsy demonstrating malignant lymphoma with a mixed population of small and large cell types. (×400).

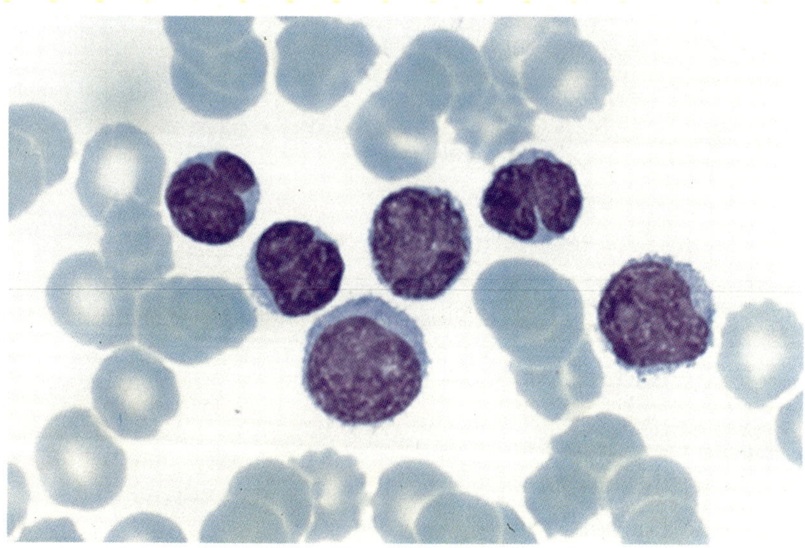

Case 12-2 Peripheral blood with small cleaved lymphosarcoma cells and larger forms with occasional nucleoli. (×1000).

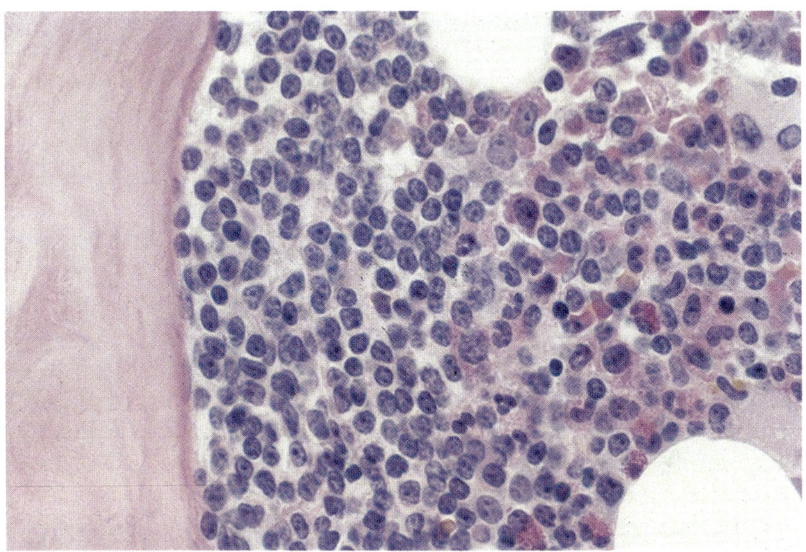

Case 12-3 Bone marrow biopsy. Focal paratrabecular involvement by lymphoma is present. (×400).

sis. The patient was started on combination chemotherapy and transferred to another center.

QUESTIONS:

1. Does the patient have leukemia or lymphoma?
2. Does the cytologic appearance of lymphoid cells in the peripheral blood correlate with the type of lesion in the lymph node biopsy?
3. Name the condition in which epithelial tumor cells circulate in leukemic proportions.

LABORATORY RESULTS:

B. *Confirmatory Results*

Cytochemistry: AEST−, BEST−, AP−, Tdt−.

Flow cytometry on circulating tumor cells: sIgM+ and sIgG+ in >80% cells. CD10+, CD19+, CD20+, CD24+, HLADR+, CD5−, CD11c−, CD13−, CD25−, CD38−.

Cytogenetics: 46XX.

Molecular genetics on circulating leukemic cells: IgH gene and κ-IgL gene rearranged. TCR-β germline. Results interpreted as consistent with clonal B-cell proliferation.

DIAGNOSIS: Lymphosarcoma cell leukemia.

DISCUSSION: The development of leukemia in patients with malignant lymphoma has been recognized since the turn of the century and was initially characterized by Sternberg in 1908 as "leukosarcoma." At that time, the three recognized forms of malignant lymphoma were lymphosarcoma, reticulum cell sarcoma, and Hodgkin's disease. The term *lymphosarcoma* was applied to malignant lymphomas of small lymphocytes, and included cases that would be presently classified as malignant lymphoma, small cleaved follicular center cell (SCFCCL); malignant lymphoma, small lymphocytic; mantle zone lymphoma; and monocytoid B-cell lymphoma. In contrast, the term *reticulum cell sarcoma* was used to describe malignant lymphoma, large cell type, and apparently all other forms of NHL. Since lymphosarcoma was most frequently observed to undergo leukemic transformation, Isaacs in 1937 introduced the term *lymphosarcoma cell leukemia* (LSCL) to better define this entity, and thereby provided a means to distinguish LSCL from CLL and reports of reticulum cell leukemia and Reed-Sternberg cell leukemia.

With the evolution of newer immunologic concepts and classifications of the NHLs, including those of Rappaport, Lukes-Collins, the Kiel classification, and the National Cancer Institute Working Formulation, sensitive immunologic methods to identify small numbers of circulating lymphoma cells (CLCs) have been developed. This has provided opportunities to better correlate the cytologic features of LSCL with other data including the type and grade of lymphoma in lymph node biopsies, cellular immunophenotype, clinical stage of disease, and survival.

Although controversial, archaic, and lacking in precision, the term LSCL is presently used to describe the leukemic phase of all the NHLs with the exception of lymphoblastic lymphoma and Burkitt's lymphoma. In this latter group, the leukemic phase is termed ALL (L1 and L2), and ALL (L3), respectively. Other notable exceptions are HTLV-I-associated lymphoma-leukemia, in which the tissue and leukemic phases of this disease frequently manifest simultaneously, and mycosis fungoides, in which circulating Sézary cells may be observed in the peripheral blood. Although cytologically atypical lymphocytes are occasionally present in the peripheral blood of some patients with Lennert's lymphoma, composite lymphomas and lymphomas of mucosa-associated lymphoid tissues (MALT), the leukemic phase of these lesions has not been well characterized, and only recently have CLCs been described in Ki-1+ anaplastic large cell lymphoma. Judging from illustrations and descriptions in the literature, we believe that cases reported hitherto as acute LSCL depict transformed lymphosarcoma cells or ALL.

Since greater than 80% of NHLs originate from clonal proliferations of B lymphocytes, it is the experience of observers in the field including Foucar et al., Said and Pinkus, and Smith et al., that most cases of LSCL encountered in practice are of B phenotype. Moreover, since SCFCCL is the most prevalent NHL, with CLCs manifesting in up to 70% of cases at some time in its natural history, it becomes apparent why the small cleaved lymphocyte ("buttock" cell) is most often depicted in the literature as the prototype of the lymphosarcoma cell. Examination of the 1937 camera lucida drawings of Isaacs, however, portray lymphosarcoma cells as large, nucleolated, and lacking a nuclear cleft. This discrepancy is in part because CLCs in any given case seldom display uniformity of size and appearance, and because not all published illustrations depicting lymphosarcoma cells are from patients with SCFCCL.

Correlation of data generated by investigators over the past 83 years is largely complicated by problems arising from differences in lymphoma terminology and by lack of uniform criteria used in establishing a diagnosis of LSCL. While some studies include cases in which occasional CLCs were detected by light microscopy, others have used more rigorous criteria and have included only those cases with associated lymphocytosis. For this reason, the authors use the designation CLC to characterize cytologically or immunologically detected lymphosarcoma cells in the absence of lymphocytosis, and LSCL when absolute lymphocytosis is additionally manifest. Such designations do appear to have clinical merit, since most patients with NHL and LSCL are observed to have a clinically more advanced stage of disease than those with CLCs.

Studies comparing the incidence of CLC/LSCL with the follicular and diffuse growth patterns of the NHL have not revealed consistent results. Nevertheless, there is a clear association between SCFCCL, a positive bone marrow biopsy, and LSCL. In the experience of Rosenberg et al. and Come et al., however, the development of LSCL in patients with SCFCCL did not appear to exert an independent effect on prognosis.

In their report of intermediate lymphocytic lymphoma, Weisenburger et al. observed LSCL in 9 of 42 patients (21%) at initial diagnosis, and in their analysis of 11 patients De-Oliveira et al. found that leukemic transformation was associated with a poor prognosis, and a median survival of less than 2 years. Immunologic studies may be of value in distinguishing problem cases, especially the CLCs of SCFCCL origin which are CD5− and CALLA+, from those of mantle zone lymphoma which are CD5+ and CALLA−.

Peripheral blood involvement in monocytoid B-cell lymphoma appears to be rare and was first reported by Traweek et al. in 1989. The total WBC count in their patient was 4.5 × 10^9/L, and 65% of circulating WBCs were considered to be monocytoid. Cytologically, such cells are indistinguishable from hairy cells but are TRAP− and CD25−. Minimal bone marrow disease was present without reticulin fibrosis, and identical clonally rearranged IgH genes were present in the peripheral blood and an involved lymph node.

The leukemic phase of malignant lymphoma, small lymphocytic, is considered by most investigators to be synonymous with CLL and does not appear to alter survival statistics. Morphologic appearances of the lymph node and bone marrow biopsies in these two lesions may be identical, making the distinction virtually impossible.

In the mixed small and large category, only a few examples of CLCs and LSCL are cited in the literature, and, as in the present case, it is apparent that the leukemic phase can manifest at initial diagnosis.

LSCL is uncommon in large cell lymphoma. In a study of 34 patients with this subtype, Smith et al. observed that CLCs could be detected up to 6 months after aggressive chemotherapy and complete remission. No CLCs were observed beyond 18 months. In a more recent report of 24 patients with LSCL and large cell lymphoma, Bain et al. report a median survival of 7 months. Sixteen cases were of B lineage and 8 were T. The prognosis was worse in the former group. Lymphosarcoma cells revealed basophilic cytoplasm, marked pleomorphism, and nuclear convolution in both phenotypes. Sixteen patients presented with lymphoma-leukemia, and we found the highly convoluted electron microscopic appearances of nuclei in their report reminiscent of Sézary cells.

While the identification of cytologically abnormal lymphosarcoma cells in the presence of absolute lymphocytosis is seldom a problem, recent monoclonal antibody studies with fluorescent-activated cell sorter analysis have succeeded in detecting small populations of cytologically normal CLCs in patients considered to be in clinical remission. Using such methodologies, Ault observed that up to 40% of patients with NHL, not suspected of having CLCs, actually did. Subsequently Ligler et al., using the relative fluorescent intensity of labeled antibodies against kappa and lambda light chains, were able to identify clonal excess in as few as 0.1% of CLCs. More recently, Lindl et al. have found that detection of CLCs by heavy chain gene arrangement studies may actually be more sensitive; and Horning et al. have found the application of Ig and TCR gene rearrangement studies using Southern blot hybridization to be a valuable adjunct in detecting minimal disease. Although absolute LSC counts as high as 63,500/mm^3 have been reported by Schnitzer et al., it is apparent that the application of immunologic methods would actually result in higher counts. Absolute lymphocyte counts in LSCL, however, tend to be lower than in patients with CLL and are found to fluctuate during the natural history of any given patient, being highest at times of clinical relapse and lowest following successful therapy. It is apparent, however, that counts seldom if ever reach proportions resulting in symptomatic leukocytosis. Therefore, in the absence of cytologic atypia, light microscopy is not necessarily a sensitive method to detect small numbers of CLCs, and no specific cytologic criteria apply to all CLCs. Irregularities of the nuclear membrane may range from shallow indentation to deep invaginations, and nucleoli are usually inconspicuous but may be prominent in larger and transformed lymphomasarcoma cells. This heterogenicity of nuclear morphology is believed to be secondary to disordered organization of nuclear proteins and the phase of the cell cycle. The cytoplasm is usually scant but may be abundant, and in cases of large cell lymphoma are devoid of any distinctive feature. Rarely, ribosome-lamella bodies have been observed, and recently, Groom et al. described Auer rod–like structures in CLCs. These appearances correlate well with the electron microscopic studies of Schnitzer et al., Said and Pinkus, and Bain et al. In practice, however, ultrastructural analysis is seldom if ever necessary to establish the diagnosis of either CLCs or LSCL.

The differential diagnosis of CLCs and LSCL includes CLL, PLL, HCL, secondary AML, and carcinocythemia. Differentiation from CLL can occasionally be a problem, and some points of comparison are listed in Table C12.1. The diagnostic features of PLL and HCL are considered elsewhere in this book. Secondary AML in patients with NHL is well documented, and recently Rosner and Gründwald gathered data on 117 cases. Differentiation from the CLCs of large cell lymphoma can be especially difficult on cytologic grounds, but can be made with appropriate cytochemical, immunophenotypic, and cytogenetic studies.

Carcinocythemia is the massive hematogenous dissemination of a nonhematopoietic neoplasm, and examples of carcinoma of the breast, small cell carcinoma of the lung, rhabdomyosarcoma, and other tumors are reported. Tumor cells are often clumped. Immunohistochemical stains, electron microscopy, and correlation of appearances with the primary tumor may be necessary to confirm the diag-

Table C12-1 Usual Differences between CLL and LSCL

	CLL	*LSCL*
Median age	59.5 years	48 years
Incidence	More frequently observed in practice	Rarer
Peripheral blood changes		
Absolute lymphocyte count	Higher. Occasionally greater than 100,000 × 10^9/L.	Lower. Usually <30,000 × 10^9/L.
Lymphocyte cytology	Small, with mature clumped chromatin and <11% prolymphocytes.	Varies with type of lymphoma. Small with notched nuclei in SCFCCL. Large and nucleolated in large cell lymphoma.
Anemia and thrombocytopenia	More frequent. Associated with advanced clinical stages.	Less frequent.
Bone marrow	Lymphocytes >30% of all nucleated cells.	Virtually all cases have a positive bone marrow biopsy.
	Variable nodular, diffuse, interstitial, or mixed patterns possible.	Focal paratrabecular, interstitial, or diffuse.
Immunologic differences	B phenotype more frequent than T.	B phenotype more frequent than T.
	CALLA−.	CALLA+ when secondary to SCFCCL.
	CD5+, CD19+, CD20+.	Identical in cases of small lymphocytic lymphoma. Variable in other types.
	sIg faint monoclonal. IgM predominantly (occasionally combined with IgD). Greater tendency to form rosettes with mouse RBCs.	sIg bright monoclonal. Selective light chain clonal excess by immunofluorescence. Lesser tendency to form rosettes with mouse RBCs.
Lymph node biopsy	Diffuse infiltrate. Small lymphocytes with rare prolymphocytes. Pseudofollicles and transformation occasionally.	Most frequently, SCFCCL.
Response to treatment and survival	Better and more predictable. Usually 72–100 months.	Worse and less predictable. Usually less than 24 months.

nosis. Cases reported in the older literature as reticulum cell leukemia and believed to be the leukemic phase of reticulum cell sarcoma would be classified presently as either HCL or monocytic leukemia. Also of interest is the report by Scheerer et al. of Reed-Sternberg cell leukemia developing in a patient with advanced Hodgkin's disease. Although the presence of circulating Reed-Sternberg cells in patients with Hodgkin's disease has been known for many years, and was found in 18.5% of 135 patients by Bouroncle, leukemic transformation is most unusual.

In summary, the clinical implication of CLCs and LSCL should not be interpreted in isolation but rather, as in this case, within the context of clinical stage and grade of the lymphoma as observed in the lymph node biopsy.

SUMMARY

Morphology	**Variable, often with small cleaved nuclei**
Cytochemistry	**AEST−, BEST−, AP−, Tdt−**
Immunophenotyping	**CD10+, CD19+, CD20+, CD24+, HLA-DR+, CD5−**
Cytogenetics	**46XX**
Molecular Genctics	**Heavy and light chain genes rearranged**
Diagnosis	**Lymphosarcoma cell leukemia**

ANSWERS:

1. In an aleukemic patient with a diagnosis of malignant lymphoma made on a lymph node biopsy, the terminology is not controversial. Likewise, in a leukemic patient with a positive bone marrow biopsy and no adenopathy, the designation *leukemia* is approriate. However, in patients simultaneously presenting lymphoma and LSCL, as in this case, the designation *lymphoma-leukemia* would also be appropriate.
2. Not necessarily. Discordant patterns of cell size in the lymph node biopsy, bone marrow biopsy, and circulating lymphoma cells are often present.
3. Carcinocythemia. This condition may develop also in nonhematopoietic mesenchymal tumors. Appearances may simulate LSCL.

BIBLIOGRAPHY

Reference Articles:

Bain B, Matutes E, Robinson D, et al: Leukemia as a manifestation of large cell lymphoma. *Br J Haematol* 77:301–310, 1991.

Bersack SR: Unusual case of cutaneous Hodgkin's disease with terminal blood stream spread. *JAMA* 126:1025, 1944.

Bouroncle B: Sternberg-Reed cells in the peripheral blood of patients with Hodgkin's disease. *Blood* 27:544–566, 1966.

Come SE, Jaffe ES, Andersen JC, et al: Non-Hodgkin's lymphomas in leukemic phase: Clinicopathologic correlations. *Am J Med* 69:667–674, 1980.

Conlan MG, Armitage JO, Bast M, et al: Clinical significance of hematologic parameters in non-Hodgkin's lymphoma at diagnosis. *Cancer* 67:1389–1395, 1991.

Dardick I, Hall R, Bailey DJ, et al: Nuclear antigens in neoplastic lymphocytes of B cell and T-cell non-Hodgkin's lymphomas. *Am J Pathol* 134:213–222, 1989.

de-Korte D, Haverkort WA, Roos D, et al: Aberrant ribonucleotide pattern in lymphoid cells from patients with chronic lymphocytic leukemia or non-Hodgkin's lymphoma. *Int J Cancer* 40:192–197, 1987.

De-Oliveira MS, Jaffe ES, Catovsky D: Leukemic phase of mantle zone (intermediate) lymphoma: Its characterization in 11 cases. *J Clin Pathol* 42:962–972, 1989.

Groom DA, Wong D, Brynes RL, et al: Auer rod-like inclusions in circulating lymphoma cells. *Am J Clin Pathol* 96:111–115, 1991.

Horning SJ, Galili N, Cleary M, et al: Detection of non-Hodgkin's lymphoma in the peripheral blood by analysis of antigen receptor gene rearrangement: Results of a prospective study. *Blood* 75:1139–1145, 1990.

Isaacs R: Lymphosarcoma cell leukemia. *Ann Intern Med* 11:657–662, 1937.

Lindl J, Lenner P, Roos G: Monoclonal B-cells in peripheral blood in non-Hodgkin's lymphoma. *Scand J Haematol* 32:5–11, 1984.

Lindl J, Johansson H, Lenner P, et al: Monoclonal B-cells in blood, in non-Hodgkin's lymphoma. Correlation with clinical features and prognoses. *Acta Oncol* 28:641–646, 1989.

Lindl J, Lindstrom A, Lenner P, et al: Immunoglobulin heavy-chain gene rearrangement in peripheral blood mononuclear cells in non-Hodgkin's lymphomas: Correlation with kappa:lambda analysis and clinical features. *Europ J Haematol* 42:134–142, 1989.

Liang R, Chan VV, Chan TK: Immunoglobulin gene rearrangement in the peripheral blood and bone marrow of patients with lymphomas of the mucosa-associated lymphoid tissues. *Acta Haematol (Basel)* 84:19–23, 1990.

Lugassy G, Vorst EJ, Varon D, et al: Carcinocythemia. Report of two cases, one simulating a Burkitt lymphoma. *Acta Cytol* 34:265–268, 1990.

Ludman H, Spear PW: Reed-Sternberg cells in peripheral blood: Report of case of Hodgkin's disease. *Blood* 12:189–192, 1957.

Mathé G, Pouillart P, Schwarzenberg L, et al: Leukaemic conversion of non-Hodgkin's malignant lymphomata. *Br J Cancer* 31:96–101, 1975.

Mintzer DM, Hauptman SP: Lymphosarcoma cell leukemia and other non-Hodgkin's lymphomas in leukemic phase. *Am J Med* 75:110–120, 1983.

Morra E, Lazzarino M, Castello A, et al: Bone marrow and blood involvement by non-Hodgkin's lymphoma: A study of clinicopathologic correlations and prognostic significance in relationship to the Working Formulation. *Eur J Haematol* 42:445–453, 1989.

O'Briain DS, Lawlor E, Sarsfield P, et al: Circulating cerebriform lymphoid cells (Sézary-type cells) in a B-cell malignant lymphoma. *Cancer* 61:1587–1593, 1988.

Rosenberg SA, Diamond HD, Jaslowitz B, et al: Lymphosarcoma: A review of 1269 cases. *Medicine (Baltimore)* 40:31–84, 1961.

Rosner F, Gründwald HW: Chemicals and leukemia. In *Leukemia,* ed 5. Philadelphia. W. B. Saunders Co., 1990, pp 271–277.

Scheerer PP, Pierre RV, Schwartz DL, et al: Reed-Sternberg cell leukemia and lactic acidosis. *N Engl J Med* 270:274–278, 1964.

Smith BR, Weinberg DS, Robert NJ, et al: Circulating monoclonal B lymphocytes in non-Hodgkin's lympnoma. *N Engl J Med* 311:1476–1481, 1984.

Sternberg C: Ueber Leukosarcomatose. *Wien Klin Wochenschr* 21:XXI, 475, 1908.

Swerdlow SH, Murray LJ, Habeshaw JA, et al: Lymphocytic lymphoma/B-chronic lymphocytic leukemia. An immunohistopathological study of peripheral B lymphocyte neoplasia. *Br J Cancer* 50:587–599, 1984.

The Non-Hodgkin's Lymphoma Pathologic Classification Project: National Cancer Institute sponsored study of classifications of non-Hodgkin's lymphomas: Summary and description of a Working Formulation for clinical usage. *Cancer* 49:2112–2135, 1982.

Traweek BST, Scheibani K, Winberg CD, et al: Monocytoid B-cell lymphoma: Its evolution and relationship to other low-grade B-cell neoplasms. *Blood* 73:573–578, 1989.

Weinberg DS, Ault KA, Pinkus GS: Circulating malignant cells in non-Hodgkin's lymphoma: Correlation with binding by peanut agglutinin. *Blood* 72:698–704, 1988.

Weisenburger DD, Duggan MJ, Perry DA, et al: Non-Hodgkin's lympnomas of mantle zone origin. *Pathol Annu* 26:139–157, 1991.

Weisenburger DD, Nathwani BN, Diamond LW, et al: Malignant lymphoma, intermediate lymphocytic type: A clinicopathologic study of 42 cases. *Cancer* 48:1415–1425, 1981.

Wong KF, Chan CS, Ng YC, et al: Analplastic large cell Ki-1 lymphoma involving bone marrow. *Am J Hematol* 37:112–119, 1991.

Yam L, Castoldi GL, Garvey MB, et al: Functional cytogenetic and cytochemical study of the leukemic reticulin cells. *Blood* 32:90–101, 1968.

Zeffren JL, Ultman JE: Reticulum cell carcinoma terminating in acute leukemia. *Blood* 15:277–284, 1960.

Review Articles:

Ault KA: Detection of small numbers of monoclonal B lymphocytes in the blood of patients with lymphoma. *N Engl J Med* 300:1401–1405, 1979.

Brada M, Mizutani S, Molgaard H, et al: Circulating lymphoma cells in patients with B and T non-Hodgkin's lymphoma detected by immunoglobulin and T-cell receptor gene rearrangement. *Br J Cancer* 56:147–152, 1987.

Foucar K, McKenna RW, Frizzera G, et al: Incidence and patterns of bone marrow and blood involvement by lymphoma in relationship to the Lukes-Collins classification. *Blood* 54:1417–1422, 1979.

Koo CH, Rappaport H, Sheibani K, et al: Imprint cytology of non-Hodgkin's lymphomas. *Human Pathol* 20:1–137, 1989.

Koziner B, Filippa DA, Martelsmann R, et al: Characterization of malignant lymphomas in leukemic phase by multiple differentiation markers of mononuclear cells. *Am J Med* 63:556–567, 1977.

Ligler FS, Smith RG, Kettman JR, et al: Detection of tumor cells in the peripheral blood of nonleukemic patients with B-cell lymphoma: Analysis of "clonal excess." *Blood* 55:792–801, 1980.

Morra E, Lazzarino M, Orlandi E, et al: Leukemic phase of non-Hodgkin's lymphomas. Hematological features and prognostic significance. *Hematologica* 69:15–29, 1984.

Said JW, Pinkus GS: Immunologic characterization and ultrastructural correlation for 125 cases of B- and T-cell leukemias. *Cancer* 48:2630–2642, 1981.

Schnitzer B, Loesel LS, Reed RE: Lymphosarcoma cell leukemia. A clinicopathological study. *Cancer* 26:1082–1096, 1970.

CASE 13

PATIENT: 37-year-old white male.

CHIEF COMPLAINT: Right flank pain.

MEDICAL HISTORY: The patient was in good health until the onset of right flank pain, 5½ weeks prior to examination by his local physician.

PHYSICAL EXAMINATION: No abnormality on physical examination, routine urine analysis, a kidney-ureter-bladder series, and chest x-ray examination. However, due to the presence of an abnormal CBC, he was referred for additional investigation.

LABORATORY RESULTS:

A. *Screening Procedure*
   WBC of 18.0 × 10^9/L with a differential of segmented neutrophils 18%, bands 2%, eosinophils 1%, monocytes 2%, lymphocytes 60% (most with plasmacytoid features), and plasma cells 17%. HGB 12.4 g/dL. HCT 0.35 L/L, MCV 91.7 fL, MCH 32.6 pg, MCHC 35.6 g/dL, RDW 14.0. Platelets 127 × 10^9/L.

HOSPITAL COURSE: The peripheral blood film revealed plasma cells with eccentric nuclei, perinuclear clearing, and abundant gray-blue cytoplasm (Case 13.1). Rarely, plasma cells were nucleolated. Following examination of the bone marrow (Case 13.2), and immuno-

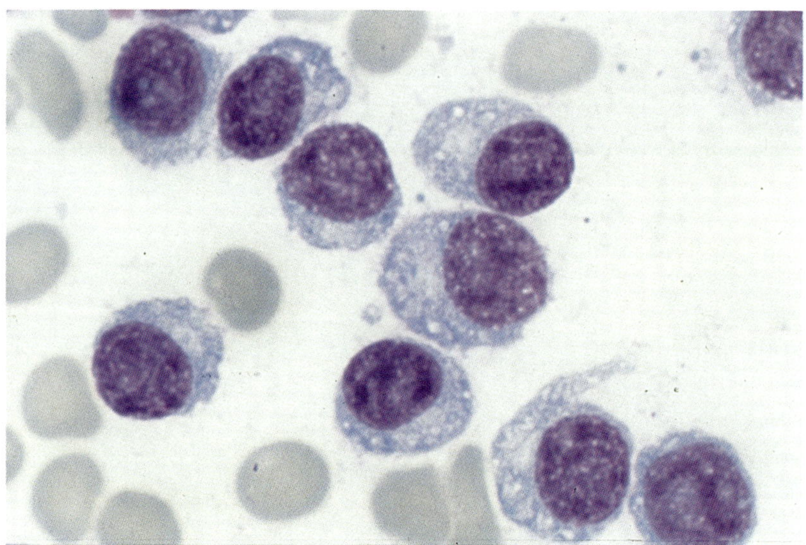

Case 13-1 Peripheral blood film with numerous plasma cells (×1000).

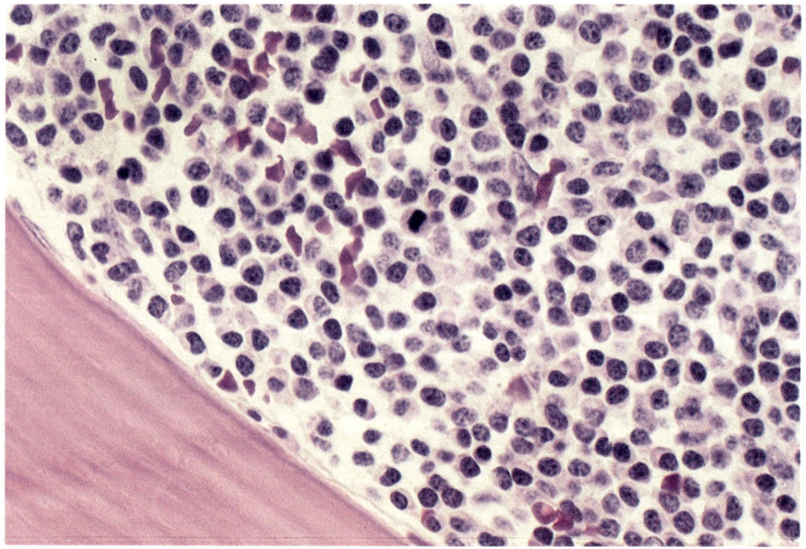

Case 13-2 Bone marrow biopsy. A diffuse plasmacellular infiltrate is present (×400).

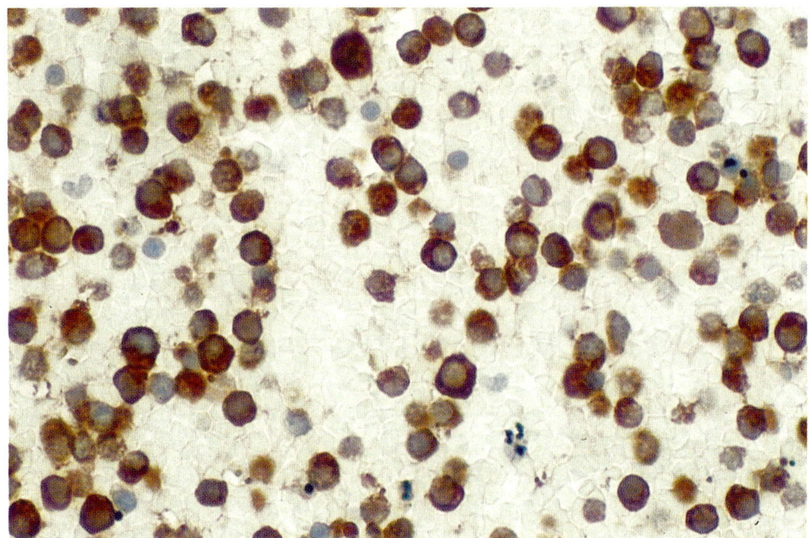

Case 13-3 Bone marrow clot section with strong cytoplasmic staining for kappa light chains. Immunoperoxidase technique (×400).

peroxidase stains for light chain excess (Case 13.3), the patient was started on Melphalan (L-phenylalanine mustard) and prednisone. He returns for regular follow-up, now 22 months from initial presentation.

QUESTIONS:

1. What lesions enter into the differential diagnosis?
2. Do greater than 10% plasma cells in the bone marrow always indicate a plasma cell dyscrasia?
3. What are Türk cells?

LABORATORY RESULTS:

B. *Confirmatory Results*

Bone marrow examination: The marrow was replaced by a diffuse infiltrate of well-differentiated plasma cells, some with lymphoplasmacytic features. Rare azurophilic cytoplasmic inclusions were observed in some plasma cells. All normal hematopoietic cells were markedly decreased, and the overall fat/cell ratio was 2:98. Plasmacellular elements constituted about 90% of all cells and were A-EST+, B-EST−, and PAS−. Dutcher bodies were absent. Immunoperoxidase staining for kappa and lambda light chains revealed virtually 100% of plasma cells staining for kappa light chain.

Radiologic examination: The initial skeletal series, chest x-ray film, and abdominal CT scan revealed no lesions. However, 2 months later, lytic lesions could be identified in the long bones, pelvis, and skull.

Clinical chemistry: Serum calcium at admission was 10.2 mg/dL. Total serum protein was 6.5 gm% with decreased gamma globulin, of 0.02g% (normally 0.68–2.1). IgG was 219.0 mg (normally 800–1700), IgA <8.0 mg% (normally 100–400), and IgM <6 mg% (normally 50–320). IgD and IgE levels were not evaluated. Albumin, alpha-1-, alpha-2-, and beta-globulin levels were normal. Serum beta-2-microglobulin was 5.5 μg/mL. Marked proteinuria of 19.9 g/24 hr was observed, and monoclonal kappa light chain was detected in the serum and urine on immunoelectrophoresis. Serum viscosity was normal.

Immunophenotyping studies: Plasma cells in the bone marrow aspirate were CD38+, CD2−, CD5−, CD10−, CD13−, CD14−, CD19−, and CD20−.

Ckytogenetics: Performed on bone marrow aspirate: 46XY.

Molecular genetic stydies: Southern blot analysis on peripheral blood: IgH and κ-IgL genes rearranged. The β-TCR gene was germline. Changes were interpreted as indicative of a monoclonal B-cell lesion (Courtesy of Jeffrey Medeiros, National Cancer Institute, Bethesda.)

DIAGNOSIS: Leukemic myelomatosis.

DISCUSSION: Plasma cell leukemia (PCL) is a rare disorder, first described at the turn of the century by Foa, Gluzinski, and Reichenstein. Both acute and chronic forms are encountered in clinical practice and may occur de novo or in association with multiple myeloma (MM). The later form of disease is known as secondary PCL when it succeeds established MM, and leukemic myelomatosis when it precedes MM or is diagnosed concurrently. Other hematopoietic neoplasms that have preceded PCL have included examples of CLL, WM, Ph^1+ CML, and CNL.

According to present consensus, a diagnosis of PCL is admissible when leukemic plasma cells account for >20% of the differential leukocyte count, or when absolute numbers exceed 2×10^9/L.

The true incidence of de novo primary PCL is unknown but is estimated by Kosmo and Gale at <1 case per million in the general population. Hepatosplenomegaly is less frequently encountered than in secondary PCL, and lymphadenopathy occurs in about 40% of patients. Widespread dissemination has been observed in autopsy studies and includes involvement of the liver, spleen, bone, kidneys, heart, lungs, and CNS.

Secondary PCL is usually a late manifestation of MM and develops in about 2% of cases. Bone pain, lytic lesions, osteoporosis, and fractures are more commonly encountered than in primary PCL. Lymphadenopathy is invariably absent.

Since circulating plasma cells are observed in the peripheral blood of some patients with MM and may terminally increase in numbers, the need to distinguish this seemingly leukemoid phenomenon from PCL is important. In a retrospective study of 794 myeloma patients, Kyle et al. observed circulating plasma cells in 17% of cases. Since the number of such cells is <20% in the differential white cell count, and $<2 \times 10^9$/L, the process is considered neither leukemic nor leukemoid but, as with circulating lymphoma cells in NHL, represents tumor peripheralization. Although some circulating B lymphocytes in patients with MM have been found to reveal Ig gene rearrangement, such cells are presently not included in the tally of circulating myeloma cells.

In both primary and secondary PCL, hypercalcemia, increased BUN, Bence-Jones proteinuria, and an M protein have been observed. However, as in this case of leukemic myelomastosis, lytic bone lesions and hypercalcemia may be absent at the time of diagnosis. All five isotypes of Ig and restricted light chain types (as in this case with kappa light chain) have been observed in PCL. In about 50% of cases, the paraprotein is IgG, and about 15% of cases are IgA-associated. IgM, IgD, IgE, light chain, biclonal, and nonsecretory types appear to be less frequently represented. Why over 25% of patients with IgE myeloma, the rarest such paraproteinemia, develop PCL remains an enigma. Hyperviscosity is rare in PCL but has been observed with the isotypes IgG and IgA and contrasts with the IgM-associated hyperviscosity of WM. Amyloidosis is uncommon.

In most cases of PCL, the total leukocyte count has varied between 20 and 100×10^9/L. Higher counts have been reported, and plasma cells have been known to constitute 100% of the differential leukocyte count. Examination of the peripheral blood smear may reveal leukemic cells with a range of cytologic appearances varying from well-developed plasma cells with eccentric nuclei, clumped chromatin, radially oriented parachromatin, a clear perinuclear hof, and abundant cytoplasm to those with lymphoplasmacytic features, nucleoli, a high N/C ratio, and blastic appearances virtually indistinguishable from those of other acute leukemias. In such cases, evaluation of the cytochemical, immunophenotypic, and cytogenetic profile can be invaluable. Rouleaux formation may be evident, and anemia, increased ESR, and thrombocytopenia are frequently present.

Bone marrow examination usually reveals a diffuse plasmacellular infiltrate that, as in this case, may virtually replace all other hematopoietic elements. In aspirate preparations, binuclearity, nucleoli, and plasmablastic features may be better appreciated. Russell bodies and erythrophagocytosis have been reported. Azurophilic needlelike intracytoplasmic Ig crystals resembling Auer rode may be present. Similar inclusions were first reported in myeloma cells by Snapper and Schneid in 1946.

Cytochemical studies in PCL reveal a positive staining reaction for AP, A-EST, and beta-glucuronidase. In some instances, Tdt, PAS, and oil-red-O activity have been reported. As in this case, immunohistochemical demonstration of clonal excess in kappa or lambda light chains by immunoperoxidase technique in paraffin-embedded sections of the bone marrow is an important part of the workup.

Recently the monoclonal antibodies PC-1, PCA-1, and PCA-2 have been effectively utilized to identify benign and neoplastic plasma cells; and Anderson et al. report that PC-1 accurately identified circulating plasma cells in two cases of PCL. CD38 (OKT 10, Leu 17) activity is also demonstrable in PCL, and in this case was of additional diagnostic value. It is also of interest that the coexpression of leukocyte common antigen (LCA) and epithelial membrane antigen (EMA) in PCL has been reported by Salter et al. Cytoplasmic Ig is strongly positive, and sIg is usually absent. Since plasma cells are terminally differentiated B lymphocytes, CD19 and CD20 are characteristically negative. Rarely, expression of FMC7 activity, which is usually present in B-PLL and HCL, has been demonstrated in PCL. Of comparable rarity is the presence of CD11b (OKM-1) activity, which is typically present in monocytes and myelocytes and is reminiscent of a similar phenomenon in some cases of MM described by Grogan et al. However, the presence of FMC7 and CD11b in PCL is of uncertain significance and may be an expression of lineage infidelity.

On electron microscopy, no ultrastructural difference separates PCL from MM. Appearances vary with the level of cellular maturity and degree of plasmacellular or lymphoid differentiation. Bilobed and segmented nuclei have been observed, and osmophilic intranuclear inclusions similar to Dutcher bodies are rarely present. A variably prominent nucleolus, and clumped chromatin with radiating heterochromatin, are usually present. In plasmablasts the chromatin may be scant and delicate with wide expanses of intervening heterochromatin. The endoplasmic reticulum is variably dilated, and polymorphic mitochondria with anomalous transverse cristae connecting the mitochondrial walls have been reported. Cytoplasmic fibrils, considered by some observers to be amyloid precursors, are present in most cases including those with blastic features. Such filaments are often concentrated in a perinuclear location. The cytoplasmic membrane may reveal a ruffled appearance with multiple buds and blebs.

Cytogenetic abnormalities in PCL most commonly include the long arm of chromosome 1, with deletions and duplications including trisomy, tetrasomy, and hexasomy. Abnormalities of chromosome 14, primarily 14q+, have been reported, as have also the translocation abnormalities t(11;14), t(8;14), and 5q35. Deletions and duplications of chromosomes 8 and 9, and less frequently chromosomes 6, 7, 16, and 17, and ring chromosomes have also been reported. Studies before and after therapy suggest that the chromosomal abnormalities in PCL occur de novo and are unrelated to therapy. It is of interest that trisomy 12, which is commonly observed in CLL, has to our knowledge not been reported in PCL.

Molecular genetic studies in PCL have revealed rearrangement of light and heavy chain genes, compatible with that of a clonal B-cell neoplasm. Sümegi et al. reported that amplification and enhanced expression of the c-*myc* oncogene was present in two-thirds of 24 patients with PCL but absent in a parallel study of 21 patients with MM.

Disorders that cytologically need to be distinguished from chronic PCL are WM, CLL, and B-prolymphocytic leukemia. In each of these conditions circulating lymphoplasmacytic cells and an M spike may be present. In WM the process is virtually never leukemic, whereas in CLL and B-PLL the absolute lymphocyte count may be less than 15×10^9/L in the early stages of disease. Nucleoli are usually more prominent in B-PLL, and intranuclear Dutcher bodies are not characteristic in this disease. In some instances, additional immunologic characterization may be necessary, and the differences usually observed are outlined in Table C13.1.

The reason for leukemic transformation in MM remains an enigma and may not primarily be a matter of marrow overload, since no cytologic, ultrastructural, labeling, or mitotic index appears to separate one disorder from the other. While the presence of the c-*myc* oncogene, cytoplasmic J chains, and a growth-promoting synergism between the cytokines interleukin-6 and interleukin-3 have been observed in some cases of PCL, their role, if any, in leukemic transformation is uncertain. Furthermore, the expression of the *bcl*-2 gene, *ras* oncogene, and common ALL antigen (CALLA) in some cases of MM but not in PCL may be of additional significance.

Table C13-1 Distinguishing Immunologic Features of Chronic PCL, WM, B-PLL, and B-CLL

Immunologic Parameter	*Chronic PCL*	*WM*	*B-PLL*	*B-CLL*
sIg	−	±	+ + +	±
cIg	+ + +	+	±	±
mRBC	−	±	±	+ + +
CD5	−	±	±	+ + +
CD10	−	±	±	−
CD19/20	−	+	±	+
CD25	−	±	−	±
CD38	+	+	−	−
FMC7	±	+	+ + +	±
PCA-1	+	+	−	−

Source: Adapted from Catovsky: Markers in B-PLL, HCL, and related B-cell leukemias. In *Leukemia,* ed 5. Philadelphia, WB Saunders, 1990, p. 643. Stone: Immunophenotypic characterization of B cell maturation. *Haematol/Oncol Clin North Am* 4:460, 1990. Silber and Stahl: Phenotype of cells in CLL and related disease. In Canellos GP (ed): *Hematology,* 4th ed. New York, McGraw-Hill, 1990, p. 1015.
Filomena and Hyun: Waldenström's macroglobulinemia. *ASCP Check Sample* 32:90-6, 1990.

Overall median survival in PCL is short and estimated at around 6 months. However, longer survivals have been reported, and as with this case of leukemic myelomatosis, residual myeloma may remain in the bone marrow despite control of the leukemic phase.

SUMMARY

Morphology	**Plasma cells**
Cytochemical and Immunoperoxidase studies	**A-EST+, B-EST−, PAS−, kappa light chain positive in bone marrow infiltrate**
Immunophenotyping	**CD38+, CD5−, CD10−, CD 19−, CD20−**
Cytogenetics	**46XY**
Molecular Genetics	**Ig heavy chain and kappa light genes rearranged**
Diagnosis	**Leukemic myelomatosis**

ANSWERS:

1. The three conditions that should be considered in the differential diagnosis of chronic PCL are WM, B-CLL, and B-PLL.
2. No. In a study of 12 healthy controls, Wintrobe demonstrated that less than 4% of hematopoietic elements in the bone marrow were

plasma cells. The kappa/lambda ratio among such normal plasma cells is about 2:1. In the plasma cell dyscrasias, the resulting plasmacytosis is monoclonal and readily demonstrable by immunoperoxidase staining of light chains in paraffin-embedded tissue. In contrast, the plasmacytosis of reactive states is polyclonal and benign.

3. Türk cells are reactive to plasma cells that are occasionally observed in peripheral blood smears. Contrary to earlier belief, they are not a sign of marrow irritation.

BIBLIOGRAPHY

Articles:

Anderson KC, Bates MP, Slaughenhoupt B: A monoclonal antibody with reactivity restricted to normal and neoplastic plasma cells. *J Immunol* 132:3172–3179, 1984.

Baldini L, Cro L, Delia D, et al: Analysis of tumor-specific immunoglobulin gene rearrangement in peripheral blood B-cells in multiple myeloma patients. *Am J Hematol* 37:1–5, 1991.

Beltran G, Stuckey W: Nuclear lobulation and cytoplasmic fibrils in leukemia plasma cells. *Am J Pathol* 58:159–164, 1972.

Bernasconi C, Castelli G, Pagnucco G, et al: Plasma cell leukemia: A report on 15 patients. *Eur J Haematol* (Suppl)51:76–83, 1989.

Brouet JC, Fernand JP, Laurent G, et al: The association of chronic lymphocytic leukemia and multiple myeloma: A study of eleven cases. *Br J Haematol* 59:55–66, 1985.

Butterworth CE Jr, Frommeyer WB Jr, Riser WH Jr: Erythrophagocytosis in a case of plasma cell leukemia. *Blood* 8:519–523, 1953.

Cai ZJ: Primary plasma cell leukemia. A comprehensive analysis of 44 cases. *Chung Hua Chung Liu Tsa Chig* 12:314–317, 1990.

Caldwell CW, Yesus YW, Loy TS, et al: Acute leukemia/lymphoma of plasmacytoid T-cell type. *Am J Clin Pathol* 94:778–786, 1990.

Catovsky D: Markers in B-PLL, HCL, and related B-cell leukemias. In Henderson ES, Lister TA, (eds): *Leukemia,* ed 5. Philadelphia, WB Saunders, 1990, p 643.

Clofent G, Klein B, Commes T, et al: No detectable malignant B cells in the peripheral blood of patients with multiple myeloma. *Br J Haematol* 71:357–361, 1989.

Durie GM, Grogan TM: CALLA positive myeloma: An aggressive subtype with poor survival. *Blood* 66:229–232, 1985.

Epstein J, Xiao H, He X-Y: Makers of multiple hematopoietic cell lineages in multiple myeloma. *N Engl J Med* 322:664–668, 1990.

Filomena CA, Hyun BH: Waldenströms macroglobulinemia. *ASCP Check Sample* 32:90-6, 1990.

Fitzgerald PH, Rastrick JM, Hamer JW: Acute plasma cell leukemia following chronic lymphatic leukemia: Transformation of two separate diseases? *Br J Haematol* 25:171–177, 1973.

Foa P: Sulla produzione cellulare nell inflammazione ed inaltri processi analoghi specialmente in cio che si riferisce alle plasmacellule. *Folia Haematol (Leipz)* 1:166–167, 1904.

Gahrton G, Zech L., Nilsson K, et al: Two translocations, t(11;14) and t(1;6) in a patient with plasma cell leukemia and two populations of plasma cells. *Scand J Haematol* 24:42–46, 1980.

Geraci JM, Hansen RM, Kueck BD: Plasma cell leukemia and hyperviscosity syndrome. *South Med J* 83:800–805, 1990.

Gluzinski A, Reichenstein M: Myeloma und leucaemia lymphatica plasmocellularis. *Wein Kin Wochenschr* 19:336–339, 1906.

Grogan TM, Durie BGM, Spier CM, et al: Myelomonocytic antigen positive multiple myeloma. *Blood* 73:763–769, 1989.

Kosmo MA, Gale RP: Plasma cell leukemia. *Semin Hematol* 24:202–208, 1987.

Koybayashi M, Miyagishima T, Imamura M, et al: Establishment and characterization of a plasma cell leukemia cell line dependent for growth on IL-6 and a bi-phenotypic subclone dependent upon both IL-3 and IL-6. *Br J Haematol* 78:217–221, 1991.

Lehndorff H: Wilhelm Türk. A prominent hematologist of fifty years ago. *Blood* 9:642–647, 1954.

Matěja F, Tichý M, Novotný J, et al: Plasmacellular leukemia with IgD paraproteinemia. *Vnitr Lek* 36:81–87, 1990.

Maynadie M, Mugnert F, Guy H, et al.: Translocations involving 5q35 may also be associated with plasma cell leukemia. *Br J Haematol* 76:156, 1990.

Moeschlin S: Macroglobulinemia Waldenström with miliary lung infiltrations and terminal plasma cell leukemia. *Acta Med Scand* 179(Suppl 445):154, 1966.

Montecucco C, Riccardi A, Mazzini, et al: DNA content analysis of peripheral blood B-lymphocytes in plasma cell malignancies. *Basic Appl Histochem* 29:275–282, 1985.

Nacheva E, Fischer PE, Sherrington PD, et al: A new plasma cell line, Karpas 620, with translocations involving chromosomes 1, 11 and 14. *Br J Haematol* 74:70–76, 1990.

Ogawa M, Preston RA, Carson MD, et al: Cytoplasmic fibrils in plasma cell leukemia. *Acta Haematol (Basel)* 56:123–128, 1976.

Osanto S, Muller HP, Schuit HRE, et al: Primary plasma cell leukemia: A case report and a review of the literature. *Acta Haematol* 70:122–129, 1983.

Pasqualetti P, Casale R, Colantonio D, et al: Contemporaneous presentation of plasma cell leukemia and multiple myeloma. Description of a clinical case with a biclonal component. *Minerva Med* 78:907–910, 1987.

Pattersson M, Jernberg-Wiklund H, Larsson LG, et al: Expression of the *bcl*-2 gene in human multiple myeloma cell lines and normal plasma cells. *Blood* 79:495–502, 1992.

Pedraza MA: Plasma cell leukemia with unusual immunoglobulin abnormalities. *Am J Clin Pathol* 64:410–415, 1975.

Petrini M, LaGioia A, Lofaro A, et al: A case of multiple myeloma with peripheral plasmacytosis. *Haematologica (Pavia)* 70:271–272, 1985.

Pilarski LM, Mant MJ, Ruethen BA: Pre-B cells in peripheral blood of multiple myeloma patient. *Blood* 66:416–422, 1985.

Polliack A, Rachmilewitz D, Zlotnick A: Plasma cell leukemia: Unassembled light and heavy chains in the urine. *Arch Intern Med* 134:131–134, 1974.

Roser FE, Gruendwald H: Multiple myeloma terminating in leukemia. Report of 12 cases and review of the literature. *Am J Med* 57:927–939, 1974.

Ruiz-Arguelles GL, Katzmann JA, Greipp PR, et al: Multiple myeloma: Circulating lymphocytes that express plasma cell antigens. *Blood* 64:352–356, 1984.

Sakai A, Kawano M, Oguma N, et al: A case of plasma cell leukemia superimposed on Philadelphia (Ph) chromosome-positive chronic myeloid leukemia. *Am J Hematol* 36:222–223, 1991.

Salter DM, Krajewski AS, Miller EP, et al: Co-expression of leukocyte common antigen and epithelial membrane antigen in plasmacytic malignancies. *J Clin Pathol* 38:843–844, 1985.

Sandberg AA, Chromosome in human leukemia. *Semin Hematol* 23:201–217, 1986.

Sataline L: Acute plasmacytic leukemia with hypercalcemia. Report of a case without bone lesions. *Ohio State Med J* 61:138–140, 1965.

Scully RE, Mark EJ, McNeely WF, et al (eds): Plasma cell leukemia. Case records of the Massachusetts General Hospital, Case 20-1987. *N Engl J Med* 316:1259–1267, 1987.

Silber R, Stahl R: Phenotype of cells in CLL and related disease (Table 114-5). In Canellos G (ed): *Hematology* ed 4. New York, McGraw-Hill, 1990, p 1015.

Snapper J, Schneid B: On the influence of stilbamidine upon myeloma cells. *Blood* 1:534–536, 1946.

Stavem P, Vandvik B, Skrede S, et al: Needle like crystals in plasma cells in a patient with plasma cell proliferative disorder. *Scand J Haematol* 14:24–34, 1975.

Stone RM: Immunophenotypic characterization of B cell maturation (Table 1). *Haematol/Oncol Clin North Am* 4:460, 1990.

Sümegi J, Hedberg T, Björkholm M, et al: Amplification of the c-*myc* oncogene in human plasma cell leukemia. *Int J Cancer* 36:367–371, 1985.

Szela S, Sciborski R, Malycha R, et al: Plasma cell leukemia in a 65 year old patient. *Wiad Lek* 43:742–745, 1990.

Sztejnhaus AR, Santos RA, de Almeida TV: Primary plasmacytic lambda chain leukemia: Report of a case. *AMB Rev Assoc Med Bras* 35:120–122, 1989.

Tominaga N, Katagiri S, Hamaguchi Y, et al: Plasma cell leukemia of non-producer type with missing light chain gene rearrangement. *Br J Haematol* 69:213–218, 1988.

Ucci G, Riccardi A, Dörmer P, et al: Proliferation kinetics of plasma cells and normal hematopoietic cells in multiple myeloma. *Cell Tissue Kinet* 20:311–318, 1987.

Ueshima Y, Fukuhara S, Narai K: Cytogenetic studies and clinical aspects of patients with plasma cell leukemia and leukemic macroglobulinemia. *Cancer Res* 43:905–912, 1983.

Undritz E: Snapper-Schneid inclusions. In *The Sandoz Atlas of Haematology*. Basel, Sandoz, 1973, p 70.

Van Den Berghe H: Chromosomes in plasma-cell malignancies. *Eur J Haematol* 51(Suppl):47–51, 1989.

West NC, Smith AM, Ward R: IgE myeloma associated with plasma cell leukemia. *Postgrad Med* 59:784–785, 1983.

Wiernik PH, Sciortino D, Paietta E, et al: Plasma cell leukemia with an unusual karyotype and prolonged survival following oral alkylating agent therapy. *J Cancer Res Clin Oncol* 113:495–497, 1987.

Wurster-Hill DH, McIntyre OR, Cornwell GG III, et al: Marker chromosome 14 in multiple myeloma and plasma cell leukemia. *Lancet* 2:1031, 1973.

Yamada K, Shionoya S, Amano M: A Burkitt-type 8;14 translocation in a case of plasma cell leukemia. *Cancer Genet Cytogenet* 9:67–70, 1983.

Yip MY, Sharma P, Mansberg R, et al: Ring chromosomes in hypodiploid and hypotetraploid clones from an elderly patient with plasma cell leukemia. *Cancer Genet Cytogenet* 47:47–53, 1990.

Review Articles:

Dewald GW, Kyle RA, Hicks GA, et al: The clinical significance of cytogenetic studies in 100 patients with multiple myeloma and plasma cell leukemia or amyloidosis. *Blood* 66:380–390, 1985.

Djaldetti M: Plasma cell leukemia: Ultrastructural aspects in diagnosis. In *Human Leukemias*. Boston, Martinus-Nijhoff, 1984, pp 309–325.

Kyle RA, Maldonado JE, Bayrd ED: Plasma cell leukemia: Report on 17 cases. *Arch Intern Med* 133:813–818, 1974.

Liang W, Hooper JE, Rowley JD: Karyotypic abnormalities and clinical aspects of patients with multiple myeloma and related paraproteinemic disorders. *Cancer* 44:630–644, 1979.

Linden MD, Fishlender AJ, Tubbs RR, et al: Immunophenotypic spectrum of plasma cell leukemia. *Cancer* 63:859–862, 1989.

Parreira A, Robinson DS, Melo JV, et al: Primary plasma cell leukemia: Immunological and ultrastructural studies in 6 cases. *Scand J Haematol* 35:570–578, 1985.

Pruzanski W, Platts ME, Ogryzlo MA: Leukemic form of immunotypic dyscrasia (plasma cell leukemia): A study of 10 cases and a review of the literature. *Am J Med* 47:60–74, 1969.

Toma VA, Retief FP, Potgieter GM, et al: Plasma cell leukemia: Diagnostic problems in our experience with 11 cases. *Acta Haematol* 63:136–145, 1980.

Wintrobe MW: Differential counts of bone marrow aspirates from 12 healthy men (Table 3-3). In Lee GR, Boggs DR, Bithell TC, et al (eds): *Clinical Hematology* ed 8. Philadelphia. Lea & Febiger, 1981, p 58.

Woodruff RK, Malpas JS, Paxton AM, et al: Plasma cell leukemia (PCL): A report on 15 patients. *Blood* 52:839–845, 1978.

Zawadzki ZA, Kapadia S, Barnes AE: Leukemic myelomatosis (plasma cell leukemia). *Am J Clin Pathol* 70:605–611, 1978.

CASE 14

PATIENT: 28-year-old black male.

CHIEF COMPLAINT: Generalized itching and scaling of skin.

MEDICAL HISTORY: The patient enjoyed good health for several months prior to admission, when he experienced generalized pruritis. This was followed some time later by scaling. Local steroid applications offered only temporary relief.

PHYSICAL EXAMINATION: Diffuse erythema and scaling of the skin present. Right axillary adenopathy noted. Liver enlarged 8.0 cm below right costal margin. Spleen tip palpable.

LABORATORY RESULTS:

A. *Screening Procedure*
WBC of 27.0 × 10^9/L with a differential of segmented neutrophils 11%, bands 2%, eosinophils 4%, basophils 2%, monocytes 8%, lymphocytes 58%, and atypical lymphocytes with convoluted nuclei 15%. HGB 14.0 g/dL. HCT 0.43 L/L, MCV 92.0 fL, MCH 31.5 pg, MCHC 35.0 g/dL, RDW 13.8. Platelets 329 × 10^9/L.

HOSPITAL COURSE: The peripheral blood film revealed small and large atypical lymphocytes, some with convoluted and cleaved nuclei (Case 14.1) and occasional nucleoli. A skin biopsy showed focal in-

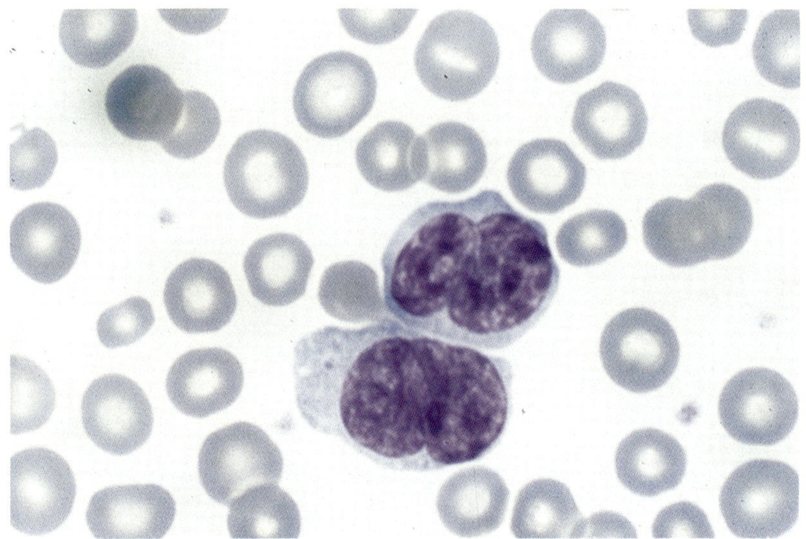

Case 14-1 Transformed MF cells (large cell variants) in peripheral blood. Nuclear irregularity and nucleoli are present. (×1000).

traepidermal collections of atypical lymphocytes with convoluted nuclei (Pautrier's abscesses). Similar cells were present in the upper dermis. The bone marrow biopsy demonstrated scattered paratrabecular and nonparatrabecular atypical monomorphic lymphoid aggregates (Case 14.2). Lymph node biopsy revealed focal architectural effacement, dermatopathic change, and infiltration by atypical lymphoid cells. The process was classified as *dermatopathic lymphadenitis; LN-4.*

During the subsequent 14 months, the patient was treated with electron beam therapy, topical nitrogen mustard, CHOP (cytoxan, adriamycin, vincristine, and prednisone), interferon, deoxycoformycin, and antibiotics. He died following the development of herpes simplex infection and adult respiratory distress syndrome.

QUESTIONS:

1. Is a skin biopsy necessary to establish the diagnosis?
2. Is cytologic evaluation of atypia a reliable means of recognizing circulating MF cells?
3. What role does the bone marrow biopsy have?

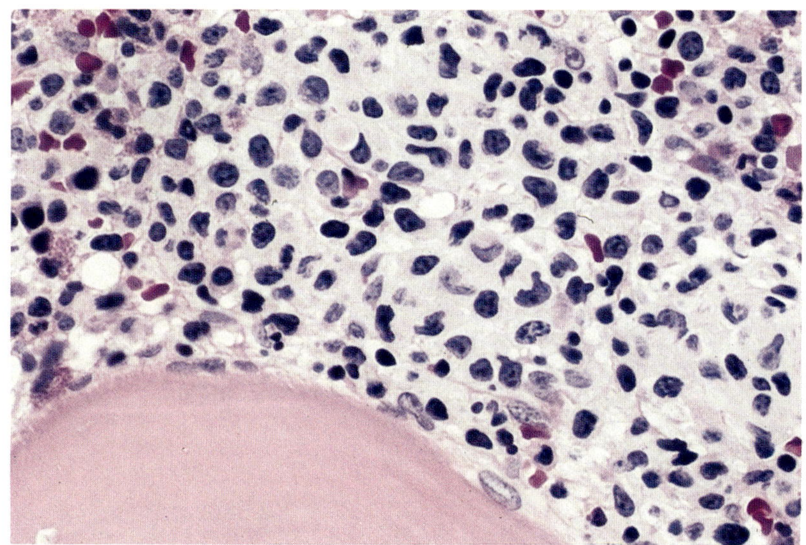

Case 14-2 Bone marrow biopsy with malignant paratrabecular lymphoid infiltrate. (×400).

LABORATORY RESULTS:

B. Confirmatory Results

Immunophenotyping studies: CD3+, CD4+, CD25+, sIg−, CD8−, CD19−, CD20−.

Electron microscopy of circulating MF cells: Highly convoluted enlarged and serpentine nuclei.

Cytogenetics: 46XY in 6 cells, and 78XY with multiple rearrangements in 9 cells.

Molecular genetic studies: Rearrangement of the TCR-β gene in circulating MF cells demonstrated on Southern blot analysis (Case 14.3).

Serologic evaluation: Viral antibodies against the HIV and HTLV-I viruses were absent.

DIAGNOSIS: Sézary syndrome.

DISCUSSION: MF is a rare T-cell lymphoma, first described by Alibert in 1806. Named after the mushroomlike facial tumors that disfigured the appearance of patients, MF was initially considered to be a skin disease. Subsequently, however, Sézary and Bouvrain

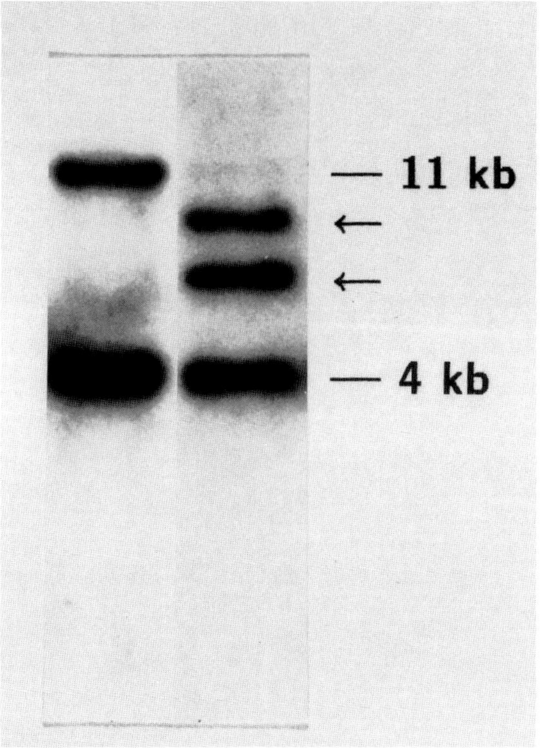

Case 14-3 Restriction fragment (Southern blot) analysis of the β-TCR gene. Genomic DNA from circulating MF-SS cells was digested with the restriction enzyme Eco RI and hybridized with a Cβ probe. The germline configuration of DNA obtained from placental tissue (left panel) is indicated with molecular size (kilobases) by dashes, and the rearranged β-TCR gene in the patient's DNA (right panel) is indicated by arrows. Courtesy of James W. Lynch, Jr., Francine Foss, Jeffrey Medeiros, and Lynne V. Abruzzo.

identified a systemic variant, which is distinguished from MF by the designation *Sézary syndrome.*

Each year about 1000 new cases of this neoplasm are diagnosed in the United States. Most patients are adults and initially present to a dermatologist. Invariably, the definitive diagnosis is first made from a skin biopsy. HTLV-I associated lymphoma-leukemia, MF and the SS are generally classified as cutaneous T-cell lymphomas; and since the latter disorders also manifest a chronic leukemic phase, their inclusion among the chronic leukemias is justified. Circulating lymphoma cells in both MF and SS are collectively referred to as Sézary cells.

Table C14-1 Risk Groups, Distribution of Lesions, and Median Survival in MF-SS

	Low	*Intermediate*	*High*
Skin lesions	Plaque disease, limited or generalized	Cutaneous tumors or erythroderma	Any type of skin infiltration
Circulating Sézary cells	Absent	Present	Present
Lymph node biopsy	LN1 or LN2	LN3	LN4
Bone marrow biopsy	Negative	Negative	Positive
Other visceral disease	Absent	Absent	Present
Median survival	12 years	5 years	<3 years

Source: Sausville, et al: Histopathologic staging at initial diagnosis of mycosis fungoides and the Sézary syndrome. *Ann Int Med* 109:372–382, 1988.
LN-1 = single and significantly atypical cells; LN-2 = small custers of atypical cells in paracortex; LN-3 = large clusters present; LN-4 = partial or total effacement of lymph node architecture.

Clinically, patients with MF progressively develop scaly pruritic skin lesions with patchy infiltrates, plaques, and tumors that may go on to ulcerate. Rarely, skin tumors may be the initial clinical manifestation (form d'emblé). In patients with MF, early in the course of disease, Sézary cells may be absent from peripheral blood. In contrast, patients with SS present with generalized erythroderma and, as in this case, usually manifest Sézary cells in the peripheral blood at the time of diagnosis. However, some overlap of clinical and laboratory features is known to occur.

In the staging system of MF and the SS (Table 14.1) developed by Sausville et al. at the Navy-NCI Medical Oncology Branch at Bethesda, Maryland, patients may be classified into three risk groups depending on the type and distribution of lesions, thereby enabling appropriate therapy. Toward this end, the role of the microscopist remains vital.

The key diagnostic feature of both MF and SS in the skin biopsy is the presence of intraepithelial collections of malignant lymphocytes (Pautrier's abscess) with convoluted and cerebriform nuclei (Case 14.4A). A similar infiltrate is present in the dermis and is most extensive in the tumor stage of disease. Following successful treatment,

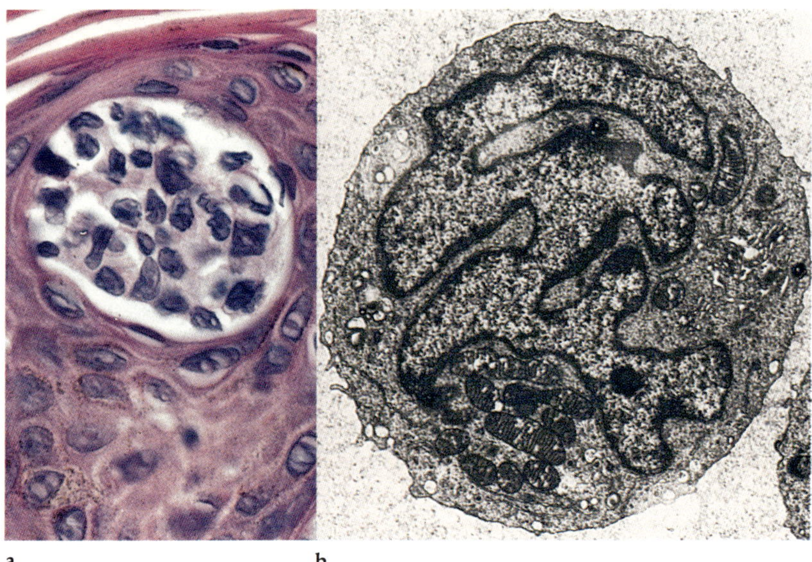

Case 14-4(a) Pautrier's abscess in the epidermis. Such lesions are not pathognomonic for MF-SS and may be seen also in adult T-cell lymphoma-leukemia. (×400, enlarged). **(b)** Electron micrograph of circulating MF cell. The serpentine nuclear configuration is characteristic. (×12,000). Courtesy of Mary Bibro.

tumor burden in the skin may be considerably diminished. The reason for epidermotropism in this neoplasm remains an enigma. Recently, however, the role of ELAM-1, an adhesion molecule for skin-homing T cells, has been considered.

In Wright-Giemsa-stained preparations of the peripheral blood, two types of Sézary cells may be observed in patients with MF or the SS. The small cell variant is comparable in size to a normal small lymphocyte and reveals a high N/C ratio, scant and essentially unremarkable cytoplasm, and a large internally convoluted cerebriform nucleus with coarse clumped chromatin. Such cells may be cytologically indistinguishable from circulating reactive small lymphocytes in patients with benign dermatoses. The large cell type, as is predominant in this case, reveals finely stippled chromatin with occasional nucleoli, cell diameters between 11 and 17 μm, and more abundant cytoplasm and may occasionally lack cerebriform nuclei. The precise cytologic distinction of these cells from reactive lymphocytes can sometimes be a problem, and under such circumstances their identity can be further ascertained by flow cytometry. Since a small number of patients on long-term chemotherapy for MF and the SS will go on to develop secondary AML, an appropriate battery of cytochemical stains and cytogenetic studies may be additionally indicated under these circumstances.

Both the small and large cell variants of Sézary cells may be simultaneously observed in the peripheral blood of patients and, when consisting of ≥20% of the circulating lymphocytes, constitute an adequate tumor burden to allow the peripheral blood to be considered to be involved. According to Schechter et al., when the large cell variant is predominant and constitutes greater than 50% of circulating lymphocytes, lymph node effacement and visceral disease can be expected. The large cell variant is indicative of transformation, a process similar to that observed in certain low-grade non-Hodgkin's lymphomas, and one that generally connotes a worse prognosis.

It will be apparent from the foregoing discussion that in the absence of a highly atypical nuclear configuration, the definitive cytologic identification of Sézary cells in routine peripheral blood smears can be difficult. Immunologic methods appear to be more sensitive, and in their assessment of the problem, Schechter et al. accepted ≥10% E-rosetting lymphocytes in cytocentrifuge samples of the peripheral blood as evidence of blood involvement. Nonetheless, it is advisable that such evaluations be performed in tandem with cytologic evaluation and flow cytometry, since the T/B lymphocyte ratio in the peripheral blood is normally about 4:1, and both CD4+ and CD8+ T lymphocytes ordinarily form E rosettes. Using flow cytometry, changes in CD4/CD8 ratios (normally about 2:1) with increased numbers of CD4+ cells would be additional supportive evidence of clonal excess due to Sézary cells. Another approach to evaluation and enumeration of Sézary cells is that recommended by Fletcher et al. These investigators found that plastic-embedded semithin sections of mononuclear cells previously separated on a density gradient were a useful adjunct to routine peripheral blood smear analysis and offered an effective means of cytologically identifying Sézary cells without resorting to electron microscopy.

Several studies have now confirmed that Sézary cells are CD2+, CD3+, CD4+, CD5+, and variably Tac+; and these findings are in keeping with their identity as T helper lymphocytes. In several cases studied by Foss et al., transformed Sézary cells have been CD7+, and Stein et al. also report Ki-1 activity in some instances. Recently, a new monoclonal antibody, CH-F42, has additionally been found to be effective in recognizing Sézary cells, as has been the presence of low-density CD24 epitopes recognized by the antibody BA-1. There is also some evidence that other T-cell subsets and lymphokine-activated killer cell (LAK cell) activity may be diminished in MF and the SS, and possibly serve as markers of aggressive disease.

The absolute Sézary cell count in most patients with MF and the SS is seldom greater than 20,000/mm^3 of blood (20.0 $\times$ 10^9/L). However, we have occasionally observed patients with counts as high as 50,000. Eosinophilia is commonly associated with MF and the SS, and is apparently the outcome of eosinopoietic factors such as interleukin-5 produced by the neoplastic T lymphocytes.

Although early studies suggested that MF and the SS seldom involved the bone marrow, more recent data, including those of Salhany et al. and Graham et al., have shown that marrow involvement may be present in up to 20% of patients at diagnosis. Other than the very rare marrow-effacing lesion, a diagnosis of MF or the SS is seldom possible from examination of the bone marrow aspirate alone. In biopsy sections, the distribution of lesions is focal and often paratrabecular, features more in keeping with involvement by lymphoma than leukemia. Lesions manifest as monomorphic lymphoid aggregates comprised of atypical small lymphocytes, with appearances similar to those observed in the skin, and with occasional interspersed larger cell forms. Aggregates vary in size. In the event of paratrabecular localization, we unequivocally interpret lesions as evidence of marrow involvement. Small, sparse nonparatrabecular aggregates lacking cytologic atypia are more likely to be interpreted as benign and reactive. Of the 180 bone marrow biopsies from cases with MF and the SS reviewed by Graham et al., 55 had lymphoid lesions. Of these, 16 were considered to be benign and 39 malignant and diagnostic of MF or the SS. Further breakdown of the malignant lesions according to localization revealed 13 to be nonparatrabecular, 6 paratrabecular, 9 nonparatrabecular and paratrabecular, 9 with lesions confined to clot sections only, and 2 with a diffuse growth pattern. As with staging of other malignant lymphomas, it is our standard practice to perform bilateral iliac crest biopsies, thereby ensuring adequate sampling.

Although the approach to expert interpretation of lymph nodes in MF and the SS has varied somewhat among different investigators, we have followed the guidelines established by Matthews and Gazdar at the Navy-NCI Medical Oncology Branch. These investigators found that since pigment mobilization and Langerhans cell hyperplasia was frequently encountered, the diagnostic prefix *dermatopathic lymphadenitis* was appropriate for affected nodes. However, they emphasized that the cell of interest was really the small atypical lymphocyte observed also in the skin and peripheral blood. Recent studies, including electron microscopy, cytogenetics, and DNA hybridization, have confirmed the identity of these cells as CD4+ malignant T helper lymphocytes. Langerhans cells can be readily distinguished from Sézary cells in such lymph nodes since the former are larger, have pale chromatin, and are S-100+. In contrast, Sézary cells are smaller, have darker chromatin, and are UCHL-1+ and Leu-22+. Assessment of tumor burden is the major determinant in the LN classification (Table 14.1) and may result in interpretive difficulty, especially between the categories LN-2 and LN-3. Rarely, Hodgkin's disease with Leu-M1+ Reed-Sternberg cells has been reported in patients with MF, and most reports of large cell lymphoma in patients with MF are apparently examples of blastic transformation.

Electron microscopic studies of Sézary cells were first reported by Lutzner and Jordan in 1967 and have been confirmed in numerous subsequent studies. The most characteristic feature by transmission electron microscopy is the hyperconvoluted serpentine nucleus, apparent in Sézary cells from the blood, lymph nodes, and skin. More recently, quantitative electron microscopy has revealed that a nuclear contour index of 7 and a nuclear profile area greater than 30 μm^2 are useful discriminants in identifying Sézary cells.

As in this case, Sézary cells have been found to demonstrate β-TCR gene rearrangement, further supporting the identity of this neoplasm as clonal and malignant. While such Southern blot DNA hybridization studies may be a valuable adjunct to flow cytometry, we have not found it necessary to identify β-TCR gene rearrangement for the sole purpose of establishing a pathologic diagnosis.

Cytogenetic studies reveal no consistent abnormality in either MF or the SS, and random aberrations are frequently present. Material from affected lymph nodes reveal anenploidy in 85% of cases; and on chromosomal banding studies, a wide range of heterodiploidy can be demonstrated. Chromosome 1 most frequently displays structural abnormalities, and numerical aberrations are most often observed in chromosomes 2, 11, and 22. Hyperdiploidy and near tetraploidy are poor prognostic indicators.

In 1987, Manzari et al. isolated a unique new human retrovirus from a continuous cell line from a CD4+, Tac− cutaneous T-cell lymphoma in leukemic phase. This virus was distinct from other human T-cell lymphotropic viruses and named HTLV-V. The role of the Langerhans cell where such viral material has been localized is presently under investigation.

Rarely, in patients with classic MF and the SS, antibodies against HTLV-I have been demonstrated. Hence, this additional means of differentiating these conditions from HTLV-I-associated lymphoma-leukemia does not appear to be entirely specific.

The histogenesis of MF and the SS remains controversial. Since both lesions demonstrate skin changes and lack bulky lymphadenopathy, it was once considered that lesions originated in the skin and involved the nodes secondarily. However, claims to the contrary are presently under investigation.

SUMMARY

Morphology	**Highly convoluted nuclei of lymphoid cells**
Immunophenotyping	**CD3+, CD4+, CD8−, CD25+**
Electron Microscopy	**Enlarged serpentine nuclei**
Molecular Genetics	**Rearranged β-TCR**
Serology	**Antibodies against HTLV-I and HIV absent**
Diagnosis	**Sézary syndrome (high-risk disease)**

ANSWERS:

1. MF and its systemic form, SS, always manifest dermatologic changes. The diagnosis is therefore invariably made first on skin biopsy.
2. Cytologic identification of Sézary cells in the peripheral blood is reliable only when significant nuclear clefting and folding are present. In the absence of these changes, identification of Sézary cells by the sheep-rosette technique is more reliable. The most sensitive means of confirming the presence of Sézary cells, however, is by establishing the presence of a clonal excess of T helper lymphocytes with a CD3+, CD4+, CD8− profile.
3. The bone marrow biopsy is an important aspect of clinical staging. Patients with a positive bone marrow, as in this case, are classified as having high-risk disease.

BIBLIOGRAPHY

Articles:

Alibert JL: Description des malides de la peau: Observees a l'hospital St. Louis et exposition des meilleures methodes suivries pour leur traitement. Paris, Barrois L'Aine et Fils, 1806, p 167.

Burke JS, Sheibani K, Rappaport H: Dermatopathic lymphadenopathy. An immunophenotypic comparison of cases associated and unassociated with mycosis fungoides. *Am J Pathol* 123:256–263, 1986.

Chu AC, Morris JF: Sézary cell morphology induced in peripheral blood lymphocytes: Reevaluation. *Blood* 73, 1603–1607, 1989.

Demtar M, Pauli G, Anagnostopoulos I, et al: A case of classical mycosis fungoides associated with human T-cell lymphotropic virus type 1. *Br J Dermatol* 124:198–202, 1991.

Fine RM: HTLV-V: A new human retrovirus associated with cutaneous T-cell lymphoma (mycosis fungoides). *Int J Dermatol* 27:473–474, 1988.

Fletcher V, Zackheim HS, Beckstead JH: Circulating Sézary cells. A new preparatory method for their identification and enumeration. *Arch Pathol Lab Med* 108:954–958, 1984.

Flug F, Pelicci P-G, Bonetti F, et al: T-cell receptor gene rearrangements as markers of lineage and clonality in T-cell neoplasms. *Proc Natl Acad Sci USA* 82:3460–3464, 1985.

Foss, F: CD7 activity in transformed Sézary cells. Personal communication, 1992.

Gilmore SJ, Bensen EM, Kelly JW: T-cell subsets with a naive phenotype are selectively decreased in the peripheral blood of patients with mycosis fungoides. *J Invest Dermatol* 96:50–56, 1991.

Graham SJ, Sharpe RS, Cotelingam JD: Bone marrow involvement in mycosis fungoides: Experience of the Bethesda Navy-National Cancer Institute Medical Oncology Branch. Unpublished observations, 1992.

Labastide WB, Rana MT, Baker CR: A new monoclonal antibody (CH-F42) recognizes a CD7− subset of normal T lymphocytes and circulating malignant cells in adult T-cell lymphoma-leukemia and Sézary syndrome. *Blood* 76:1361–1369, 1990.

Long JC, Mihm MC: Mycosis fungoides with extracutaneous dissemination: A distinct clinicopathologic entity. *Cancer* 34:1745–1755, 1974.

Lynch JW, Linoilla I, Sausville E, et al: Prognostic implications of evaluation for lymph node involvement by T-cell antigen receptor gene rearrangement in mycosis fungoides. *Blood* 79:3293–3299, 1992.

Manzari V, Gismondi A, Barillari G, et al: A new human retrovirus isolated in a Tac-negative T-cell lymphoma/leukemia. *Science* 238: 1581–1583, 1987.

McNutt NS, Heilbron DC, Crain WR: Mycosis fungoides. Diagnostic criteria based on quantitative electron microscopy. *Lab Invest* 44: 466–474, 1981.

Merlo CJ, Hoppe RT, Abel E, et al: Excutaneous mycosis fungoides. *Cancer* 60:397–402, 1987.

Mulshine JL, Carrasquillo JA, Weinstein JN, et al: Direct intralymphatic injection of radio-labeled ^{111}In T101 in patients with cutaneous T-cell lymphomas. *Cancer Res* 51:688–695, 1991.

Peters MS, Thibodeau SN, White JW, et al: Mycosis fungoides in children and adolescents. *J Am Acad Dermatol* 22:1011–1018, 1990.

Picker LJ, Kishimoto TK, Smith CW, et al: ELAM-1 is an adhesion molecule for skin homing T cells. *Nature* 349:796–799, 1991.

Pirrucello S, Lang MS: Differential expression of CD24 related epitopes in mycosis fungoides/Sézary syndrome. A potential marker for circulating Sézary cells. *Blood* 76:2343–2347, 1990.

Salhany KE, Cousar JB, Greer JP, et al: Transformation of cutaneous T cell lymphoma to a large cell lymphoma. *Am J Pathol* 132:265–277, 1988.

Salhany KE, Greer JP, Cousar JB, et al: Marrow involvement in cutaneous T-cell lymphoma. *Am J Clin Pathol* 92:747–754, 1989.

Sausville EA, Worsham GF, Mathews MF, et al: Histologic assessment of lymph nodes in mycosis fungoides/Sézary syndrome (cutaneous T-cell lymphoma): Clinical correlations and prognostic import of a new classifications system. *Human Pathol* 16:1098–1109, 1985.

Scheffer E, Meizer CJLM, van Vloten WA, et al: A histologic study of lymph nodes from patients with the Sézary syndrome. *Cancer* 57:2375–2380, 1986.

Simrell CR, Boccia RV, Longo DL, et al: Coexisting Hodgkin's disease and mycosis fungoides. *Arch Pathol Lab Med* 110:1029–1034, 1986.

Slater DN, Rooney N, Bleechen S, et al: The lymph node in mycosis fungoides: A light and electron microscopy and immunohistochemical study supporting the Langerhans cell–retrovirus hypothesis. *Histopathology* 9:587–621, 1985.

Stein H, Mason DY, Gerdes J, et al: The expression of the Hodgkin's disease associated antigen Ki-1 in reactive and neoplastic lymphoid tissue: Evidence that Reed-Sternberg cells and histiocytic malignancies are derived from activated lymphoid cells. *Blood* 66:848–858, 1985.

Stolz, W, Schmoeckel C, Burg G, et al: Circulating Sézary cells in the diagnosis of Sézary syndrome: Quantitative and morphometric analysis. *J Invest Dermatol* 81:314–319, 1983.

van der Loo EM, Crossen J, Meijer CJLM: Morphologic aspects of T-cell subpopulations in human blood: Characterization of the cerebriform mononuclear cells in healthy individuals. *Clin Exp Immunol* 43:506–516, 1981.

van der Loo EM, van Juijen GNP, van Vloten WA, et al: C-Type virus-like particles specifically localized in Langerhans cells and related cells of skin and lymph nodes of patients with mycosis fungoides and Sézary's syndrome. *Virchows Arch B, Cell Pathol* 31:193–203, 1979.

Vonderheid EC, Van Scott EJ, Wallner PE, et al: A 10 year experience with topical mechlorethamine for mycosis fungoides: Comparison with patients treated by total skin electron-beam radiation therapy. *Cancer Treat Rep* 63:681–689, 1979.

Vonderheid EC, Sobel EL, Nowell PC, et al: Diagnostic and prognostic significance of Sézary cells in peripheral blood smears from patients with cutaneous T-cell lymphoma. *Blood* 66:358–366, 1985.

Whang-Peng J, Lutzner M, Edelson R, et al: Cytogenetic studies and clinical implications in patients with the Sézary syndrome. *Cancer* 38:861–867, 1976.

Weiss LM, Wood GS, Hu E, et al: Detection of clonal T-cell receptor gene rearrangements in the peripheral blood of patients with mycosis fungoides/Sézary syndrome. *J Invest Dermatol* 92:601–604, 1989.

Willenze R, Scheffer E, Meijer CJLM: Immunohistochemical studies using monoclonal antibodies on lymph nodes from patients with mycosis fungoides and Sézary syndrome. *Am J Pathol* 120:46–54, 1985.

Wood GS, Hong SR, Sasaki DT, et al: Leu 8/CD7 antigen expression by CD3+ T cells: Comparative analysis of skin and blood in mycosis fungoides/Sézary syndrome relative to normal blood values. *J Am Acad Dermatol* 22:602–607, 1990.

Wood NL, Kitces EN, Blaylock WK: Depressed lymphokine activated killer cell activity in mycosis fungoides. A possible marker for aggressive disease. *Arch Dermatol* 126:907–913, 1990.

Review Articles

Dmitrovsky E, Mathews MJ, Bunn PA, et al: Cytologic transformation in cutaneous T cell lymphoma: A clinicopathological entity associated with poor prognosis. *J Clin Oncol* 5:208–215, 1987.

Kemme DJ, Bunn PA: State of the art therapy of mycosis fungoides and Sézary syndrome. *Oncology* 6:31–42, 1992.

Lutzner MA, Jordan HW: The ultrastructure of an abnormal cell in Sézary syndrome. *Blood* 31:719–726, 1968.

Matthews MJ: Surgical pathology of mycosis fungoides and Sézary syndrome. In Jaffe ES (ed): *Surgical Pathology of the Lymph Nodes and Related Organs.* Philadelphia, W. B. Saunders, 1985, pp 329–356.

Rappaport H, Thomas LB: Mycosis fungoides: The pathology of extracutaneous involvement. *Cancer* 34:1198–1229, 1974.

Sausville EA, Eddy JL, Makuch RW, et al: Histopathologic staging at initial diagnosis of mycosis fungoides and the Sézary syndrome. *Ann Intern Med* 109:372–382, 1988.

Schechter GP, Sausville EA, Fischmann AB, et al: Evaluation of circulating cells provides prognostic information in cutaneous T cell lymphoma. *Blood* 69:841–849, 1987.

Sézary A, Bouvrain Y: Erythrodermic avec presence de monstreuses dans le derme et le sang circulant. *Bull Soc Fr Dermatol Syphilogr* 45:254–260, 1938.

Vonderheid EC, Lawrence W, Diamond MD, et al: Lymph node histopathologic findings in cutaneous T-cell lymphoma. *Am J Clin Pathol* 97:121–129, 1992.

Whang-Peng J, Bunn PA, Knutsen T, et al: Clinical implications of cytogenetic studies in cutaneous T-cell lymphoma (CTCL). *Cancer* 50:1539–1553, 1982.

INDEX

DATE DUE

SEP 25 '97			
FEB 18 '99			
MAR 24 '99			
NOV 29 '99			
JUN 15 2000			
MAR 16 2001			
OCT 20 2003			
JUL 19 2004			
APR 10 2007			
APR 14 2009			

GAYLORD PRINTED IN U.S.A.